FACING EUGENICS

Reproduction, Sterilization, and the Politics of Choice

Facing Eugenics is a social history of sexual sterilization operations in twentieth-century Canada. Looking at real-life experiences of men and women who, either coercively or voluntarily, participated in the largest legal eugenics program in Canada, it considers the impact of successive legal policies and medical practices on shaping our understanding of contemporary reproductive rights. The book also provides deep insights into the broader implications of medical experimentation, institutionalization, and health care in North America.

Erika Dyck uses a range of historical evidence, including medical files, court testimony, and personal records, to place mental health and intelligence at the centre of discussions regarding reproductive fitness. Examining acts of resistance alongside heavy-handed decisions to sterilize people considered "unfit," *Facing Eugenics* illuminates how reproductive rights fit into a broader discussion of what constitutes civil liberties, modern feminism, and contemporary psychiatric survivor and disability activism.

ERIKA DYCK is Canada Research Chair in the History of Medicine and an associate professor in the Department of History at the University of Saskatchewan.

Facing Eugenics

Reproduction, Sterilization, and the Politics of Choice

ERIKA DYCK

UNIVERSITY OF TORONTO PRESS
Toronto Buffalo London

ISBN 978-1-4426-4416-8 (cloth)
ISBN 978-1-4426-1255-6 (paper)

Printed on acid-free, 100% post-consumer recycled paper with vegetable-based inks.

Library and Archives Canada Cataloguing in Publication

Dyck, Erika, author
Facing eugenics: reproduction, sterilization, and the politics of choice /
Erika Dyck.

Includes bibliographical references and index.
ISBN 978-1-4426-4416-8 (bound). – ISBN 978-1-4426-1255-6 (pbk.)

1. Sterilization (Birth control) – Social aspects – Alberta – Case studies.
2. Sterilization (Birth control) – Alberta – History – 20th century – Case studies.
3. Reproductive rights – Canada – Case studies. I. Title.

HQ767.7.D93 2013   363.9'70971230904   C2013-905958-X

University of Toronto Press acknowledges the financial assistance to its
publishing program of the Canada Council for the Arts and the Ontario Arts
Council.

 Canada Council   Conseil des Arts
for the Arts   du Canada

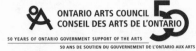
ONTARIO ARTS COUNCIL
CONSEIL DES ARTS DE L'ONTARIO
50 YEARS OF ONTARIO GOVERNMENT SUPPORT OF THE ARTS
50 ANS DE SOUTIEN DU GOUVERNEMENT DE L'ONTARIO AUX ARTS

University of Toronto Press acknowledges the financial support of the
Government of Canada through the Canada Book Fund for its publishing
activities.

This book has been published with the help of a grant from the Canadian
Federation for the Humanities and Social Sciences, through the Awards to
Scholarly Publications Program, using funds provided by the Social Sciences
and Humanities Research Council of Canada.

Contents

Acknowledgments

When I originally imagined writing a book about eugenics, I thought I would either unearth a series of coercive and heinous medical surgeries or, conversely, be stonewalled by the lack of information. What I ended up finding was something entirely different. I was amazed by the evidence available through regular archival channels, literature, newspapers, and journals, and often surprised by the information these documents contain. Eugenics in Alberta, I found, did not follow a singular track, and it did not affect people uniformly. Some embraced sexual sterilization surgery as an empowering image of self-control and reproductive autonomy. Others concealed their hysterectomies from their public personas but railed against the rampant and unbridled fertility of families considered feeble minded. I quickly realized that those most often absent from the official historical picture were the very ones who had experienced sterilization first-hand. This book aims to put those individuals at the front of the picture and, through them, allow us to appreciate the multiple ways in which eugenics has shaped individual bodies, families, and cultural ideas about reproductive rights.

I am indebted to the many people and organizations that helped make this book possible, and I am solely responsible for any of its shortcomings and weaknesses. Generous and courageous archivists helped me sift through mountains of material, and guided me through reference lists to tease out the coded lists and indexes that housed some of the most valuable materials for this project. I am especially grateful to Raymond Frogner, whose knowledge of the Provincial Archives of Alberta and extreme generosity at the University of Alberta Archives made much of this material available. The Provincial Archives of Alberta has an incredible reading room and a challenging organizational system; thank you, Wayne Murdoch, for helping me to navigate through both and for understanding the spirit of the project. Harvey Krahn at the University of Alberta's Department of Sociology provided insights from his experiences with the eugenics files that he reviewed for the legal cases; his assistance has been invaluable. Staff at the Red Deer and District Archives, the City of Edmonton Archives and the Glenbow Archives in Calgary, Dennis Slater at the Calgary Health Services Archives, John Stewart at the *Red Deer Advocate*, and John Court at the Centre for Addiction and Mental Health Archives in Toronto, all contributed to this project through their assistance and knowledge of their collections.

Throughout the project I was the fortunate recipient of various funds, beginning with seed money from the University of Alberta's Killam Foundation, which helped me to secure a standard research grant from the Social Sciences and Humanities Research Council of Canada. The Community University Research Alliance funds provided support for hiring students, and through my conversations with them regarding their research into eugenics in western Canada, my own thinking on this topic has been much enriched. Much of the funding was directed towards the undergraduate and graduate students who helped locate documents, chase up references, photocopy materials, and, in some cases, painstakingly take photographs of documents and index them. I am indebted to the amazing team of students who helped me through this journey. Beginning during my time at the University of Alberta, I thank Pat Farrel, who became my eyes in Toronto when I could not be there, and Eric Lizée, whose encouragement and knowledge of the Alberta Archives system helped more than he knows to keep me focused on the topic. When I relocated to the University of Saskatchewan in 2008, I encountered a new crew of talented students: Michael Kirkpatrick, Rachel Malena, Mathew Mossey, Paul Rowe, Erin Spinney, and Heather Stanley. I am especially grateful to Leslie Baker, Sheila Gibbons, and Amy Samson, all of whom have since carved out their own original projects in the history of eugenics; through our conversations and their careful studies I came to appreciate new ways of thinking about the topic and was challenged to rethink many of my conclusions. My writing group at the University of Saskatchewan saw unpolished and unclear drafts of chapters, and helped me to see through the confusion and towards a more careful articulate analysis. Thank you, Simonne Horwitz, Mark Meyers, and Lisa Smith, for helping me see my way through this project. Special mention in this group is reserved for Valerie Korinek, who has served as my mentor in many ways since I moved back to the University of Saskatchewan after many years; she has encouraged me all the way, including reading the entire manuscript and providing me with thoughtful and critical advice that substantially improved the work. Other colleagues also guided me through specific sections: Justin Bengry, Molly Ladd-Taylor, Maureen Lux, and Larry Stewart all made this a stronger book through their thoughtful suggestions. Len Husband at the University of Toronto Press invited me to work with him and ultimately coordinated reviews from three anonymous referees; I hope I have done their suggestions justice. Editorial assistance from Wayne Herrington and Barry Norris helped see this book through to publication, and made it a better read, while Natalie Neill created the index.

I need to make a special point about my involvement with the Community University Research Alliance, Living Archives on Eugenics in Western Canada, headed by Rob Wilson at the University of Alberta and run by Moyra Lang. This integrative initiative not only introduced me to a talented group of scholars interested in the history of eugenics, but, importantly, it has provided the framework for working with the community and raising public awareness about mental health, disability, and eugenics in a contemporary setting. Through this program we have run summer internship programs for undergraduate students, who gain valuable research skills and, more significantly, have the opportunity to work directly with survivors of the eugenics program and to appreciate the impact that historical research is making on public education campaigns and on the way in which we talk about and understand the legacy of eugenics and the challenges people with disabilities face. My own interns, Shannon Coleville, Justin Fisher, Keith Flysak, Rachel Malena, Kristina Rissling, Laura Shaw, and Amanda Shea, have all made exceptional contributions to this process. This experience has been incredibly valuable, and it has enriched my perspective on this history while reinforcing the desire to place sterilized individuals at the centre of analysis. The team overseeing that project is large and evolving, but I would like to acknowledge the bravery of Judy Lytton, Leilani Muir, and Nick Supina III, who remain at the project's heart. Nicola Fairbrother, Colette Leung, Claudia Malacrida, Natasha Nunn, Dick Sobsey, Bruce Uditsky, Gregor Wohlbring, Mark Workman, and all the other members and students who have played important roles in bringing this history into current conversations; I am grateful to them for being involved in this important work.

My colleagues in the study of the history of eugenics and medicine were unquestionably supportive as I embarked on the project, and they helped me to grow into it as I began seeking feedback. Thank you to Ian Dowbiggin, Jana Grekul, Harvey Krahn, Molly Ladd-Taylor, Paul Lombardo, Angus McLaren, Pat Prestwich, Christabelle Sethna, Susan Smith, and Paul Weindling for answering my detailed questions and providing me with additional resources when I floundered. Members of the Manitoba-Ontario-Minnesota-Saskatchewan consortium on Medical History, the Society for the Social History of Medicine, the American Association for History of Medicine, and my local colleagues patiently listened through earlier presentations and provided helpful corrections and comments.

Finally, without my family this book would never have come to completion. They supported me through the process even when sometimes it meant dinner was late or came out of a bag so that mom could stay at the office. John, my partner and inspiration, helped me to imagine my way through the project and encouraged me to see it to the end even when it seemed impossible. I am truly grateful to him for his love and sense of humour. Felix, our son, was born part way through the writing of this book. His early arrival, at only twenty-five weeks' gestation, meant that we spent four months together in the hospital as I watched him transform behind glass from a struggling fetus into a tiny little boy. He was only one pound at birth, and three pounds later he came home in what seemed like doll's clothes. Those four months are now a blur, and Felix is now a busy and thriving big brother to our daughter Amelia, whose arrival was considerably less complicated. For their love and encouragement I am indebted to my parents, Penny and Phil, siblings Lyndon, Alana, and Susan, and John's family – Gary and Michele, Ken and Marcia, David and Kinda and Ruby – who welcomed me into the fold; all found the time to distract me from my children so that I could write. Without this extensive network of support this book would still be just an idea.

About the Cover

"Portrait and Perception" (The Eugenics Dimension) (2005), Nick Supina III. Courtesy of University of Alberta Art Collection.

Cover image description:
This painting represents a piece of Alberta's eugenics history. Leilani Muir, as a young girl, stands in the foreground casting a long shadow

over the scene. Her paper dress displays drooping flowers, wilting in shame at the macabre scene. Her ballet pose mirrors the flowers on her dress; her arm extends gracefully and beautifully but lacks energy as she holds this position. Immediately behind her is a ghostly image of a car, representing the way that she and many children were dropped off at the Provincial Training School by their families or guardians. Behind the car looms the administration building of the Michener Centre, or Provincial Training School, in Red Deer, where trainees like Leilani were brought before the Eugenics Board and recommended for sexual sterilization. As toxic as the eugenics institution was, Leilani – the young barefoot woman in a canvas, standard-issue dress – received some genuine empathy from the nurse who greeted her. Below the scene, at Leilani's feet, the disembodied heads of Albertan premiers John Brownlee, William Aberhart, and Ernest Manning smile, with the latter two embracing a demon-like figure. Emily Murphy's face, wrought with agony for her influence in promoting the eugenics program, calls out from between the United Farmers of Alberta premier and the two Social Credit figures, helping to represent the split in parties but also their shared views on eugenics. The cloud hovering over the administrative building symbolizes the judgment that hangs over this scene, and serves as a reminder of the skewed brands of pseudo-Christianity that course through this history.

Nick Supina III, a professional fine artist, has painted many images depicting a social justice theme. His particular interest lies in illustrating the plight of people who have been misunderstood on account of intellectual and learning disabilities.

FACING EUGENICS

Reproduction, Sterilization, and the Politics of Choice

Introduction

Alberta distinguished itself in Canadian eugenics history as having the longest and most aggressive sexual sterilization policy in the country. Its eugenics program opened with the passage of the Sexual Sterilization Act in 1928, the first such law in Canada. British Columbia followed suit in 1933, but Alberta significantly out-sterilized its western neighbour:[1] over the course of its existence, the Alberta eugenics program recommended sexual sterilization surgeries for 4,725 individuals, and ultimately performed operations on 2,822 people; by comparison, British Columbia operated on nearly 200 individuals. Recommendations for Alberta's surgeries came from an appointed Eugenics Board and fell into five categories: psychotic patients; mental defectives, which included individuals with arrested mental development for congenital or acquired reasons before the age of eighteen; neurosyphilitic patients who did not respond to treatment; patients with epilepsy, psychosis, or mental deterioration; and individuals with Huntington's Chorea disease. The Board approved sterilization surgery when its members determined there was a "danger of the transmission of any mental disability or deficiency to offspring, or a risk of mental injury either to such persons or to the progeny if sterilization were not carried out."[2]

The program from its beginning targeted individuals considered "feeble-minded" or "mentally defective," often relying on intelligence tests and behavioural observations by psychologists and medical officials who categorized children and adults as "imbecile," "idiot," and "moron" – terms that generically referred to a sliding scale of mental deficiency and lowered or defective intelligence. "Morons" were often considered the most dangerous because they could pass at times for individuals of "normal" intelligence, but, according to eugenicists, they made poor parents and were likely to pass on both genetic and social defects to their children.

Throughout this book I explore people who fell into these categories, and I often rely on the language used at the time to describe people's mental and intellectual capabilities. As other historians have argued, to fail to use such language when we examine the history of intellectual disability runs the risk of forgetting the consequences of being so labelled. I thus decided to retain such terms in my historical study, not to reinforce their hurtful applications, but to remind us of their history. Although I eschew further use of quotation marks around these labels in the remainder of the book, I hope readers will interpret them in their historical context.

Although several provinces considered passing eugenics laws, only British Columbia and Alberta implemented such a program, as did thirty US states and dozens of countries, including India, Germany, Sweden, and Japan.[3] Eugenics and sexual sterilization programs took different forms in these places, but their widespread application suggests that these ideas were not confined to particular regions or ideologies.

Alberta's eugenics program remained in effect for forty-three years, long after many other jurisdictions had abandoned the idea. The act was formally repealed only in 1972, after allegations that it had not maintained sufficient genetic information to make informed decisions and that it infringed upon human rights, particularly in cases where consent had not been obtained.

Over that time, the politics of sterilization changed considerably, with eugenics fading in the shadow of the Holocaust and sexual sterilization gaining prominence as a contraceptive act of choice. Indeed, sterilization historically has been entangled with dark elements of eugenics alongside more activist expressions of reproductive choice. Alberta's eugenics program maintained an official policy of sexual sterilization surgery for women and men deemed incapable of responsible parenthood. It also created opportunities, however, for healthy and, arguably, resourceful, and more empowered women and men to challenge these laws and to negotiate access to medically sanctioned birth control in the form of surgical operations. By considering these goals of the eugenic program in tandem, I hope to understand how operations such as tubal ligations (salpingectomies), hysterectomies, and vasectomies were foisted upon certain people and denied to others. Considering these operations alone risks equating the surgery with an expression of power, but by historically contextualizing sexual sterilization operations one begins to see past the incisions and into a deeper portrait of reproductive politics, including seeing sterilization as a form of resistance.

The complicated and controversial history of sexual sterilization has engaged policy makers, religious authorities, medical professionals, women, men, and families in contests over reproductive rights. Historically, these debates have pitted feminists against non-feminists, Catholics against non-Catholics, while socialists and fascists have made strange bedfellows. Sterilization often invokes images of draconian policies, involuntary procedures, or institutionalized medicine, all suggesting political power over marginalized bodies. Over time, however, those bodies have fought back and complicated the cultural meaning of sterilization. The language of choice emerged amid human rights campaigns tied to various social movements, notably second-wave feminism; perhaps less notably, however, patient and mental health consumers also embraced choice as a defiant expression of autonomy. The shifts in language and application nonetheless have applied unevenly across time and gender; reproductive autonomy and its moral trappings remain a deeply contested arena despite legislative reforms and medical triumphs that have improved reproductive rights and health. In this book I look at some of the women and men whose bodies bear the scars of these debates.

Eugenics Comes to Alberta

By the time Canadians came to debate the merits of eugenics, the idea had already taken root in other countries. In 1883 Francis Galton, cousin of Charles Darwin, coined the term "eugenics" to mean "nobility in birth." Galton's work combined nineteenth-century trends in biostatistics and biological medicine, and helped to produce the new science of heredity.[4] The burgeoning field of study attracted attention from a wide array of scientists, policy makers, philosophers, and social reformers across the political spectrum, many of whom had a long-standing interest in population control. The possibilities captivated reform-minded enthusiasts who sought scientific solutions to a range of problems associated with urbanization, disease, poverty, moral degeneration, immigration, and race suicide. The development of eugenics societies provided significant intellectual credibility to such ideas and popularized eugenics as a progressive response to the growing pains associated with modernity.[5] As historian Marius Turda explains, "a quintessential modernist response to threats of cultural and biological collapse, eugenics located the individual and national body within a specifically scientific discourse, one whose legitimacy stemmed from its preoccupation with improving the racial qualities of the population and protecting its health."[6] As Turda describes, the collusion of interests in racial purity, healthy societies, and nationalism appealed across a broad spectrum of interests and regions and captivated attention as part of a natural component of nation building and modernization.

During the early phases of the eugenics movement, advocates used mathematical studies of degeneration to support the claim that defects in judgment, behaviour, intelligence, and morality were in fact hereditary. Such studies attempted to calculate the risk and social cost of inheriting mental and moral defects by surveying and studying subgroups within the population – primarily the criminal and the impoverished – and measuring the number of progeny falling into these categories, either through assumptions about biological defects or environmental influences. Although the biological science behind these studies remained vague, a growing number of reports indicated that biological and social factors taken together produced a disproportionate number of mental defectives and criminals, who were also often considered mentally defective on account of their poor judgment, with noted concentrations in specific populations. This observation brought the problems of human behaviour and its social organization under the scientific and medical gaze in a way that appeared politically effective and constructive, especially through an associated emphasis on preventing the growth of this element of society. In some ways, efforts aimed at curbing this trend were even regarded as humanitarian. Moreover, these kinds of studies brought medical, philosophical, and political minds together in pursuit of meaningful improvements in social organization and modern civilization. The language of the early studies borrowed heavily from the kind of rhetoric that emphasized progress and praised eugenics programs as a civilizing intervention.

Eugenicists often described their campaigns using organic metaphors, such as a garden that requires weeding or a tree that needs pruning. Eugenics and sterilization programs differed, however, in what they identified as weeds and what tools were best suited to do the weeding. In Britain, eugenics societies concentrated on class conflict and poverty as the main social pollutant, whereas US programs more often characterized race as the offending social toxin in need of cleansing. Canadian gardens seemed more susceptible to foreign weeds: immigration posed eugenic questions in the early part of the century in a manner that fused elements of class, race, and intelligence, using "foreigner" as convenient shorthand for undesirable. As eugenic gardens took root in different cultural soils, the process of weeding revealed different priorities and social tensions as different varieties jockeyed for space in the proverbial garden. At the heart of eugenics programs, however, lay a desire to exert power and surveillance over families that did not suit the national or regional plan – and although eugenics emerged as a transnational ideology, its expression was more regional in character.

The concept of eugenics crystallized some of these broader agendas into a coherent set of arguments backed by science and aided at times by financial expediency. In Britain, as historian Angélique Richardson explains, eugenics focused on the urban poor, and assumed a clear class dimension in its articulation of population control.[7] British eugenicists also more often embraced tools of deportation and segregation as a way of controlling this undesirable segment of the population. American eugenicists, by comparison, more often tended to reinforce racial differences, developing studies of anthropometry – biological sciences aimed at studying the physical attributes associated with different racial typologies.[8] The thirty US states that passed eugenics laws also took different approaches. Indiana took an early lead by implementing sterilization legislation in 1907; Georgia's entry in the field came as late as 1937. California adopted an accelerated pace, ultimately sterilizing over 20,000 individuals, far more than any other North American jurisdiction. Some southern states, including North Carolina, Virginia, and Georgia, registered sterilizations in the thousands; others, including South Carolina, Alabama, and Mississippi, each recorded hundreds of sterilizations. The repeal of these state laws also bears a patchwork of regional variations: changes came in New York and New Jersey as early as the 1920s, while sterilization laws remain in force in Washington and Mississippi.[9]

Alberta's program contained traces of British and US approaches, but the province developed its own subtle variant. The barometer of fitness in Alberta rested more specifically upon notions of mental ability, intelligence, and potential for responsible parenthood. Intelligence arose as a key variable in decisions about mental and physical fitness alongside social value, and was often grafted onto other criteria, including race, ethnicity, and class or poverty. It also conveniently applied to a largely immigrant population as a way of discussing ideal family values through the lens of intelligence and public health.

The early applications of eugenics discourse worldwide focused primarily on marginalized populations, including poor communities and institutionalized groups of individuals deemed mentally ill, defective, or criminal. Studies measured, and later predicted, the inheritability of defective qualities. The notion of defects, however, included a wide range of behaviours and symptoms that increasingly were medicalized in an attempt to gauge heredity. This development was not entirely reductionist: the interplay between biology and the environment was well recognized, challenging investigators to consider more carefully definitions of defect and the process of inheritance. For example, alcoholism suggested that individuals might suffer from biological defects that caused their bodies to metabolize alcohol in defective or dysfunctional ways. Regardless of the pathology of the behaviour, however, alcoholic parents were also considered ill equipped to raise children; improper supervision and care contributed to the development of adults with maladapted reasoning, judgment, and morality.

The results of these studies captivated the attention of reformers more so than did the actual causes, which minimized the desire to disaggregate inheritability into biological and social constituents. The movement gained momentum in the late nineteenth and early twentieth centuries, culminating, as many scholars contend, in the German-led Holocaust of the Second World War. The scale and severity of Nazi eugenics programs publicized dramatically the dire consequences of eugenics thinking and its potential for manipulation, especially along racial and ethnic lines.[10] Eugenics programs applied in this targeted way and on such a large scale brought universal condemnation. The war altered the context of eugenics science, forging a strong connection between it and genocide in the popular mind for decades to come.[11]

The Holocaust also changed the direction of the eugenics movement, including the language used to describe it, and later its historical legacy. Most studies of eugenics have focused on the period leading up to or culminating in the Second World War. More recent studies have begun to look beyond this period to trace the movement into the post-Holocaust era and to show how eugenics science and mental hygiene movements adapted in response. This temporal division has created a somewhat artificial distinction between the kinds of practices and policies in use before and after 1945. In fact, despite changes in vocabulary, a number of more traditional eugenics programs persisted after the Second World War.[12]

Alberta's was one such program. In hindsight, its early eugenics policies might be cause for embarrassment or scorn. In Canada during the 1920s and 1930s, however, Alberta was the envy of several other jurisdictions that had failed to establish similar policies – indeed, most Canadian provinces entertained debates about the need for them. Parties across the political spectrum drummed up support for policies to help reduce the expense to the public of impoverished but fertile elements of the population. After the First World War, middle- and upper-class decision makers and reformers promoted a more homogeneous vision of Canadian society, one that had not formed under the allegedly liberal immigration policies of the first part of the twentieth century. For Alberta, eugenics offered an appealing solution to the growing problem of social and moral decay by promising to support stricter immigration policies, while focusing on the internal make-up of western Canadian society and even promoting invasive measures to ensure that the so-called unfit members of society were not capable of reproduction.

Implemented at the end of the 1920s, Alberta's eugenics program was part of a growing wave of support for mental hygiene programs, many linked to ideas about nationalism and healthy, even ideal, societies. Some of its major proponents were progressive reformers, including early feminists, socialists, and health activists. The eugenics program helped to put Alberta on the international map for its forward planning and efforts at social reform. Among these were advances such as extending to women the right to vote and to hold political and judicial offices, as well as significant strides in health care. These milestone achievements and the legacies of individual reformers remain tempered, however, by harsher elements tied to eugenics.

Alberta boasted some of the strongest first-wave feminists. The "Famous Five" made a name for themselves throughout the 1910s and 1920s as social and political reformers, and helped prairie women gain a number of celebrated firsts, including suffrage, election as a Member of the Legislative Assembly (Alberta), senator, and judge. They promoted a specific kind of Anglo-Saxon values, but their vision, like that of the Ku Klux Klan, included restricting the rights of families that did not share this genetic heritage. The Famous Five were vocal proponents of eugenics, sexual sterilization, and restrictive marriage laws – indeed, they were the key motivators of Alberta's original Sexual Sterilization bill. Their unwavering support for women's rights was based in some measure on emphasizing the inferior qualities of non-Anglo-Saxons. With the complicated mixture of feminism and racism, more commonplace during the early twentieth century, these women are now remembered as difficult heroes and curious villains.[13]

Eugenics attracted not only individuals identified as progressive, left-leaning reformers. Social and fiscal conservatives also saw the potential benefits, particularly as the Great Depression encouraged prairie politicians and voters to exercise financial prudence and to develop economically efficient social programs to help establish a modicum of social security. Individuals and families exhibiting mental illness, disability, and so-called mental defective or unfit behaviour became a source of concern in a society preoccupied with designing healthy, working, and prosperous communities. Individuals who did not contribute to these goals became targets for reform through institutional or more direct means. Eugenics programs provided some of the more direct means for channelling resources or, in this case, for reducing the alleged social and financial burden of future care by limiting the reproductive capacity of individuals who were considered a genetic threat to the aspirations of a healthy society. Eugenics, or the aggressive application of modern population control measures, emerged for some people as a reasonable solution to a realistic set of modern challenges.

By the 1930s the financial argument for such a program intensified as the Depression took hold. Unsurprisingly, western Canadians expressed more support than their eastern counterparts, as the prairies suffered the most extreme and prolonged consequences of the economic downturn and since the four western provinces had been promoted as key destinations for new immigrants in the recent past. As the population swelled, local politicians and middle-class reformers increasingly adopted nativist attitudes and began to resent the influx of immigrant groups that appeared unable to assimilate into the Anglo-Saxon, largely Protestant West.[14]

Although similar support for eugenics could be found in central and eastern Canada, western Canadians articulated these views more strongly, and were able to generate consensus on the topic. In some cases new political organizations held strong commitments to single issues in defence of Anglo-Saxon, Western values. These organizations assumed a variety of guises that spread widely across political and social scales. The Ku Klux Klan, for example, which expanded into Canada from the US South, flourished in Alberta and Saskatchewan in the 1920s, adapting its message in Canada to express a fervent antipathy towards Catholics, Jews, and non-whites.[15]

Religious movements erupting in western Canada also helped to fuel the anti-"Other" rhetoric that lay at the heart of eugenics values. Social gospellers, temperance reformers, members of the Prophetic Bible

Institute, Baptists, Mormons, and others found fertile pulpits in the Canadian West, and added their sermons to the cacophony of voices offering explanations and justifications for charity, exclusion, segregation, and deportation aimed at those who did not seem to fit with their vision of Canadian society. Gradually these voices harmonized in a chorus of political support for more stringent restrictions on immigration policy, along with a narrowing focus on controlling the existing population. Despite their significant theological differences, these religious organizations had some common ground on eugenics. Not all supported eugenics programs, but facets of eugenics appealed across a wider set of factions in western Canada and allowed for a more coordinated body of support than could be secured in other parts of the country.[16]

Alberta's reformers found particular expression in the creation of a new political party: the United Farmers of Alberta, which came to power in 1921 through the combined interests and frustrations of disempowered farmers and labourers.[17] The main sources of their disenchantment with the current power structures resided in Parliament in Ottawa and in the financial districts of Winnipeg and Toronto. Together these faceless levers of power culminated collectively in antagonistic western attitudes towards the East and helped to foster a regional identity in the West. The United Farmers remained in power until unseated in 1935 by another new party, Social Credit, which in turn held onto government until 1971.

Part of the United Farmers' initial success depended on its bringing women into the political fold. Women were formally admitted to the party as full voting members as early as 1914, and in 1916 the United Farm Women of Alberta was established. In many ways the women's wing, which included the Famous Five, functioned as an advisory to the main party, especially on issues considered specific to women or family. For instance, this wing was crucial for initiating bills on marriage, inheritance, and family allowances, and instrumental in forwarding the sexual sterilization issue.[18] Once these debates solidified into proto-bills, they carried the force of the women's association in the caucus chambers and, ultimately, at the ballot box. The Sexual Sterilization Act was discussed at length and approved by the women's wing before it landed on the desks of the male representatives, and the initial reading of the bill in 1927 consequently met with little resistance. Within two years, the program was in place, and a powerful group of supporters were in position to ensure its implementation.

Alberta's passage of the Sexual Sterilization Act is in some ways remarkable, requiring as it did a delicate constellation of unlikely supporters, from feminists to social gospellers to farmers, each seeing in eugenics a plan that would bring salvation to their cause. The Great Depression then helped to fuel the program by stressing the financial imperative of reducing government expenditures, including on psychiatric hospitalization, and emphasizing the superior moral values of a homogeneous Anglo-Saxon society. Under these conditions, the program flourished.

Then, in 1935, a new party came to govern it. Within two years of coming to power, the Social Credit Party, led by William Aberhart and later by Ernest Manning, strengthened the Sexual Sterilization Act by expanding its mandate and removing the need to collect informed consent in cases where the individual was considered mentally defective, a categorization based on a psychometric test or the assigning of an intelligence quotient based on oral and sometimes written exams. Candidates whose overall scores fell below 70 were considered defective and thus ineligible to provide consent or incapable of doing so. This change set Alberta's eugenics program apart from those of other North American jurisdictions that had established consent procedures; many strengthened or added such procedures after the Second World War, but Alberta never formally revisited the consent issue before the program was abolished in 1972.

Under Social Credit the combination of an expanded and somewhat more liberal mandate also coincided with a shift away from a eugenics program built around ideals of social morality to one organized along principles of financial benefits to the province and justified by medico-scientific theories about heredity, mental deficiency, and intelligent parenting. In Social Credit's early years, which began at the height of the Depression, government reports emphasized the potential savings a eugenics program would produce for the struggling province. Reducing the costs associated with maintaining individuals in institutions or hospitals played a key part in these discussions, and helped to shift the target population away from particular immigrant groups per se and towards groups that relied on government support. Chief among these were residents of charitable or government-supported institutions, including single mothers, children with disabilities, patients in psychiatric facilities or asylums, and, although the evidence is more difficult to substantiate, Aboriginal and Inuit men and women who came into contact with provincial authorities.

The shift in focus from Anglo-Saxon values to those guided more specifically by concerns of welfare, even when those concerns were couched in the language of class or race, brought other players into scope after the Second World War. The province then developed a greater reliance on the medical community, which served in some ways as gatekeepers to institutions, and on Indian agents, who functioned as conduits to both the First Nations population and the federal government. Chapter 2 attempts to shed light on the contentious and precarious roles race and welfare elements played in cases involving Aboriginal, Inuit, and Métis candidates for sexual sterilization. The 1937 changes to the Sexual Sterilization Act also placed greater pressure on the psychiatric community to distinguish among hereditary cases of degeneration, long-term disability and its cost to government, and the relationship between sexual sterilization and sexual activity. Thus, the medical community in general and psychiatrists in particular were empowered under the law to identify potential candidates for sterilization. As historian Amy Samson points out, however, this shift to a different set of authorities had a domino effect, as it then engaged new levels of professionals and key parties – nurses, social workers, teachers, and even parents – in a more comprehensive and normalized matrix of surveillance over people deemed unfit for normal citizenship.[19]

As its own records reveal, in the 1940s the Eugenics Board grew increasingly aggressive in its attempt to reduce the financial burden on government, which they believed was caused in part by the need to pay for hospitalization and long-term institutionalization for defective members of society. Buoyed by reports from California, where, within the first decade of operations, over two thousand individuals had been sterilized – a number that increased tenfold by the 1960s[20] – the Alberta administrators believed that a similar program in their province would drastically minimize expenditures and reduce the defective population by as much as 30 per cent in one generation. California had projected savings of $2 million in institutionalization costs with the removal of a single generation of defectives.[21]

Cost-saving measures appealed to an Alberta government struggling with economic downturns and ideologically opposed to government-built infrastructure.[22] Despite changes in international law and reproductive medicine as the twentieth century wore on, the Eugenics Board successfully pressured the provincial government to expand its capacity to authorize the sterilization of individuals deemed mentally defective. The close-knit objectives of both the Board and the government meant that – regardless of changes in medical ethics, reproductive medicine, eugenics science, and the growth of the welfare state, eventually including medicare – eugenics in Alberta gradually moved further and further away from accountable medical or ethical practices.

Although informed consent arose as a key component of ethical conduct in the course of the Nuremberg war crimes trials, from which an international code of medical ethics evolved in 1947, Alberta's policy makers never reinstated provisions for informed consent in cases where individuals were already institutionalized and considered mentally defective. The Eugenics Board justified the 1937 amendment removing informed consent provisions by arguing that obtaining consent had slowed down the sterilization program and imposed greater costs on the public, since selected individuals remained wards of the government until the surgery was completed. As well, under the new provisions, discharge from an institution could be granted after only the Board had evaluated a patient. Guided by financial concerns as opposed to international or medical advice, sterilizations proceeded well into the Cold War period, although they fell off the public radar, remaining confined largely to an institutionalized and, at times, orphaned population.

The removal of informed consent provisions not only placed Alberta outside the international mainstream; it also angered patients who later discovered that they had been sterilized without their knowledge. In the 1960s, as the program continued, it was combined with other health system reforms, including the establishment of a publicly funded health care system and the closure of long-stay psychiatric hospitals and an end to institutionalization. As patients entered a transformed health care system as clients, they were also expected to take on more responsibility as consumers of a new health care regime. Psychiatric patients, especially those who had spent the majority of their lives in institutions, were expected to find housing in communities and to rely on institutions only for medications and short-term care. Patients who then discovered that they had been sterilized began questioning the wisdom of a policy that deemed them incapable of providing intelligent consent to an operation, while expecting them to live in communities, find a job, fill in government forms, and participate in civil society as rehabilitated, normal citizens. Fuelled by human rights campaigns and the development of second-wave feminism and patients' rights organizations, some of these individuals began challenging the government's authority over institutionalized and deinstitutionalized bodies.

Another key aspect of the eugenics issue was reproductive rights. Already, by the end of the Second World War, middle-class married women outside institutional settings began seeking sexual sterilization as a form of birth control, a development that affected the eugenics program in ways policy makers and medical professionals had not anticipated. Authorities responded by trying to restrict access to sterilization and threatening to hold surgeons liable for sterilizing allegedly healthy, intelligent women. Despite the hesitancy of male authorities, some middle-class women pressured their doctors to perform sterilizing surgery to put an end to their child-bearing ability. Alberta served as an important location for these practices since its eugenics law permitted surgery that opened the door, if only a crack, to more voluntary operations. Since contraception remained illegal in Canada until 1969, this small early opportunity encouraged women to demand a broadening of the definition of health risks and an extension of health autonomy to reproductive wives.

The reproductive husband, on the other hand, seemed to escape detection in the frame of either eugenics or birth-control debates in the post-war period. Although men and boys were sterilized under the eugenics program, subsequent historical interpretations of the program have tended to reinforce the way that women were targeted. Masculinity and appropriate boyish behaviour, nonetheless, attracted attention from medical professionals interested in policing the boundary between normal and abnormal behaviour. In Alberta, the main proponent of that research, Dr Leonard J. Le Vann, was also superintendent of the Provincial Training School for Mental Defectives, later renamed the Michener Centre. Le Vann was engaged in a number of experimental studies to demonstrate a relationship among mental deficiency, degeneration, and schizophrenia. Based on gendered interpretations of behaviour and the pre-existing link between assumptions of hyperactivity and boys, Le Vann relied on experiments with institutionalized boys and young adults. This experimental culture went hand in hand with the eugenics program, and continued to characterize children and adults with disabilities within a category of feeble-mindedness.

Middle-class married men did not pursue vasectomies as a form of birth control en masse until the late 1960s and early 1970s. Vasectomy surgery was well understood among medical professionals by the turn of the twentieth century, but its use remained primarily confined to institutional populations as part of population control exercises, which were more in keeping with traditional sterilization and eugenic practices. Men's health risks did not necessitate vasectomies to relieve concerns such as those faced by women – namely, ovarian and cervical cancers. For married women, sexual sterilization promised emancipation from

the burden of unwanted reproduction. For middle-class men, the vasectomy suggested a challenge to masculinity or an affront to manhood.
Over the course of the Cold War, however, those attitudes changed. As
birth control became a more openly discussed topic, and especially as
women's contraceptive methods came under public scrutiny, the vasectomy emerged as a safer, cheaper, and arguably more efficient option for
middle-class family planning.

The comparatively quiet history of the sexual sterilization of men,
both in institutional settings and within middle-class families, has resulted in assumptions that eugenics programs more often targeted
women and that birth-control advocates, feminists, family planners,
and eugenicists were all cut from the same cloth. A closer reading of the
history, however, challenges these assumptions: not only were boys
and men subjected to a broad range of experiments related to eugenics
and sexual sterilization; married men also expressed their desire for
voluntary sterilization differently than did women. The experiences of
such men show that the relationships among family planning, eugenics, and feminism were more complicated.

Sexual sterilization surgeries in Alberta took two distinct paths after
the Second World War. Operations associated with eugenic measures
remained confined to institutional and quasi-institutional settings, such
as the Provincial Guidance Clinics, set up to siphon candidates into the
mental health system, or schools and communities where teachers and
parents identified children as likely suspects for mental deficiency.[23]
Eugenic sterilizations continued to rely on the idea that certain individuals were a genetic risk to the population and that, moreover, candidates for these surgeries were incapable of responsible parenthood
regardless of their genetics.

Conversely, sexual sterilization among middle-class families represented a permanent solution to the challenge of unbridled fertility.
Families that had expanded to or beyond their financial and emotional
capacity increasingly resorted to creative methods of obtaining physician-assisted, permanent contraception. By the middle of the twentieth
century tubal ligations and vasectomies became widely popular operations, used by both sexes and across the socio-economic spectrum, although not without controversy. The operations aimed at curbing
motherhood for women considered unfit had been ushered in by maternal feminists, but later became part of the armour second-wave feminists wore to shield their right to reproductive autonomy. Men, who
signed the bills, performed the surgeries, and deciphered the fit from

the unfit, remained quietly unreflective when it came to their own sexual sterilization, perhaps owing to the long-standing view that reproduction was a woman's issue. It was not until the safety of the oral
contraceptive and the inefficiencies of the tubal ligation became patently apparent that the vasectomy arose as an appropriately masculine response to the challenges of modern life and fertility control. Bringing
men into the equation also altered the context of decision making when
it came to family planning.

Even as sterilization became intertwined with debates over personal
autonomy and human rights for middle-class families, institutionalized
individuals continued to be subjected to these operations with little regard for their place within these broader social and cultural changes.
Women such as Doreen Befus, who spent most of her life in the
Provincial Training School at Red Deer, became incensed by the challenges deinstitutionalized people faced. Following her release into the
community, Doreen began publicly to question the cultural paradox
that separated ability and disability and that applied different degrees
of choice to people according to those inflexible categories.

This questioning persisted, and in the mid-1990s survivors of the
Alberta sexual sterilization program sued the provincial government.
Leilani Muir was the first, and hers was the only case that went to trial,
which she ultimately won. The Muir trial helped to realign the history
of sexual sterilization with eugenics, and reminded Canadians of the
more coercive origins of that practice. Leilani, though, also represented
a different way of thinking about the issue. The existence of the surgery
itself was perhaps not the problem, but the way in which it was applied
revealed deep divisions in the reproductive choice that was available to
different people. By the 1970s the language of autonomy and choice
had become important parts of human rights discourse, wrestling independence away from a more patriarchal or patronizing welfare state.
Cultural understanding of sexual sterilization had also transitioned
into the language of pro-choice during this period, if only for certain
quarters of society.

The dual paths of sterilization, however, had not yet been reconciled
by the 1970s, and the language of choice moved front and centre in the
explosion of debates on abortion. The decriminalization of abortion in
Canada coincided with the repeal of the Sexual Sterilization Act in
Alberta in 1972. The timing of these two separate events is indicative of
the changing climate of reproductive rights in the latter half of the
twentieth century. The responses in Alberta, however, also suggested

that the two issues remained intimately related. As it became clear to Albertans that the eugenics laws no longer suited the late-twentieth-century context, concerns over abortion laws heated up. Many of the same players emerged in these debates, and several of the same issues arose. Would the "right" people seek out abortions? Would middle-class professional women use abortions to limit family size? Would young, poor, or marginalized women avoid abortions and over time contribute to changes in the population? The debates raised a number of well-worn issues reminiscent of 1920s eugenics discussions while introducing new alliances and a new vocabulary to use as shorthand for polarized stances on reproductive rights. Pro-life and pro-choice advocates jockeyed for the upper hand in an increasingly intense contest over the moral authority to promote one vision over the other.

In this book, I offer a social history of sexual sterilization and the politics of reproductive choice in Alberta. I examine the experiences of men and women who came into contact with sexual sterilization, both willingly and unwillingly, and I hope to add to the growing field of research in medical history by a particular focus on the history of eugenics, mental illness, disability, and institutionalization. I also consider how ideals of gender and sexuality affected these policies and how the program shaped the discourse on healthy morals and reproduction throughout the first three-quarters of the twentieth century. Although I focus on Alberta, that province's history provides insights into reproductive rights, medical experimentation, institutionalization, and health care, with broader implications for Canadians and others more generally.

Canadian historians writing about eugenics tend to focus on the period before the end of the Second World War, a time when discourse about sexual sterilization formed part of social reform movements, including elements of maternal feminism.[24] The Leilani Muir trial in the 1990s unearthed valuable evidence and situated Alberta's program within a larger international context, which has prompted historians to look at eugenics beyond the first half of the twentieth century. Chief among those authors is Jana Grekul, whose doctoral dissertation at the University of Alberta appeared in the wake of the Muir trial.[25] Indeed, prior to Grekul's sustained study, few articles and no books had appeared about Alberta's eugenics program.[26] Grekul, applying a sociological approach to the topic, examines the statistical evidence underpinning Alberta's program to show how the target groups had changed over time while the Eugenics Board's membership remained relatively static. Stemming from that dissertation, Grekul has also examined the role played by gender, arguing that the program institutionally and culturally targeted women.[27]

Other Alberta-based researchers have likewise contributed to our understanding of the provincial fascination with eugenics from different disciplinary perspectives. Several studies have focused on the legal history of the program, including Timothy Christian's 1974 honours thesis, which remains a key and often-cited study of the legislative debates surrounding the Sexual Sterilization Act and its various amendments.[28] Legal scholar and health law expert Tim Caufield has explored the complicated relationship between genetic research and ethics and, with Gerald Robertson, an expert in mental health law, has examined the human rights dimensions of the Alberta program.[29] Some of the scholarship on this topic has concentrated on pointing out the follies of the past. For instance, psychologist Doug Wahlsten's work has exposed the short-sighted or historically naive activities of the University of Alberta's psychology department in its celebration of the former head of the Eugenics Board, J.M. MacEachern.[30] Journalist Jane Harris-Zsovan, in a similar vein, has pieced together a series of government documents and newspaper articles to present a titillating and shocking exposé into Alberta's eugenics history by emphasizing how little is truly known about this program.[31]

Scholars in the United States have already begun to extend their studies into the post-war period, often finding that the evolution of eugenics programs became more complex on encountering second-wave feminism, Planned Parenthood, and lobbying efforts for access to then-illegal contraceptives. Scholars such as Wendy Kline, Rebecca Kluchin, Molly Ladd-Taylor, Paul Lombardo, Johanna Schoen, and Alexandra Minna Stern have considered sterilization more broadly, moving it beyond its direct association with eugenics programs.[32] Instead, they see it as part of the history of public health in the United States, which merges ideas about access to health care with human rights, poverty, racism, power, feminism, and state authority. Their studies draw particular attention to the ways in which eugenics fulfilled implicit state goals by targeting specific populations. Their race, class, gendered, and disability analyses, however, also reveal modes of resistance within these communities. Johanna Schoen, for example, shows how women deliberately used such policies to their advantage in an effort to gain safe medical access to a form of birth control, while avoiding detection from their (sometimes abusive) husbands. Their work provides an important counternarrative to another body of eugenics literature that focuses on Germany, Japan, or

South Africa and emphasizes the genocidal consequences of eugenics policies; these authors also show how eugenics programs were adapted to fit the growth of the welfare state in Canada and the United States. Such studies move beyond the formal application of eugenics to trace the changes in language and attitudes that accompanied cultural transitions in reproductive politics. Alberta's program provides an ideal opportunity for examining those changes in Canada.

The absence of consent provisions in sterilization cases involving individuals deemed mentally defective also demands further attention. Paul Lombardo's comprehensive study of the landmark US legal precedent *Buck v. Bell* provides critical legal historical context for understanding how juridical concerns about consent crept into eugenics policies in the United States, and suggests ways that US programs adapted to the new international ethics landscape.[33] Alberta, however, did not follow suit, instead continuing to justify its policy on financial grounds.

Internationally, studies of eugenics in the post-war period have been much more extensive, focusing on developments within broader medical, ethical, and legal debates over birth control, health care access, reproductive technologies, and disability. Chief among these works is Daniel Kevles's definitive study of the history of eugenics science, which looks at how Darwin and his contemporaries articulated a biological explanation for human behaviour and how those theories offered a framework for eugenics programs. Other notable scholars such as Gunnar Broberg and Nils Roll-Hansen discuss how some Scandinavian social democratic governments continued to justify such policies after the Second World War, while Pauline Mazumdar considers debates on both sides of the political spectrum in the field of human genetics in her study of the British Eugenics Society.[34]

This volume is a social history that locates the Canadian experience within these broader trends while focusing on how these issues played out for individual Albertans. Rather than concentrating on specific government responses to Alberta's Sexual Sterilization Act, I follow individuals through the eugenics program to show the effects of these policies or ways of medical thinking on real lived experiences. For example, in Chapter 2 I discuss the case of "George Pierre," a Treaty Indian and a pseudonym for a real patient who was recommended for sterilization, and expose how the change in consent policy affected Aboriginal patients who were brought before the Eugenics Board.

Documented cases of middle-class married women who sought legal access to sexual sterilization in Alberta are more difficult to find. Women seeking sterilization immediately following a Caesarean-section birth, or after pleading with their obstetricians or convincing them of the health risks posed by future births, appear between the lines of text by physicians concerned about their legal liability; Catholic voices also expressed outrage at the practice, indicating the likelihood of its performance. Men as subjects are even more difficult to locate in these records, but they slowly made their way into the debates as they reinserted their masculine role in family planning.

Reproductive technologies and pre-natal screening gave rise to new kinds of discussions about choice. Ruth Schwartz Cowan, for example, has published a defence of genetic screening using a historical analysis to demonstrate its social value.[35] Ian Dowbiggin's examination of sterilization during the Cold War revisits old debates in light of new technologies and medical knowledge, and concludes that global policies of population control during the Cold War contributed to a birth dearth.[36] He considers how conceptions of human rights, reproductive rights, and second wave feminism intersected in the latter half of the twentieth century to give rise to new challenges in population control. In stark contrast to these perspectives, the growing interdisciplinary field of disability studies problematizes categories of ability and disability in ways that re-evaluate the ethics of reproductive technologies, genetic screening, hereditary medicine, and even historical examinations of mental deficiency.

These studies repoliticize eugenics within the history of medicine, science, and technology, and offer critical complexity to the examination I undertake in this book. However, I add a new dimension to the dynamic debates now under way by focusing on Alberta's program, the largest and longest-standing sterilization policy in Canada and the only one in Canada or the United States to remove the need for informed consent. Because it spanned over forty years in the middle of the twentieth century and witnessed the rise of new reproductive technologies, second-wave feminism, increased secularization, and the decriminalization of abortion, Alberta's eugenics program needs to be considered against the backdrop of these contemporaneous important developments. As a result, in this book I seek to explore elements of consent, choice, sexuality, masculinity, and feminism as they concerned the individuals who faced the Eugenics Board or, conversely, as those who sought access to sexual sterilization operations were denied access. By concentrating on individuals and their experiences with sterilization, my approach refocuses the discussion on the area of social, cultural, and patient-centred medical history.

The substantive chapters move away from the political and legal machinations of the policy itself and concentrate instead on individual cases or examples that came in contact with the Sexual Sterilization Act. I selected these cases to demonstrate different aspects of the program, in temporal, gendered, and medicalized terms. The gender balance in the chapters is an effort to mirror somewhat the distribution of cases represented in the Eugenics Board files. Women outnumbered men, by approximately 58 per cent to 42 per cent. The distribution of men and women in the program shifted over time: men were equally or over-represented in the program between the First and Second World Wars, then women returned as the prime targets of sterilization after the Second World War, and remained so until the Act was repealed in 1972.

In Chapter 1 I examine the case of Mrs Nora Powers, who was picked up by the provincial police in 1924 for vagrancy and suspected prostitu-tion. She had been seen in an alley in the small town of Claresholm talking to a "Chinaman." Nora's rather extensive file in the Provincial Archives of Alberta follows her activities through various institutions and agencies, then briefly monitors her at her farm home with her hus-band and children before she was returned, it seems willingly, to a women's institution for further observation. Her case introduces a num-ber of important players in the establishment of the Sexual Sterilization Act, as Nora comes into contact with judges, medical authorities, and three members of Alberta's feminist elite – Louise McKinney, Emily Murphy, and Irene Parlby – who judged her case. Nora's case predates the eugenics legislation, but it illustrates the concerns of contemporary women's groups about Anglo-Saxon values and the kinds of surveil-lance measures that were put in place to monitor Alberta families dur-ing this period.

Chapter 2, as noted, introduces George Pierre, a Treaty Indian who was recommended for a vasectomy. The details of his experience un-folded through the words recorded by his Indian agent and Eugenics Board officials. His case engaged officials across jurisdictions in a discus-sion about Aboriginal sterilization and consent. Within the Eugenics Board files his case occasioned a prolonged discussion about race, state responsibility, and sexual aggression, which disappeared once a prece-dent for these cases was established in the 1930s. That case, however, was explored in detail while other cases provided context for examining the treatment of Aboriginal patients. Using the example of George Pierre, I maintain a focus on individuals who came into contact with the Act without resorting to a description based on statistics or generalizations.

In so doing, I explore broader categories of race, Aboriginal status, federal-provincial responsibilities for Indian health services, and the medical responses to Aboriginal health, poverty, and presumptions about their intelligence and capacity for responsible parenthood.

In Chapter 3 the focus moves away from institutionalized individuals, who represented the majority of cases that fell under the purview of the Eugenics Board, and towards a set of rather different cases illustrating the double standards of contraceptive morality as they were applied to middle-class married women in the 1940s and 1950s. Irene Parlby emerges as an unlikely character seeking sterilization. Parlby had been president of the United Farm Women of Alberta, an ardent first-wave feminist, and supporter of eugenics. Over the course of her short political career, however, she developed cysts on her ovaries and eventually received a hysterectomy at the recommendation of her gynecologist. Her correspondence with her feminist friends on the prairies indicated that other ambitious women like her had also had hysterectomies, usually for health reasons, but that ultimately left them unable to bear children. Some concealed their surgery as a shameful reminder of their inability to become mothers; over time, however, more and more married women sought this operation as a way to control their reproductive lives. Parlby and others might inadvertently have helped to pave the way for women seeking surgical solutions to their fertility.

The women in Chapter 3 emerge from the pages of medical records, religious newspapers, and letters to physicians. During the 1940s and 1950s a number of articles appeared in the *Canadian Medical Association Journal* as well as in the *Alberta Medical Review* indicating that, while so-called unhealthy women had access to sexual sterilization, in the form of hysterectomies, healthy women were restricted from such operations. Married women who sought access to physician-assisted sterilization, or vasectomies for their husbands, were denied because eugenics authorities and the majority of the medical community deemed such aggressive family planning immoral. The response of the Catholic Church in western Canada was even more condemnatory, as it moved to position itself in these debates with a firm grasp on reproductive moralities, the sanctity of life, and an increasingly central role in mental health services. National medical publications singled out Alberta as a possible location for such surgeries, and the number of women demanding such operations spiked in somewhat unlikely settings such as Lethbridge, where a surgeon's reputation for performing hysterectomies gained momentum and the number of women receiving them blossomed overnight.

Chapter 4 begins with the outraged reflections of Ken Nelson, who, in the 1990s, stood on the steps of the Alberta Legislative Building as the government announced that it would not compensate sterilization victims. Ken Nelson had been sterilized as a boy living at the Provincial Training School for Mental Defectives in Red Deer. I then look at a number of different male experiences, newspaper accounts, the personal records of one psychiatrist involved in these cases, and medical editorials that shed light on the connections between masculinity and sterilization. Although more women than men were sterilized, men did not escape from the shadow of eugenics science. Men were more often recommended for sterilization, particularly during the early years of the program, and boys became routine subjects for experimentation based on notions of appropriate youth and adult male behaviour. Dr Le Vann, the superintendent of the Provincial Training School, performed clinical experiments on the children under his care in an effort to establish a genetic link between mental deficiency and mental illness. The implications of his theory had the potential to expand the justification for routinely sterilizing a larger portion of the psychiatric population without requiring the consent of these individuals.

Healthy men living in middle-class families, in contrast, faced different challenges regarding modern masculinity. While their female counterparts brandished contraception as a badge of freedom, the vasectomy potentially undermined masculinity and contributed to a different set of concerns regarding modern family planning. By the late 1960s, however, the rates of professional and middle-class men seeking vasectomies increased dramatically and, with them, the social meaning of male sterilization and its relationship with modern masculinity shifted. In the second half of Chapter 4 I examine this shift in attitudes towards vasectomies and consider how it fits into the broader cultural changes in reproductive politics.

Doreen Befus's story unfolds in Chapter 5. Her extensive records are a rare example of a patient-oriented archival collection, including eleven boxes of materials donated by Doreen herself. Her story comes alive in these records as they reveal her experiences as an orphaned twin of a single mother who was a Russian immigrant in Red Deer, Alberta. Doreen grew up in a series of institutions, spending significant time at the Provincial Training School for Mental Defectives throughout the 1940s and 1950s. There, she was sterilized without her knowledge or consent, and was released from the institution only in the late 1960s as part of a growing wave of depopulating mental hospitals. In the community Doreen began her search for her biological family and along the way became a strong advocate for patients' rights. She earned work as a caregiver for several families, where her chief responsibilities were taking care of other people's children. Her detailed description of these jobs indicates how she began to question the right of government to decide who had the capacity to judge moral maternal qualities. Her case speaks to a host of similar cases in the Eugenics Board files concerning the rights of patients outside of the institution. In particular, Doreen's life experiences offer insight into the plight of patients after they left the institution and confronted the reality of their social roles as previously alleged unfit members of society.

In Chapter 6 I look at the voluminous extant records of Leilani Muir, the only person successfully to have sued the Alberta government in the 1990s for wrongful sexual sterilization. Her operation occurred in the 1960s while she was institutionalized, based on an IQ rating below 70 that inaccurately ranked her in the moron category of intelligence. Her case exposes the legal history of the eugenics program in Alberta, and offers a rare glimpse into the reflections and political activism that grew out of Leilani's determination to discuss publicly issues of reproductive rights, human rights, and government's abuse of authority over individuals deemed disabled or defective. Leilani's records are the largest collection of documents on a single eugenics case, and include extensive correspondence with lawyers in Canada and abroad who eventually aided her in what is a landmark legal decision in Canadian human rights. Importantly, Leilani's experiences provide reflections on reproductive choice and the changing context of disability activism and reproductive rights discourse evident by the 1990s.

Chapter 7, the final substantive chapter, is about a real patient whose pseudonym, given to her by the charge nurse who entered her case notes, was Jane Doe. Jane was fifteen years old when she arrived at the Foothills Hospital in Calgary nearly twelve weeks pregnant and requesting an abortion. The prohibition on abortion relaxed in 1969 when the federal government introduced an amendment to the Criminal Code. Meanwhile, Alberta's Sexual Sterilization Act remained in place for another two years. Jane's case merges with ongoing discussions about reproduction and choice, and explores how the legacy of eugenics continued to shape discussions about reproduction, autonomy, and consent into the 1970s and 1980s in Alberta. Rather than usher in a new era of language describing reproductive rights and choices, the public discourse on abortion returned to an older set of attitudes that refocused the blame on women, combined elements of sexuality with accusations of immorality, and questioned the viability of abortion for middle-class women while sanctioning them along with the sterilization of women considered to be less desirable mothers, including those who were either young or disabled. The implications of these accusations refocused medical attention on women as the guardians of reproductive morals, which justified resurrecting medical control over women's bodies.

Stepping back from the individual cases, I consider the effect that successive policies and practices had on reproductive rights, genetic research, and government, medical, and religious authority, as well as elements of resistance, autonomy, and the expression of civil liberties within these trends. I begin addressing eugenics as it comingled with notions of virtue that were tied to first-wave feminist ideals of citizenship. The book ends with the bittersweet victory of pro-choice feminists who successfully lobbied for safe access to medical abortions but continued to be chastised for contributing to the modern version of race degeneration. I also attempt to recognize the myriad ways in which civil liberties tied to reproduction affected families and individuals. Successes achieved by some women neither trickled down to all women nor were they celebrated uniformly. Historical examples help to paint a much more complicated picture of reproductive rights, at the heart of which lies a more fundamental set of concerns about medical authority, human – both men's *and* women's – rights, and the contested nature of progress itself.

Chapter One

Vagrancy, Violence, and Virtue: Nora Powers

On 12 May 1924, according to the Alberta police, Mrs Nora Powers ran away from her farm, leaving behind her husband and five children. A local police officer, Sergeant Hidson, later arrested her in the nearby southern Alberta town of Claresholm. He reported that he had charged Nora because he had caught her engaging in "immoral behaviour," which he ascertained after following her up an alley where she had been observed accompanying a "strange man" into a "Chinese rooming house." The man, under police questioning, admitted that he had bought Mrs Powers dinner and ice cream, then proceeded to have sex with her.[1]

Nora sat in jail for a few days before appearing before a judge and pleading guilty to the charges of vagrancy and prostitution. She received a six-month jail sentence. The deputy attorney general reported that Nora was likely "defective mentally, with the result that she is a sex pervert."[2] In the Fort Saskatchewan Prison, just outside of Edmonton, Nora communicated with her husband William by letter. William wrote that he wanted a divorce. Distressed by this news, Nora wrote back, promising to behave properly if he permitted her to return home. Somewhat reluctantly, William conceded: "Sure, I will let you come home any time you like. But I hope this will be the last trouble you will be in. I can't figure out how you got into this mixup."[3] He added that the children missed her and wanted her to come home.

Unfortunately for Nora, patching up her relationship with her husband was not enough to release her from jail. From the outset her case straddled both the criminal and the medical worlds, and provided ample evidence for authorities to explore opportunities beyond jail time. Although Nora did not appear to want her jail sentence changed, others did. The president of the Woman's Christian Temperance Union (WCTU), Louise McKinney, later a member of the Famous Five, visited Nora in jail and subsequently pleaded with the attorney general to have a psychiatric examination scheduled for her. McKinney felt that the arresting officer had missed a few details about Nora's situation. She in fact had nine children, not five, and one had recently died in childbirth. This situation alone might necessitate a psychiatric examination, since Nora might have been suffering from emotional stress following the death of her child. Similarly, the financial anxieties owing to the upkeep of nine children might have driven her to seek additional income or to behave out of self-despair in combination with a pre-existing low intelligence that allegedly made her incapable of making better decisions. Any of these scenarios might have warranted a psychiatric assessment, according to contemporary practices, but the legal authorities remained reluctant to take this route.

McKinney framed the case as one involving a woman with a mental deficiency, which served as the underlying reason for her poor judgment, and strongly urged the attorney general to reconsider Nora's case as a medical one rather than a criminal one. She wrote: "her mental deficiency seemed to cause her to veer towards immorality," and went on to suggest that Nora might be suffering from a mental disease, such as "nymphomania or excessive venereal impulse which is a symptom of her weak mindedness. A gaol seems hardly the place for such a woman." Moreover, a woman of sound mind, she maintained, would have pleaded not guilty. The attorney general seemed convinced by this justification, and recommended that Nora be sent for a psychiatric examination.[4]

Nora remained in jail while the provincial authorities reviewed her case. Before consulting her, the attorney general made arrangements for the jail's physician to monitor her behaviour until a psychiatric assessment could be scheduled. The physician agreed that Nora might be suffering from a mental disease, and recommended therefore that she be transferred to the Provincial Mental Hospital at Ponoka. Before any such transfer, however, a psychiatrist visited Nora and reported that he "observed no evidence of insanity," meaning that Nora should instead stay at the jail because her problem was criminal, not medical.[5]

McKinney, again acting on behalf of the WCTU, was not satisfied with this result, and demanded that the authorities carefully reconsider Nora's mental state before leaving her in jail to serve out her sentence. McKinney maintained that Nora had been pushed towards criminal behaviour due to underlying medical and psychological factors that impaired her judgment. The matron of the jail agreed, describing Nora as "dazed and nervous. For several days she was anxious to be allowed to work rather than be in confinement ... She appears to be a little simple minded, but is a good worker, willing and anxious to please, personally she is very clean and tidy and so far has shown no sign of any bad habits. She is very anxious to get back to her husband and children and promises to do better when released."[6] The matron's statement offered further evidence to support Nora's good character, her concern for her family, and her cleanliness, all of which combined to support a neat package of favourable values. These women authorities, it seemed, did not see Nora as a criminal to be cast beyond the rehabilitative reach of the system, but as a woman with a fragile mental condition who, with some assistance, could return to a relatively normal family life – or, at worst, as in need of public support and sympathy for her distress and mental deficiencies that prevented her from coping with stress in a more socially acceptable way.

The combined pressure of these two middle-class women eventually convinced the attorney general to order a second psychiatric assessment, which concluded that Nora was somewhat "weak minded but [the examiner] could not find evidence of insanity of Nymphomaniac tendency." Like the prison matron, the psychiatrist described Nora as someone of "clean and tidy appearance and bright manner but her intelligence is only fair. She is a good worker but is restless and impulsive and her emotions are poorly controlled."[7] The psychiatric interpretation fell short, however, of a convincing diagnosis that might have transferred Nora to the provincial mental hospital, and she would remain in prison for the duration of her sentence. Here the archival records of Nora's case end.

Nora's story, based on a real person, has been pieced together using records from the attorney general's office and the provincial police. Her experience offers a glimpse into the conditions women, mothers, and poor families faced in Alberta in the 1920s when confronted by legal, medical, and political authorities. Alberta, like other western jurisdictions, clamoured to develop a strong, healthy society in the wake of the First World War. Its strength rested upon the quality of its citizens in character, hygiene, socio-economic status, and morality. Within this framework, poor and immigrant families came under scrutiny for their potential contributions to or detractions from this goal. Although Nora's experience helps to illustrate the conditions leading up to the establishment of the eugenics program, its circumstances are historically specific. Eugenics and reproductive politics changed over time as legal, political, social, and medical forces refined attitudes towards population control and fertility in the province. The eugenics program was one particular aspect of this broader attempt to use medico-legal power to shape Albertan families in the first half of the twentieth century.

Although we do not know what ultimately happened to Nora, her case exhibits some typical features of the social and moral concerns in circulation in the 1920s. In particular it struck at the heart of contemporary debates about the criminal versus mentally defective behaviour of lower-class citizens, which often resulted in a disproportionate focus on immigrants and poor families. Within this climate social reformers embraced the rising tide of eugenics theories that had begun percolating throughout North America, applying them to their own communities in the hope of securing a better moral and economic future.

Eugenics and Politics in Alberta

In 1921 Albertans elected an untested political party, the United Farmers of Alberta (UFA), to lead it through the post-war period of reconstruction. UFA Historian Bradford Rennie describes the party as a movement that combined the interests of famers and labourers into a coherent articulation of progressive pursuits. He argues that, "at the heart of this movement culture [sic] were feelings of community; a sense of class opposition; assumptions about gender roles and traits; commitment to organization, cooperation, democracy, citizenship and education; a social ethic; religious convictions; agrarian ideology; and collective self-confidence."[8] Together these values, coupled with strong regional roots in rural Alberta, gave strength to the UFA.

Part of that strength derived from the active role women played in the organization and, consequently, in the way women were elevated to the status of "mothers of the race."[9] Women leaders in the organization exhibited a version of maternal feminism that was conditioned in part by agrarian values. As Sheila Gibbons has argued, for these feminists suffrage emerged as an important but secondary focal point behind their more prescient campaigns for health and maternal welfare. Suffrage emerged as a natural extension of farm women's views of partnership within the family farm enterprise, but the politicization of motherhood arose as a more sophisticated rallying point for agrarian feminists.[10] United Farm Women of Alberta (UFWA) members, including activists such as the WCTU's McKinney, kept maternal issues on the political radar, and brought considerable public attention to concerns of race degeneration.

Prior to the 1921 election the UFA had already established itself as a political party with concerted interests in areas of public health and social ethics. In 1918 members asserted at their annual convention that "the insane and feeble-minded constitute a source for a large proportion of the paupers, criminals and prostitutes of Alberta."[11] At the end of the war they seized upon the opportunity to build a new, healthier post-war society. As Rennie explains, "[f]earing that the soldiers' sacrifices might be in vain, farmers concluded that governments must create a new society through prohibition, health care, eugenics, social welfare, and progressive taxation."[12] Moreover, "farmers feared that because of the war the 'race' was losing 'its strongest and most physically fit,' and [the UFA/UFWA] endorsed eugenics solutions to keep Canada racially virile."[13]

As political architects of a progressive Alberta, the UFA worked steadily towards implementing policies that would mould Albertans, native and immigrant alike, into an ideal society. As its plans unfolded, the party increasingly incorporated elements of eugenics into its social planning. Eugenics discourse in Alberta knitted together threads of maternal agrarian feminism, nativist concerns about so-called problematic immigrants, and escalating fears of an infectious form of mental deficiency that would spread through the population. Together these elements culminated in a eugenics movement that gained political traction within the UFWA, which then helped to give eugenics a legislative presence.

Although the Sexual Sterilization Act would not be passed until 1928, the seeds of Alberta's eugenics program were sown in the 1910s and 1920s, when people like Nora came to the attention of local authorities. These early beginnings reveal some of the ways in which the idea of progress was drenched in the language of eugenics and how, in this Canadian version of an international trend, agricultural and class interests framed the discussions. The Alberta chapter in the international story of eugenics borrowed ideas from US and European experiments, but the province ultimately tailored its program to suit its own ideals of good and bad citizens: eugenics on the Canadian prairies targeted immigrants and people deemed mentally deficient. Where race had played a formative role in shaping programs south of the border, in Alberta the focus was more often on the "undesirable" ethnic traits of eastern European immigrants. Poverty or even class-based ideals played key roles in the program's development, particularly through the conflation with poor judgment, criminal activity, and large families. Together these characteristics contributed to the construction of feeble-mindedness or mental deficiency or defectiveness in ways that stretched these categories beyond their medicalized boundaries and married social and biological theories of degeneracy with progressive visions of a healthy nation.

As the UFA suggested, there was a strong relationship between mental deficiency and criminality. Consequently, issues of social justice and the state's responsibility to protect its upstanding citizens relied on a careful interpretation of that relationship. The political distinction between criminal and mentally defective behaviour frequently boiled down to an issue of responsibility, where the former reflected intent and the latter could be excused as a matter of disease. Both categories, however, purportedly were ballooning out of control and threatening the stability of progress and social order in the province. Both necessitated intervention by social reformers and the provincial government in an effort to promote a healthy, morally progressive society. The social distinction between the two categories, however, hinged upon a set of nativist and elitist ideals that reinforced negative attitudes towards particular immigrant families and poverty.

Within this context intelligence emerged as a suitable demarcation of rights, albeit one infused with the language of class values. Weak-minded or mentally deficient individuals were considered incapable of making good decisions on the basis of their mental disease or lowered intelligence. Concerns for character, work habits, and sexual behaviour seemed to guide such assessments, as in Nora's case. The process of determining a person's mental state, which affected the terms of confinement and later human or reproductive rights, involved a complicated mixture of factors. The designation of mental competence functioned like a hinge that could swing towards ensuring individual rights and responsibilities, even if responsibility meant jail time, but in the other direction mental *in*competence prioritized the province's objectives over the rights of individuals. Mental illness conveyed a different kind of sentence, one that removed an individual's capacity for legal responsibility and replaced personal rights with state guardianship. Shrouded in the language of philanthropy, the provincial government of 1920s Alberta moved forward with plans to build a stronger, healthier society by eradicating mental deficiency and thus creating a more responsible citizenry.[14] Although the specific language and application of eugenics changed over time, the spectrum of responsibility remained a key feature of discussions about reproductive autonomy. Responsibility, whether determined through intelligence, behaviour, emotional, physical or psychological strength, age, sex, or resources, often formed the backbone of decisions that vacillated between reproductive autonomy and protection.

In Alberta the process of formalizing eugenics and codifying the specific language of reproductive protection was helped along initially by women's associations, especially the UFWA, which had an abiding interest in political reform, including suffrage, and the promotion of women's rights through marriage, inheritance, and custody laws. This growing cluster of issues soon became associated with the rise of maternal agrarian feminism, which found champions in Alberta. A vocal and active women's movement on the Canadian prairies promoted eugenics as an extension of the campaign to improve maternal circumstances and bring political attention to family values. Alberta feminists often merged maternal with agrarian politics in a manner that provided subtleties both in terms of women's professional roles and as mothers familiar with the language of animal husbandry and the rigours of farm life, including cultivation cycles, hereditary concepts, and genetic variation. Consequently, agrarian feminist values were interlaced with threads of eugenics theories.[15]

As early as 1923 the UFWA approved a motion to introduce a sexual sterilization law that would target individuals considered feeble minded.[16] Over the next several years the women's branch of the United Farmers continued to press male politicians for an act to curb rampant reproduction by individuals who were "morons," a term reserved for those with a very low intelligence quotient and considered incapable of learning. The UFWA stressed the importance of more stringent screening at the point of entry to Canada as well as among families already settled in Alberta that were considered of low-grade intelligence,[17] claiming that morons were a "drain on the physical, mental and economic resources"[18] and that "many of the criminal offences against children are committed by persons who are of low mental development."[19] UFWA activists lobbied the provincial government to acknowledge the argument for the genetic causes of mental deficiency, claiming that "feeble-mindedness is hereditary in about 80% of cases."[20]

Feminists, however, were not the only supporters of eugenics in Alberta. The ideas underpinning a eugenics outlook came from a more disparate set of perspectives that tended to value middle-class, Anglo-Saxon virtues over the poor, the non-English-speaking, and women of loose morals or untidy habits. The women's movement did not create these perspectives, but, in an effort to improve the position of women, capitalized on the rising tide of antipathy towards marginalized groups within western Canadian society.[21]

Although some aspects of Nora's case are well preserved in the archival records, smaller fragments of other cases that made their way to the attorney general or the premier's office, or came to the attention of police officials, highlight similar themes and illustrate some of the ways in which contemporary attitudes laid the foundations for the introduction of the eugenics program. Social reformers encouraged the Alberta government to craft a more forward-thinking response to perceived moral problems. Their views were influenced by the rising international popularity of eugenics and the local manifestations of a mental hygiene movement that directed political and social attention to the public health arena and found expression in a receptive political movement.

The focus of these early discussions concerned families and their social place in disproportionately infecting the moral stock of the nation. Eugenics programs later targeted individuals for their contributing roles in this process, but the early manifestation of eugenics discourse in western Canada looked to more systemic challenges, including immigration, education, and citizenship. Family histories and racial or ethnic characterizations borrowed from the language of disease and contagion to describe the need to quarantine and ultimately expel the allegedly diseased segments of society. In the early part of the twentieth century, reformers believed that western Canada was falling ill to a plague brought by immoral and unsavoury immigrant families whose crass customs and unbridled fertility threatened to overwhelm more progressive ideals for the region.

Nams, Jukes, and Kallikaks

The manifestation of a mental hygiene movement in Canada took some of its cues from British and US studies that had already developed more sophisticated ways of measuring the downstream social effects of unchecked mental deficiencies. The British reformers focused most of their attention on the rampant growth of the working classes and, using Malthusian logic, considered the scarcity of resources and the environmental influences of multigenerational poverty on an increasing segment of the population.[22] US researchers, combining statistical and genealogical data, similarly produced family studies that showed an increase in mental defects and moral degeneration within multiple generations of a single family.[23] Some of these studies became famous for their exposés of feeble-mindedness and the collateral damage it wreaked on communities and local economies.

One example, by eugenicist Charles Davenport, focused on a family called Nam, living in a rural area of New York State known pejoratively as Nam Hollow. Davenport, a professor of biology and supporter of Mendelism,[24] began his research with a single couple and traced their progeny through several generations to arrive at a population involving over 800 individuals within the Nam clan. By following the relations and habits of this family, Davenport reported that the group included "232 licentious women and 199 licentious men, and only 155 chaste women and 83 chaste men. 54 have been in custodial care either in asylums or county houses, 24 have received outdoor aid, and in addition private aid has been given to them by charitable persons for years. 40 have served terms in state's prison or jail. There are 192 persons who use alcohol in extreme quantities, ie., are sots."[25] Davenport emphasized both the inheritability of undesirable characteristics and the toll such qualities took on state resources by confining members of this family in prison or supporting them through various charitable means. Moreover, he claimed, the family engaged in several illegitimate and some consanguineous relationships, which amplified the degree of defects observable physically and mentally. His liberal application of the term "hereditary" suggested direct and even blood links between generations in terms of their taste for alcohol or propensity to law breaking.

In an attempt to use his study as a call to social action, Davenport compared the scourge of the Nams to an outbreak of the bubonic plague, implying that breakaway members of the family were likely to infect New York City: "Not a few cases are known where harlots from the hollow have become prostitutes in the cities, even in New York, and the tendencies to commit arson, assault and burglary have gone with the individuals which they tenant to remote parts of the country."[26] Playing upon the urban-rural divide and fears of an epidemic of immorality, Davenport's study helped to galvanize support for more direct intervention with respect to the unchecked fertility of less desirable elements of American society.

Other studies drew similar conclusions. In 1874 sociologist Richard Dugdale conducted an investigation of the Juke family of upstate New

York after observing their overrepresentation in local jails and poor-houses. Dugdale emphasized the role of the environment and how it interacted with the bloodline inheritability of characteristics.[27] He none-theless concluded that both environmental and inheritable causes of degeneracy necessitated intervention or regulations to prevent such defectiveness from affecting American society.

In 1912 psychologist Henry Goddard added a study in this vein on the Kallikak family, this time focusing more concertedly on the plight of feeble-minded individuals. Although Goddard was later criticized for crudely altering the images in his book to give people blank, expres-sionless faces or angry dispositions, he initially drew substantial atten-tion to the links between feeble-mindedness and degeneracy.[28] Goddard emphasized the connections between intelligence and strong moral values in an effort to steer the focus towards individuals considered feeble minded, morons, imbeciles, and idiots. Such people, he felt, did not exhibit a level of intelligence that might allow them to know right from wrong. For example, he suggested a young woman raised in a low-intelligence household would not experience the realities of the outside world and, therefore, would be "prey to the designs of evil men or even women and would lead a life that would be vicious, immoral, and criminal, though because of her mentality she herself would not be responsible."[29] Feeble-minded people, he argued, had neither the ge-netic pedigree nor the social graces or behavioural skills necessary to raise responsible children. With moral reformers jockeying for position on this debate, Goddard helped to provide a clear target group whose future infertility might reduce the numbers of feeble-minded people in subsequent generations.

Canadian reformers also contributed to such family studies. Most in-famously, T.C. Douglas, future Co-operative Commonwealth Federation (CCF) premier of Saskatchewan, wrote his 1933 master's thesis on the "Problem of the Subnormal Family," adopting an approach similar to that of Goddard, Davenport, and Dugdale. Rather than examine a fam-ily per se, however, Douglas used a combination of the British focus on the lower classes and the US preference for family studies, identifying a small number of women considered subnormal and tracing them and their offspring over multiple generations. Douglas, too, emphasized the social and financial costs of unchecked fertility among members of what he termed subnormal categories, which he meant to include the feeble minded or mentally defective, those exhibiting low moral standards, families subject to "social disease," and those who had become a public charge.[30] He then recommended a multifaceted approach that took into account both environmental and hereditary influences and that considered the community's obligation to address these problematic families. He stated: "We must consider the causes that have produced this social phenomenon in modern society. Without knowledge of these underlying causes, our approach will be largely hypothetical."[31]

Douglas's focal point was his own community of Weyburn, Saskatchewan, from which he selected several hundred people out of the town's small population of about five thousand whom he classified as indigents chronically dependent on charity. He started with a group of twelve "immoral or non-moral women," categories he defined as follows: "by immoral I mean common prostitutes, and by non-moral I mean women who are mental defectives, and have no knowledge of right or wrong, but who are used for immoral purposes by their husbands or others."[32] By tracing the progeny of these twelve women through two generations, Douglas identified two hundred people: the original twelve had ninety-five children collectively, who in turn had one hundred and five children; the birth rate among this group thus was 7.9, compared with the average rate of 3.1 for the rest of the community.[33] Analysing the intelligence levels, disease states, and criminal activity of this larger group of people, Douglas concluded by recommending curbing the rapid rate of reproduction within such subnormal elements of society.

As his US counterparts did decades earlier, Douglas found instances of consanguineous relations in the small community setting – particularly where its "subnormal" members remained socially segregated from the rest – that seemed to amplify some of the problems. A group of boys from this Weyburn group had formed a gang that engaged in delinquent activities, while the girls tended to deviate from sexual norms, including seeking abortions or having illegitimate children. Douglas argued that the risk of such activities spreading to schoolmates or other members of the community was higher in a smaller community where exposure to these individuals was more difficult to limit.[34]

Douglas departed slightly from most US researchers, however, in elaborating on the environment as both a cause and an effect of subnormal behaviours. He suggested that the state, the religious community, and the education system needed to work together to address the problems, along with laws restricting marriage among subnormal groups, enforcing their segregation from the community, promoting sexual sterilization, and decriminalizing birth control.[35] In particular, segregating children in special classrooms tailored to their learning needs struck Douglas as a progressive move with benefits for both the subnormal group and "normal" children who might be held back by their being surrounded by less capable peers: "the teacher tends to think the child obstinate and ungovernable when the pupil is really just desperately behind the rest of the class."[36] Segregating children in this manner, Douglas suggested, might help children of all intelligence levels gain the confidence and self-esteem to participate in mainstream society with a suitable set of skills coupled with good morals and law-abiding behaviour.

As for sexual sterilization, Douglas deferred to modern advances in medical science that made it possible to reduce the risk of reproduction without affecting an individual's ability to engage in sexual activity. He regarded these advances as meeting the criticism levelled at steriliza-tion laws that had not taken the basic human need for sexual expression into account. He suggested that the medical profession could be trusted to determine the best candidates for sterilization surgery, although he added: "only those mentally defective and those incurably diseased should be sterilized. Many subnormal families whose intelligence is not of a high order are capable of raising useful citizens."[37] Greater empha-sis, he argued, should be placed on decriminalizing birth control and educating families about it, believing that many in fact might embrace such measures to improve their economic and social standing. He none-theless recognized the paradox of contemporary birth control: "The re-markable thing about modern society is that while those economically capable of rearing children practice birth control, those in a state of pov-erty are deprived of the necessary information."[38]

Douglas's solution to the challenges posed by the increase in subnor-mal families rested primarily with religious authorities. He criticized the churches of all denominations for not providing more guidance to subnormal families and helping them integrate into the broader com-munity. "The task of the church," he maintained, was "to find an outlet for their social desires. To help them to play their parts as parents, as children, as citizens, and as human beings."[39] It is perhaps unsurprising that Douglas, a student of divinity at a Baptist university, would argue for churches to play a greater role in addressing the problems of the subnormal family, but the emphasis he placed on acceptance and inte-gration distinguishes his study from those of some of his predecessors. He concluded that the church "can call men into a new relationship of affection by her democratic spirit of equality, she can give to these socially repressed individuals the opportunity for social expression and recognition."[40] He believed in the inherent human desire for self-reflection and improvement, and recognized the role that the church played in that process: "nothing can lift these people faster than their own evaluation of themselves."[41]

Although Douglas was later criticized for such views, his thesis captured some of the reformist views on the issue as it was understood in Canada at that time. He abandoned his stance on sexual sterilization, some claimed, after learning of the events in Germany during the Second World War;[42] more recent partisan critics have cited Douglas's thesis as proof that Canada's future father of medicare subscribed to elements of dark or misguided science.[43] Despite his support of sexual sterilization, however, his thesis emphatically favoured a more empowering outcome for the majority of individuals within his subnormal framework. The combination of invasive and embracing techniques used to address fears associated with social degeneration was consistent with the ways progressives adopted eugenics theories in western Canada before the Second World War.

Canadian mental hygiene reformers fit within a broader international movement of intellectuals and activists interested in testing eugenics theories of social degeneration, the heredity of delinquency and criminality, and the associations between "mental abnormality" and "illegitimacy, prostitution, and dependency."[44] The Canadian National Committee for Mental Hygiene (CNCMH), formed in 1918 with a mandate to survey facilities and programs across Canada that catered to the mental health needs of the population, developed in some measure as a result of the goodwill, volunteerism, and spirit of social reform that had taken hold among middle- and upper-class Canadians at the turn of the century and merged with the eugenics movement.[45] The CNCMH investigated the current state of mental health facilities and immigration policies, along with the state of public education and prison populations in each province. Its provincial mental hygiene surveys later served as a baseline for the introduction of social and moral reforms aimed at reducing the numbers of individuals in the asylum and prison populations.

The CNCMH had as its underlying agenda a plan to reduce the number of people in asylums, believing that these institutions were outdated and expensive. It thus proposed medical examinations of immigrants and Aboriginals and broadening the term feeble minded to include criminal behaviour, prostitution, vagrancy, and unemployment.[46] Psychiatric hospitals, or asylums, and prisons emerged as the two key institutions in need of attention and possibly reform. The CNCMH encouraged a public health movement predicated on assessing the severity of mental health problems across the country.[47] Although it formed part of an ethos of progressivism, its focus was not on individuals in need of mental health services. Rather, the mental hygiene movement maintained an interest in the collateral socio-political consequences of unchecked mental diseases and the scourge or spread of feeble-mindedness, which tended to reinforce class and ethnic values. Fundamentally, like their US counterparts, these Canadian reformers believed there was a strong correlation between mental abnormalities, or levels of intelligence, and criminal or immoral behaviour, and likened these categories to a social disease or epidemic that threatened to infect mainstream society. Families in the lowest categories of intelligence tended to have more children, which alarmed reformers and fuelled their argument that such families were poised to overwhelm the ranks of the intelligent.

Although the national committee attracted men and women who were chiefly interested in preventing further social and moral degeneration, the mental hygiene movement assumed different forms across the country. In Alberta, the committee's mandate stipulated that "the aim of the movement is to study individuals in such a way that their weaknesses and strengths can be determined, and with this as a preliminary measure, to formulate treatment and training that will be productive of the best social results."[48] The statement was characteristic of the manner in which the movement combined elements of psychometrics, or intelligence ratings, with medical and social issues to justify targeting families with lower intelligence quotients or those deemed mentally abnormal for contributing to contemporary social ills.

In its mental hygiene survey, the Alberta branch of the CNCMH attempted to categorize individuals and predict their value or, conversely, their cost to society based on the severity of their abnormality or deviation from middle-class values. The survey suggested that "[a] mentally defective individual is one who through failure of brain development never reaches the adult standard of intelligence and personal control. Three sub-groups are generally recognized – idiots, imbeciles and morons." The survey went on to state, "[i]n other words, once a mental defective always a mental defective. The question might then be asked if treatment is of any avail. In answer the point should be stressed that although mental defectives cannot be made whole as far as brain capacity is concerned, it is nevertheless true that the majority of morons [sic] can attain fairly successful life in the community when suitable training and supervision are instituted."[49] These reformers did not recommend an aggressive eugenics or sterilization program for everyone, nor did they suggest building larger or more asylums and prisons to segregate abnormal or criminal members from the mainstream society. Rather, they attempted to devise a more sophisticated triage approach that allowed people to be siphoned into different treatment, rehabilitation, or penal institutions based on the prognosis associated with their deficiencies. Such a classification system relied upon up-to-date medical and statistical research informing these divisions and predicting outcomes.

One underlying concern of the mental hygiene movement was the potential problem posed by liberal immigration policies. The rather open-door policy that had been in place in Canada at the turn of the century had startled reformers who felt that other countries were using Canada as a dumping ground for unwanted members of their society, including individuals who exhibited mental defects, who were considered insane, or who were unable to work due to physical or mental deficiencies.[50] The Alberta provincial survey reported, in relation to immigration, that "[i]t is particularly desirable to reject the insane and mentally deficient because they often prove a greater menace than any other group." It further claimed that, "[i]n other words, immigrants have contributed more than their fair share to the insane and feeble-minded population, and to other undesirable groups."[51]

This attitude was reflected in the political rhetoric of the day, and entrenched in the anti-immigrant sentiment found throughout western Canada. Perhaps most famously, J.S. Woodsworth, later the founding leader of the CCF, published a treatise in 1909 on the "problem of the immigrant" called *Strangers within Our Gates*, in which he claimed that "this little book is an attempt to introduce the motley crowd of immigrants to our Canadian people and to bring before our young people some of the problems of the population with which we must deal in the very near future."[52] Woodsworth was tapping into fears of "race suicide" – that the better classes would be subsumed by the lower classes, who tended to have larger families and who were thought to contribute disproportionately to contemporary social problems.

Woodsworth outlined a veritable hierarchy of races and ethnicities based on their capacity to assimilate to the most desirable cultural traits of Canadian society. Non-white races fell at the bottom of the list, and non-English-speaking immigrants came second to native English families, with more subtle rankings based on virtues such as thrift, temperance, and work ethic. For example, southern Italians ranked lower than those from the north, with Woodsworth claiming that "most of the diseased and criminal Italians, who have given their compatriots such an unenviable reputation in America, have been shipped from Naples by the police authorities."[53] More generally, he suggested that immigration posed a serious challenge to Canadians: "English and Russians, French and Germans, Austrians and Italians, Japanese and Hindus – a mixed multitude, they are being dumped into Canada by a kind of endless chain. They sort themselves out after a fashion, and each seeks to find a corner somewhere. But how shall we weld this heterogeneous mass into one people? That is our problem."[54]

Although Woodsworth wrote from his vantage point in Winnipeg, Albertans shared similar views, and looked to their provincial government to act upon allegations that foreign experiences conditioned immigrants to transgress Canadian law. The letters Alberta premiers received throughout the 1920s offer a window into such attitudes, which were folded into contemporary mental hygiene campaigns. In 1924, for example, the enforcement branch of the provincial liquor control board reported that it had searched the farm of a Mr J.A. Lamontagne on suspicion of his owning distilling equipment and had determined that Lamontagne was indeed making and selling moonshine. The enforcement officers further found that the man was a returned soldier from Kentucky and that, "being a Kentuckian he is no doubt well versed in the art of trade of making moonshine."[55] In this instance the man's foreign origin trumped any consideration of his status as an English-speaking immigrant, and his intemperate qualities ultimately overwhelmed any further consideration of his good morals.

Another case from the same year reinforced the view that Americans were not immune to this kind of treatment. About a man from Los Angeles who tried to homestead in Alberta and had experienced several bad harvests, a neighbour wrote to the police claiming he was "mentally unbalanced" and was carrying a revolver and a knife. In the letter his neighbour stated: "One day he will appear fairly rational and the next his talk is impossible to understand. He has the delusion that his neighbours want to hunt him out of the country. There is no foundation for this as they pity him and try to help him when he tries to do something to help himself … He is getting on the people's nerves and before anything untoward happens I take the liberty of reporting his state to you."[56] A police officer investigated, but the man did not appear violent or criminal and no weapons were found on him. Although the man exhibited no personal signs of insanity, the officer discovered that his mother and sisters had spent time in psychiatric institutions, and concluded that he might "become insane at any time." Furthermore, he added, "I consider [the man] to be a very undesirable type of settler, and I would suggest that he be deported if it is possible to do so."[57] Delusional or not, the man was justified in fearing that his neighbours were conspiring against him and seeking to have him deported. The case reinforces the connection between illness, family, and finances, as his supposed undesirability became linked to his presumed genetic predisposition in combination with his poor farm returns.

In another case, a man named Wallace complained to the police that the Ku Klux Klan was after him, but his neighbours believed he was mentally unbalanced. The subsequent police report indicated that, "on the night of the 13th instance Wallace left Rogers' Ranch in a very unusual manner, wearing suit of underwear, a shirt, overcoat and cap."[58] Upon closer scrutiny, the police found that two other men staying at the ranch had chased Wallace. They dropped all charges, but kept Wallace under surveillance. The silence in the official record raises questions about sexuality, temperance, and general masculine ranch culture, and draws attention to the ways in which conventional values were policed during this period.

A 1926 case involved a man caught on suspicion of causing an explosion on the front lawn of a judge's home. The police found a monogrammed cigarette lighter in the debris, and traced it to an Italian man, a Mr Cantazzi, "who is a suspicious character and evidently capable of being the perpetrator of the outrage." The police, following up on this lead, searched Cantazzi's house for liquor and evidence of his participation in the explosion. Inside they found "various figures emblematic of Farmer Members, Judges, Attorney Generals [sic] and others, with various implements of destruction including bombs and fuses."[59] The Italian anarchist movement reached a fever pitch in the United States during the 1920s, and whether Cantazzi had been part of that transnational campaign or the provincial government feared that Cantazzi represented the anarchists' moving into Canada, his actions prompted a swift response.[60] The combination of his Italian origins, anarchist leanings, and threatening behaviour branded Cantazzi as a dangerous man at large. The evidence collected from his home also suggested that his acts had been premeditated and therefore not the result of an abnormal mental condition. Nonetheless, the conflation of ethnic background and mental stability continued to shape his identity, and although Cantazzi emerged as a political radical, his mental capacity came under scrutiny, with the government justifying his confinement as a mental health intervention.

Among the variety of cases that caught the attention of Alberta premiers, those of Ukrainian immigrants attracted a concerted and disproportionate concern. A 1921 report by the provincial Department of Public Health identified Ukrainians as having a particularly difficult time assimilating Canadian values. Recognizing that most Ukrainian families in Alberta had been "victims of the most abominable social system the world has seen" under the communist regime, the report also claimed that the Ukrainian language and customs put these families at higher risk of feeble-mindedness and made them more susceptible to disease: "the districts are not well supplied with medical men, add to that ignorance, and you have an ideal soil for the spread of venereal disease."[61] Moreover, the fact that Ukrainian women often worked in the fields alongside the men, though laudable for its display of work ethic, attracted criticism for their supposed neglect of their domestic duties, including rearing children.[62] The home, the report averred, was a key ingredient in the development of good Canadian citizens. This observation justified an aggressive focus on educating parents about social and mental hygiene and dissipating the cloud of ignorance that was thought to dilute assimilation strategies aimed exclusively at school children.[63] Lectures and sermons directed at Ukrainian parents attempted to convince them that they "are not mere 'foreigners,' but that they form an integral part of this great Dominion, and that they must share its responsibilities as well as privileges. Once they catch the flame of enthusiasm, they will consider it their sacred duty, as Canadian citizens, to conserve their own health and the health of their children."[64]

Perhaps unsurprisingly, the government's focus on health and immigration created an atmosphere of fear and suspicion. As public health nurses and government officials visited regions to police the situation, they soon found that immigrant families were reluctant to admit to any health problems.[65] Officials nonetheless distributed copies of the provincial Health Act, and enlisted local reeves and councillors to identify health problems among immigrant communities. Some regions reported strong compliance with the law, especially the Health Act, but others raised concerns. In district 514, for example, a cursory investigation had revealed no disease, but "[t]he people do not understand English, I was unable to talk to them. Where children were at home I made an attempt to explain things. They merely grin and think the law is very foolish. Those people understand but one law – the law of force."[66]

The Department of Public Health report came down particularly hard on the living habits of eastern Europeans: "The foreign element, called collectively Russian although including Galician, Pole, Austrian and all other nationalities from that section of Eurasia, has no conception of the meaning of the word sanitation."[67] The report described the filthy conditions that families lived in, mixing livestock and children and the resultant exacerbation of health problems. Here again, the department recommended the use of force to achieve compliance among this motley group of undifferentiated Russians: "Inspectors can be developed who will enter the houses and force sanitary conditions upon these people, who now menace the health of the whole province by their disgusting habits of life."[68] It is unclear what specific measures officials intended to use to force a change in habits, but the use of inspectors, who later included public health nurses, to investigate homes alongside the force of the government to legislate action, created a culture of surveillance.[69]

The issue of mentally defective immigrants raised alarms with the Department of Public Health. In 1924 the minister, upset with the insufficient mechanisms in place to prevent unhealthy immigrants from entering Canada, wrote to the premier complaining that medical examinations were overly cursory at the point of entry: "Several medical officers are sealed in a room and endeavor to pick out defective persons as these people march past."[70] Furthermore, he argued, this practice had resulted in a large number of foreign-born individuals residing in the Provincial Hospital for the Insane. Canadians, for example, represented 49 per cent of the provincial population and 27 per cent of patients in the asylum, while immigrants from the British Isles, Europe, and the United States, although they represented 17, 14, and 18 per cent of Alberta's population, respectively, were a disproportionately higher 25, 24, and 22 per cent of asylum patients.[71] The minister further complained that the situation had resulted in significant expense for the government as it waited for deportation cases to be processed – noting, for example, the cases of "colored imbeciles for whom the Department has been paying for two years and is still unable to get any action in respect of deportation."[72] The minister felt that, at the very least, the federal government should compensate provinces for the expenses associated with cases that slipped through the medical examinations at the point of entry.

Indeed, a few months earlier the head of the nursing branch of public health had given the premier a list of undesirable families in Alberta that had passed the medical examiners undetected and that should be deported as potential public charges. A woman whose husband had deserted her was described as "incapable of supporting herself and children, one of whom was a suspect mental defective, and it was deemed cheaper to return her to her relatives in England than to allow her to remain here."[73] Thus, having children suspected of being or deemed feeble minded was enough to put an entire family at risk of deportation.[74]

The threat of deportation, however, applied not only to families with potential mental deficiencies, but also to those who were destitute. The Department of Public Health was responsible for paying the hospital fees of recent immigrants who were incapable of working or who had lost their jobs, and kept a running total of these expenses, which it forwarded to the premier to help bolster the case for deportation. One case involved the McConnell family, from England, whose father had aggravated an old war injury during his first year trying to farm. The doctor who examined him recommended that he find a new vocation, given the permanent damage to his hands from his injuries. At that point McConnell sought relief for his wife and child while he searched for another job. The province filed deportation papers, but McConnell managed to find work in Edmonton, whereupon the department put his case on hold and forwarded its details to the premier for further consideration.[75]

Such cases thus reflected the twinned concerns of unemployment and expenses related to health care costs borne by the government, which made immigrant families targets for deportation to reduce the burden on government and, by association, healthy native-born taxpayers. Even families that had resettled in Alberta from other provinces became the subject of complaints by those responsible for their health bills.

Although escaping stereotypes about foreigners and the threat of deportation, destitute Métis families, too, were the subject of concerns in police files about their character and work ethic. In one case a Métis man had not worked for some time, having chosen instead to care for his ill wife and two small children. The police officer investigating the family's application for relief advised the man to leave his wife and children with relatives and seek employment, although he also gave the family a voucher for five dollars worth of groceries.[76] The officer offered no comment on the habits of Métis families, unlike many other cases that relied on assumptions about race or nationality to guide the characterization of individuals who came to police attention.

In another case police investigated a woman whose husband had left her and taken their two children. "She has now an illegitimate child about one and one-half years old and does not seem to have any sense in regard to morals and has different men to her shack. The city has provided her a shack and also meals, but, in her state of mind this will have to be done away with at once."[77] The Provincial Mental Hospital at Ponoka was already overcrowded, however, and would not take the woman; moreover, no suitable facilities existed for the illegitimate child.

Parents often bore the brunt of the blame for neglecting children considered defective. In such situations medical officers appeared more sympathetic, and institutionalization was deemed a progressive, humanitarian option. In one severe case, police discovered a twelve-year-old girl in a grain bin. Upon examining her, a doctor described the girl as "dreadful, the child's general appearance is that of an undersized, starved, diseased, sickly imbecile," and suggested that, with proper care and nutrition, she might recover somewhat from her condition: "I believe this is not a case of insanity, but of rickets with complications arising out of the dreadful conditions the child has been kept in. It would be a crime for the state to leave the child to the unintelligent negligence of the father and stepmother."[78]

Individuals with low intelligence were also the target of those who were concerned about the dangers of degeneration and feeble-mindedness. One case that came across Premier Brownlee's desk in 1929 involved a man with serial convictions for "vagrancy, assault, damage to property, drunkenness and supplying liquor to Indians."[79] Rather than having him spend more time in jail, the perpetrator was sent to the Provincial Mental Hospital at Ponoka for a psychiatric assessment. The doctor there reported that the man had no clear signs of mental abnormalities, but did exhibit low intelligence. After the man underwent two more stints of jail and two more psychiatric examinations, the psychiatrists remained firm in their assessment that he did not exhibit any true mental symptoms and was aware of his actions. In his last examination, however, he had explained that he had behaved badly hoping that his actions would result in his transfer from the Lethbridge jail to the mental hospital at Ponoka. The attorney general and his staff at this point concluded that no further action needed to be taken towards the man: he was clearly in control of his actions and was therefore responsible for his behaviour, and deserved jail time rather than hospital treatment.

Questions of competency and responsibility became critical criteria for determining which institution best fit the crime. In a telegraph sent to the premier, Alberta MP Henry Spence tried to provide some clarity on a case that, like that of Nora Powers, straddled both jail and hospital. A man convicted of murder was tried before a judge who suspected that the man might, in fact, be insane and therefore in need of a hospital sentence. The expert witnesses, presumably psychiatrists, called upon to examine the man agreed that he was subnormal, but nonetheless believed he had sufficient appreciation of his actions and should receive jail time.[80] After four separate assessments the conviction stood, and the accused was transferred to prison.

In another instance a Mr Barclay protested the decision to confine his wife to the Hospital for the Insane, and blamed the government and the police for breaking up his family. In his letter he described how authorities had questioned him and his wife several times at their house before deciding that Mrs Barclay should be placed in the hospital. She was now refusing to return home because, Mr Barclay believed, she assumed he had been behind the decision to confine her. Instead, as part of her treatment, she was transferred to the home of a lawyer, where she did domestic chores. Mr Barclay was now outraged that his wife was not receiving care with her own family. Upon investigating the case, the deputy attorney general insisted that Mrs Barclay had admitted that she had been on the edge of a nervous breakdown before being sent to the hospital and that she had improved outside the influence of her husband, concluding that "Mr. Barclay, though a hard worker and of good habits, is a bit queer."[81] When questioned by the police, the couple's seventeen-year-old daughter claimed her father was abusive towards her and her mother and that her mother's imminent nervous breakdown had offered her an escape from a troubled marriage. The attorney general, however, agreed to let the family work out its differences, as no criminal activities further complicated the issue. The case nonetheless illustrates how important these institutions had become for mediating family disputes, as well as for detaining individuals for criminal or immoral activities.[82]

Confining children to institutions almost invariably involved the family. In a 1924 case of a boy deemed mentally defective, the attorney general reported that the hospital would assume custody of the boy only if the father could provide the requisite fee for his upkeep, which amounted to $15 per month.[83] In an inverse case a mother who became a candidate for insanity, according to police, risked losing custody of her children, her ability to care for her children resting on the decision of a psychiatrist as to whether she required institutional care or was free to remain at home.[84] The woman had come to the attention of authorities after repeatedly attempting to stay at an Edmonton hotel despite having no money. At first the hotel keeper tried to take matters into his own hands by hiring her as a housekeeper in exchange for allowing her and her two children to stay at the hotel, but he soon began to regard her as strange and depressive. At that point the police became involved, and found her a domestic position with a suitable family. The woman continued to deteriorate, however, and the family feared she was on the brink of a nervous breakdown due to her obsessive worrying. Further investigation revealed that she had been married to a soldier who had gone to the United States after the war instead of coming home to his family. He had corresponded with his wife for a short time, then ceased all communication when he learned that she had been in trouble with the law while he was away. The police report stated that "the woman is not dangerous either to herself or others at the present time but is very apt to become so shortly and mental treatment at this stage may prevent her becoming a permanent charge on the Government."[85]

Even where individuals were not well suited to institutional care, the government intervened in cases where the family was concerned about a member's feeble-mindedness. A mother grew anxious about the fate of her thirty-six-year-old son, who had inherited property and assets but whose low intelligence risked his losing it all and having to resort to relief. The police magistrate who examined the case reported: "I wish to make it quite clear, that according to the present evidence before me the man is not dangerous, the trouble is, that he is not capable of managing his own affairs, and he is dispensing of his estate amongst unscrupulous persons who are taking advantage of his mental weakness."[86]

A young boy suffering from "dementia praecox" – literally, early onset dementia, later understood as schizophrenia – told police that he had "a special 'calling' to Christianise the sinful city of Edmonton."[87] The boy was too young, however, to stay at the mental hospital in Ponoka and was not a danger to himself or others, which also excluded his being confined in jail. In another case a grandfather brought an "incorrigible" boy to the attention of the police after the boy's parents allegedly had failed to take responsibility for his actions. The police officer investigating the case decided, however, that the problem lay with his parents and the poor environment they provided the boy. After questioning the boy, the officer stated that "he appeared to be quite bright and I do not think he could be adjudged insane. All he requires is proper attention and some children to play with, of his own age, also food that is more suitable to him than that provided on the farm. There is no doubt about it that the child is sick and requires attention and as long as he remains where he is, he cannot get it."[88] In such cases police officers judged the mental fitness of children before directing them towards or away from medical attention, thus reinforcing the close resemblance of criminal and defective behaviour.

The mental health campaign as it manifested itself during the 1920s continued into the Depression, but by then it became entangled with rising concerns about communism and government attempts to curb the red scourge. Circulars from workers' organizations across Canada made explicit the links between the mental hygiene campaign and government efforts to imprison or deport communist sympathizers during a period of unprecedented labour unrest. One such pamphlet explained that the Toronto police had detained a Ralph Spooner after he had established an organization called the Workers Education Association of Canada. Spooner described a series of events, including his incarceration in different custodial institutions, torture and beatings by guards, and imprisonment in the Mental Hospital of Ontario, which he regarded as the worst of all institutions. In a last plea for assistance from his fellow workers, he said that on 1 March 1932 he had been deported to the United States "as an alleged dangerous maniac not desired in Canada." He further added that he was there placed in a Roman Catholic insane asylum to "prevent my continuing work on behalf of suffering humanity, and for the social and economic progress, and betterment of Canadian people." Although his journey through the asylum and jail systems began in Toronto, Spooner was ultimately deported from Edmonton, and appealed to local Alberta workers to help fight this abuse of power.[89]

Although such statements undoubtedly elaborated the gruesome details, providing a hyperbolic tale to galvanize support for the workers' organization, there was more to Spooner's claim than conspiracy. The police who seized the circular also forwarded to the Alberta premier a list of known communists on relief, indicating their country of origin, the date they had arrived in Canada, and additional remarks, usually indicating their willingness to work. The list overwhelmingly contained men from countries such as Poland, Lithuania, Germany, Czechoslovakia, Hungary, and the Soviet Union (mostly Russia and Ukraine). The arrival dates ranged from 1925 to 1929,[90] suggesting that many might have entered Canada with experience of living under communism. It is unclear how many of these men later served time in provincial jails or asylums, but the evidence suggests that the government used both kinds of institutions to control activities it deemed threatening.

Mothers of the Race

These kinds of cases brought attention to the family values and morals of Albertans and focused political attention on domestic issues. Concerns regarding custody, illegitimate children, spousal abuse, negligence, and destitution repeatedly appeared in the files and demanded the government's intervention. Passionate speeches by leading members of the UFWA appealed for women to have a role in politics, in particular to add moral authority to the political culture in general and to extend legislative discussions to domestic issues. UFWA members linked campaigns for women's rights – defined chiefly as suffrage, property ownership, and inheritance – with what they identified as a pressing need to develop policies governing communities at the familial level. UFWA president Irene Parlby and leading party activists such as Emily Murphy, then chief magistrate for the Edmonton courts, articulated a desire for policies that emphasized the importance of family law and provided the province with legal means to intervene in family affairs. In part, their demands stemmed from broader concerns about the rights of women in Alberta and in Canada more generally. For example, they argued that, without the right to property ownership, single mothers often were left with few financial options in the event of absentee or delinquent fathers. Further observation of the jails, mental hospitals, and infirmaries convinced feminist reformers that women bore the brunt of the burden of disease, poverty, and delinquency due to the combination of limited political rights and inherently weaker constitutions, which made them more susceptible to disease.

These early feminist reformers linked poverty and reproduction even more explicitly with feeble-mindedness, and eugenics became a significant part of their campaign in Alberta, embracing the ethos of eugenics as a progressive approach to improving the province's families.[91] Eugenics discourse, however, became linked with women's rights in a manner that privileged middle-class family values. The reformers first targeted their sisters in the working and lower classes, suggesting that these women were disproportionately responsible for social degeneration. The Committee for Social Hygiene reported that, "of unmarried mothers 85 per cent are feeble minded and should not be allowed to go on reproducing their kind. Mrs. Murphy had little sympathy with maukishly [sic] sentimental folk who shed tears over these people. Sterilization is being urged to prevent the crime which allows the insane to bring into existence innocent victims."[92] Moreover, placing such women in institutions was considered costly and inefficient. Drawing attention to the breakdowns in the homes, Miss Bradford, the secretary of the Social Service Council of Canada, "estimated that one-fifth of the total relief is directed towards mental deficients [sic] and 50 per cent of the school population are mentally deficient … Control of the problem, Miss Bradford felt, must be effected through control of procreation and special training and protection for deficient's [sic]."[93]

UFWA president Parlby delivered a speech in 1924 directly on mental deficiency and prostitution in which she spoke of the grave concerns surrounding the subject and the urgent need for the public to consider its role in assuaging the calamitous effects of prostitution, illegitimacy, drunkenness, and criminality on society. To that end, she recognized that modern society assumed that people considered mentally deficient required care and support: "then it seems only reasonable that those who have to carry the added taxation to provide this care should be interested in learning all they can about it, and have a word to say as to how they wish the problem handled."[94] Parlby cited US family studies on the Kallikaks and Nams as further proof of the inheritability of mental deficiency. The role of the community, she argued, was to distinguish carefully between categories of deficiency on the basis of danger, weakness, and malicious intent. Feeble-minded individuals, for example, were not necessarily suited for institutional care but were overly susceptible to the suggestions of others and easily fell prey to conniving influences. The main problem, she continued, remained the high birth rate among people in the defective category, for which she recommended regulation of marriage, segregation of all mental defectives, and sterilization: "Curious, is it not, that we cull our flocks and herds, allowing only the finest and most physically perfect to breed, and yet when it comes to the human race we allow the mating of the most diseased and imperfect both mentally and physically?"[95] She concluded with a special plea to women: "as women, as mothers of the race, we should be considering this subject very seriously indeed. We should have every sympathy for those who are so unhappy as to have brought defective children into the world, through perhaps no fault of their own, except that of marrying into an unwholesome stock, a fact of which may have been in entire ignorance, at the time of marriage. Our sympathy, however, should not allow sentiment to blind our commonsense."[96] Parlby's comments demonstrate her commitment to eugenics, but also reveal the agricultural basis of her politics and, in this case, her arguments for sterilization.

In a newspaper editorial, judge, author, and fellow UFWA member Emily Murphy made the point even more forcefully: "The remedy is obvious. It is a matter of humanity. Insane people are not entitled to progeny."[97] Two years later this sentiment would form the basis of the law that health minister George Hoadley claimed could be boiled down to an issue of "sterilization or segregation."[98] Segregation, however, meant institutionalizing individuals in long-stay facilities paid for by the government. He pointed out that "hundreds of thousands of dollars were being spent on this class of people that would be far better spent on the well. The province ... could do everything within its power to see that as few as possible feeble minded people come into the world." Moreover, he claimed, the majority of the individuals admitted to institutions for the insane were foreign born: "seventy per cent of those in Canada's hospitals are not born in the dominion while the total foreign born population of Canada is only 53 per cent."[99] Fiscal concerns, coupled with nativist and race-class purity attitudes, were certainly not unique to Alberta or to the United Farmers, but local political support for these sentiments made it easier for the party to implement legislation to this effect than was the case in other provinces.

Succumbing to these persuasive arguments, in 1928 Alberta passed the Sexual Sterilization Act, Canada's first such legislation. Newspaper accounts of debates in the provincial legislature indicated that concerns over the bill did not actually include opposition to the policy itself, but focused on the manner in which the governing party introduced it.[100] Historian Bradford Rennie suggests that, in addition to tapping into international trends, the impetus for this policy represented the unique blend of maternal feminism and agrarian democracy that existed in the UFA.[101] Both the party and the UFWA gave political expression to a deeper set of fears about race suicide and moral degeneration, and Albertans moved forward with plans to improve their society by weeding out those who appeared to contribute less and cost more.

The early Alberta eugenicists framed their discussions around concerns about immigration and the working-class lifestyle, which they deemed less refined, unhygienic, and unintelligent. By the end of the 1920s, as the province moved forward to implement the Sexual Sterilization Act, those values became institutionalized. Within a few years, however, circumstances were to change both politically and economically, and the eugenics program shifted under the weight of fiscal demands. Although the program retained its focus on foreigners during its first decade, changes to both the program and its targets indicated that eugenics philosophy had more far-reaching implications. The program did not develop specific policies targeting Aboriginals, for example, despite recognition on the part of health officers that First Nations reserves exhibited some of the worst hygienic and cultural conditions in the province. In the next chapter, I consider how these communities fared in the context of eugenics, and examine the absence of official language regarding Aboriginal health in eugenics legislation.

Chapter Two

Race, Intelligence, and Consent:
George Pierre

George Pierre was diagnosed with catatonic schizophrenia and deemed mentally defective when he was admitted to the Provincial Mental Hospital at Ponoka in the early 1930s. The details of his case are limited – there are no records of his own or his family's views on his condition and no specifics concerning his behaviour leading up to his committal. It is even unclear if this was his first admission to the mental hospital or if his admission on this occasion resulted from serial problems or a chronic health condition. The case file also does not explain whether his hospitalization was voluntary or coerced or, if the latter, the source of the coercion, such as family members, medical authorities, or the police. There is also no mention of violence on the part of George Pierre, although violent acts of individuals to themselves or others remained an important criterion in the Mental Diseases Act necessitating hospitalization. All we know for certain is that George Pierre was one of several Aboriginal males who came before the Eugenics Board and was approved for sexual sterilization during a critical moment in the program's history.

What distinguishes his case from those of the other men who received vasectomies for eugenics purposes was the inclusion of his Indian agent in the discussions about George Pierre's consent for the operation. Because he lived in reserve territory in northern Alberta, the responsibility for his health care fell to the federal government. His agent therefore appeared as a suitable authority capable of granting consent in this case, just as consent was sometimes received through the provincial attorney general for children who were wards of the government. Rather than assign blanket consent to his and other Aboriginal cases, however, George Pierre's agent used the opportunity to question the intent of the program, raising a number of concerns about the potential for racial profiling. More bluntly, he warned members of the Eugenics Board that, before proceeding with any such surgeries on Aboriginal people, the sterilization decisions had better be guided by sound clinical reasoning, not racial stereotypes.

"George Pierre," in fact, is a pseudonym that I assigned to a real case that came before the Eugenics Board in 1937. Neither his voice nor that of any other Aboriginal patient who came before the Board throughout this period or later is recorded in the extant documents. As a result, I rely on evidence drawn from medical, legal, and political discussions about the plight of Aboriginal people with respect to Alberta's eugenics program. Unlike the eastern European immigrants who were clear targets of mental health campaigns throughout the early part of the program, the case against First Nations and Métis communities is more difficult to substantiate, as high-level discussions in political or medical circles did not include specific language urging the Eugenics Board to focus on such communities. Aboriginal people could not be deported, which required a different approach with respect to their integration into Albertan society. First Nations and Métis people made up only 2.7 per cent of the province's population in the 1920s and 1930s, and many such families lived away from the urban centres and thus outside the direct surveillance of local eugenicists and public health officials, which might account in part for their absence from the early eugenics discussions.[1]

Another reason Aboriginal and Métis people do not appear in these discussions might be that, as medical historians and anthropologists have suggested, officials assumed that such populations were in a state of natural decline, an assumption that bears out some of the features of the social Darwinian thinking that was in circulation at the time. The notion of a "dying race" likely contributed to an attitude among reformers and eugenicists that, through the combined effects of assimilation and a high rate of mortality, Aboriginal people were already engaged in a more natural eugenics exercise, one better understood through theories of social Darwinism.[2]

As successive generations of First Nations people persevered on reserves – despite poor health, sanitation, and social conditions – and confronted the painful realities of colonialism, the relationship between eugenics and Aboriginal bodies developed in a more complicated fashion. Although Aboriginals largely escaped formal eugenics policies through most of the Alberta program, elements of eugenics philosophies were woven into assimilation strategies. Only in the late 1960s, when the Aboriginal population no longer seemed to be in decline, did public health officials shift the focus dramatically with concerted attention aimed at sterilization in these communities. By that time the social context of sterilization had shifted to denote a more empowering practice, but the application of such surgeries to marginalized communities remained reminiscent of older attitudes towards population control, and continued to rely on coercion.

The idea that Aboriginal people did not fall under the gaze of early eugenicists because reformers believed that these communities were already succumbing to race degeneration is a controversial interpretation. Some scholars have claimed that the Alberta eugenics program in fact disproportionately targeted First Nations and Métis people. For example, Yvonne Boyer, in a graduate thesis in the Faculty of Law at the University of Ottawa, reports that these people were considered part of the "wrong" social group, a claim she bases on a 2010 news article in the *Lethbridge Herald*.[3] Although the claim might have some validity, Boyer fails to produce historical evidence to support it.[4] Boyer even extends this allegation by suggesting that residential schools might have been involved in sterilizing First Nations students in western and northern Canada. Although residential schools provided an additional layer of surveillance of Aboriginal children, and consequently could have directed at least some to the eugenics program or even overseen operations on their own, the link between these schools and the eugenics program has not been demonstrated, and the broader historical context suggests that Aboriginal children were not targeted in this direct way until the late 1960s, with a noticeable rise of Red Power and the growing visibility of resilient Aboriginal communities on the Canadian landscape. This interpretation does not negate the reality that Aboriginal families underwent coercive sterilization surgeries, but it does suggest that its history is more complicated, if even more insidious.

Similarly, in a thesis submitted to the Faculty of Education at Lakehead University, Paul Primeau argues that, during the Leilani Muir trial in the mid-1990s, the court produced evidence from mental health reports supporting the view that "there were systemic biases in the operations of the Board. Female natives were most likely to be sexually sterilized."[5] Primeau also cites the findings of Timothy Christian, whose undergraduate honours thesis at the University of Alberta shows that, although individuals of Aboriginal or Métis descent constituted merely 3.4 per cent of Alberta's population, they represented 25.7 per cent of the sterilization cases, particularly in the final years of the program.[6] Primeau concludes that such statistics reveal an inherently racist bias in the eugenics program. Indeed, his evidence is compelling, and combined with other historically sensitive studies of childbirth, hospitalization, and colonialism, helps to illustrate some of the ways in which concepts of race comingled with presumptions about intelligence and mental hygiene. By locating these figures along a temporal scale, however, the spike in Aboriginal sterilizations and their timing becomes difficult to ignore. For nearly forty years the eugenics program did not appear openly to target First Nations or Métis communities, which makes all the more startling the dramatic increase in sterilizations that occurred in the final years of the program.

More recently, Karen Stote has argued in a PhD thesis that Aboriginal women "were the most prominent victims of the board's attention,"[7] and suggests that "[t]hose in Canada most likely to fit this categorization [of feeble-mindedness] and on whom Alberta's legislation was disproportionately applied were Aboriginal peoples; more specifically young Aboriginal women." She too cites Christian's undergraduate essay as proof of this claim.[8] Although Stote stretches her analysis well beyond the Alberta program and offers convincing evidence to support the tidal wave of coercive sterilizations in the late 1960s and 1970s, she does not substantiate the argument that this policy went back to the origins of the program.

The persistence of such claims, however, requires a more careful contextualization of the complicated collusion of colonialism and eugenics. It is also not to suggest that Aboriginal people were not sterilized, or even targeted at times by eugenics policies, but rather to emphasize that the relationship between eugenics philosophies and Aboriginal people was perhaps even more insidious. Based on the belief that the Aboriginal population was already in a state of natural decline, eugenicists did not need to expend energy or resources focusing on speeding that process along. In the second half of the twentieth century, as it became evident that this population was not in decline, the cultural meanings behind sexual sterilization had shifted, and in many ways were freed from the formal program. By the late 1960s sexual sterilization carried with it images of feminism and notions of empowerment that were then brought into Aboriginal communities and presented to Aboriginal women as modern and progressive. Many of the women approached in that manner were not recorded in the eugenics files because most of those sterilizations took place outside the reach of the official policy, although the coercive nature of these operations is difficult to ignore.

Medical anthropologists and social workers have attempted to bring to light some of the experiences of First Nations and Inuit people through ethnographic research that taps into the oral histories of Aboriginal women in Northern Canada. For example, in the 1980s John D. O'Neil revealed a number of cases, primarily of women, who were sterilized without their knowledge or consent in the 1960s and 1970s. One woman recalled: "The only other time I was sad like this was when I found out I couldn't have any more children. They did a hysterectomy in Churchill [Manitoba], but I didn't know about it. I am still angry about that."[9] These operations often coincided with treatment for other complaints, from depression to tuberculosis or cancer, and were not explained to the women by the southern physicians who performed the surgeries. Oral interviews uncovered these clandestine experiences, exposing some of the gritty realities of medical encounters shrouded in colonialism and progress.

Although Alberta's official eugenics program did not explicitly identify Aboriginal people as candidates for sexual sterilization, the language of ideal citizenship relied on racialized hierarchies conceptualized within a broader colonial framework. The Alberta arm of the eugenics movement seized upon intelligence and mental ability as arbiters of human worth, while, conversely, mental deficiency raised the spectre of degeneracy. Intelligence, as middle-class social reformers had constructed its cultural value, was equated with whiteness, the English language and Western customs, middle-class values, thrift, and hygiene. In the early phases of the eugenics movement, however, targets of racial profiling tended to be eastern Europeans. Timothy Christian, in his 1974 undergraduate thesis, argues that, "once the link between sexual immorality and mental deficiency had been formed in the public mind it was but a short step to introduce the notion that East European immigrants were the chief contributors to mental illness." He suggests that "the racial antipathy of the Anglo-Saxon majority toward Slavic immigrants provided a ready vehicle for popularizing the sterilization proposal."[10] Race, at this time, applied widely and negatively to anyone who did not visibly conform to the mainstream Anglo-Saxon image.

Despite an explicit focus on eastern European immigrants, who were 16.0 per cent of the population and 21.3 per cent of the sterilization cases, Aboriginal and Métis patients also appeared among those approved for sterilization from the beginning of the program. Although this combined racial group represented only 2.5 per cent of the Alberta population according to census data, Christian found that it made up

8.2 per cent of the sterilization cases by the program's end.[11] Moreover, there was a dramatic increase in sterilizations among these populations in the final three years of the program, from a comparatively low rate of 3.6 per cent to 25.7 per cent, the highest rate of any racial group.[12] Christian's analysis is all the more important since he conducted his study before the government destroyed 80 per cent of the eugenics records; it also bolsters the claim that, by the 1960s, attitudes towards sterilization and Aboriginal peoples had shifted significantly.

In the 1990s Jana Grekul, Harvey Krahn, and Dave Odynak, sociologists from the University of Alberta, revisited the statistical evidence in the eugenics files and discovered that the Aboriginal population, which the Eugenics Board identified as "Indian, Metis, half-breed, treaty, and Eskimo[,] ... hovered between 2% and 3% of the total" population.[13] Yet this group of people represented 6 per cent of sterilizations that took place over the program's forty-three years. While these researchers do not tease apart the rate of sterilization over time as Christian does, they nonetheless find that Aboriginals appear disproportionately in the eugenics files, which they argue can be accounted for in part by the power dynamics involved in the sexual sterilization program. Aboriginal patients were more often diagnosed as mentally defective than were non-Aboriginals, and intelligence quotients (IQs) assigned to these individuals routinely ranked them below the acceptable rate of so-called normality. Patients with such an IQ ranking who appeared before the Eugenics Board were also less likely to appeal the Board's decision or to refuse it in the first place, either because they did not understand the process or lacked the information they needed to defend their case.[14] Aboriginal women fared the worst, and in this regard shared the gendered bias against non-Aboriginal women.

As these quantitative studies demonstrate, the relationship between eugenics and Aboriginal status is complicated. It is difficult to extract meaning from these cases based on the numbers alone, especially as more subtle or even subversive elements of racism crept into the equation when IQs were routinely used as a barometer of human value. The experiences of Aboriginal patients in the health care system were made more difficult by a complicated set of rules and regulations that crossed political and religious boundaries and created new layers of authority and discipline over their bodies.[15] Concerns about health care costs and decision making, including consent, occupied federal and provincial officials in debates over responsibility for an "Indian problem," one characterized sometimes by policies of segregation and at other times by assimilation. In addition, medical and mental hygiene officials claimed that Aboriginal and Métis communities were disproportionately filthy, that their inhabitants were more often than not diseased, and that such people clung to superstitious customs that frequently exacerbated unhealthy conditions. Such officials also regarded indigenous medical men or women as purveyors of misinformation and practitioners of unscientific and ineffective rituals. Consequently, mental health emerged as a contested site for Western versus indigenous beliefs, provincial versus federal responsibilities, and Anglo-Saxon versus Aboriginal values.

Medical historians similarly emphasize how colonial medical encounters increased surveillance over First Nations families and borrowed the language of modern scientific medicine to justify aggressive health interventions, leaving people in these communities more susceptible to spending time in institutions. Some such encounters were carried out ostensibly under a program of assimilation, but relied on policies of segregation and substandard health care based on racialized assumptions about biological inferiority. Maureen Lux, for example, examines a separate Indian Hospital that the federal government built to contain the spread of tuberculosis in First Nations communities in Alberta. The treatments in the hospital, however, differed from those in non-Aboriginal hospitals, serving instead to institutionalize and control a population under the banner of progress. She states: "the characterization of Aboriginal communities as unrepentantly backward and roundly infected reinforced the superiority of white colonizers, justifying further isolation and repression."[16] Her study highlights the profound racism, informed by turn-of-the-century biology, that influenced medical approaches and treatments divided by race. Such critical examinations illustrate the way in which health and illness emerged as sites that called for progressive intervention. Colonizers praised the potential imbued in modern medicine to augment the so-called civilizing mission by bringing health to the Canadian North, while Aboriginals often suffered by being removed from their communities to obtain hospital care. Policies of segregation, isolation, and fundamental changes in diet and lifestyle caused more serious permanent damage, and outweighed the benefits of access to modern Western medicine.[17]

Given the destruction of most of the Eugenics Board's records, a comprehensive retroactive analysis of historical racial categories is no longer possible. Racism certainly played a critical role in the Alberta eugenics movement, but it also merged in subtle and complicated ways with ideas about mental capacity, intellectual prowess, work ethic, and assimilability.[18] Aboriginal lives were already under government surveillance, so mental hygiene programs in these communities assumed different political meanings. As mental health officials increasingly relied on measures of intelligence as an indicator of human value, the customs and practices of Aboriginal communities ranked lower, reinforcing a connection between non-Western health practices and inferior intelligence and emphasizing the superiority of science-based Western medicine. Thus, a more complicated story, set in a post-colonial context, is required to explain the ways in which Aboriginal people were ignored, disciplined, scrutinized, and ultimately sterilized along eugenics lines in Alberta. In this chapter I do not employ voices from the Aboriginal community but instead rely upon textual evidence, primarily from the Alberta government and the medical community, to gauge how public officials and medical authorities viewed Aboriginal reproduction within the context of eugenics. This approach sidesteps potentially conspiratorial allegations and concentrates on situating the medical views of bodies, reproduction, sexuality, and the implications of these views with respect to Aboriginal citizenship.

The case of George Pierre adds crucial context to the history of Aboriginal experiences, in part because it runs contrary to the perception that government officials simply approved sexual sterilization in an effort to curtail reproductive capabilities within these communities. George Pierre's case serves as a further reminder that the relationship between eugenics and Aboriginals in Alberta was anything but simple. The Eugenics Board minutes in his case suggest, in fact, that local and federal Indian agents shared some concerns about the Board's capacity to run roughshod over Aboriginal patients – indeed, George Pierre's agent took extra steps to safeguard his right to consent. His case indicates that, at least during the first two decades of the program, immigrants and lower-class families bore the brunt of the eugenics movement, while the federal government offered a modicum of protection to Aboriginal families, which had not yet become particular targets of the formal program.

The Health of the Race

In the period leading up to the introduction of the Sexual Sterilization Act, Alberta conducted a number of medical surveys to determine the health status of its communities. One striking observation emerged. Although early social reformers focused on immigrants as the primary carriers of disease and degeneration, a closer look at the predominantly Aboriginal population in the northern region of the province showed legislators and medical authorities that poverty and illness were more endemic in these communities than they had realized. Concerns about the health of the Aboriginal population raised new issues. Who was responsible for public health costs associated with this population? With deportation not an option, as it was with immigrants, how might local public health officials address the substantial health needs of the Aboriginal population? How could social reformers begin to curtail the allegedly twinned problems of poor health and poor work ethic? Surveys indicated that the Aboriginal population did not match envisioned social ideals, and that their assimilation into mainstream Canadian society was critical. However, attempts to address health concerns with Western medicine conflicted with indigenous practices and exposed deeply held cultural tensions, which further exacerbated government concerns about the need to press on with plans for cultural assimilation.

One such survey conducted in the late 1920s exposed the severity of the situation in the province. Surveyors used such terms as sick, poor work ethic, unsanitary, and ignorant to describe individuals, rarely identified by name, living in these communities. The reports capitalized on differences framed in racial terms to promote the need for discipline, intervention, and education to protect and modernize this segment of the population – in short, health status emerged as a convenient proxy for promoting a modernizing, civilizing agenda. Areas of both physical and mental health garnered attention and became important arbiters of progress.

Surveys routinely identified the overrepresentation of disease among the Aboriginal population, compounded, as historians have noted, by malnutrition, poverty, and cultural demoralization.[19] These factors appeared in the reports as endemic in Aboriginal communities, especially on northern reserves, and sometimes were blamed on carelessness or ignorance. For example, in describing maternity cases, a surveyor emphasized the lack of discipline and hygiene on the part of expectant and new mothers: a newborn child "is nursed whenever it cries, and is removed [from a moss bag] once or twice a day and given a dry rub, never a bath ... Even at two and three years of age children are put to the breast when they cry or are frightened. They are never punished and never washed."[20] In this and other excerpts, hygiene, cleanliness, and discipline arose as a set of distinctions between white and indigenous health practices that were framed in terms of inferior and superior intelligence.

Historian Maureen Lux also shows how Aboriginal midwives held es-
teemed positions in the community for their knowledge of the birthing
process and for aiding women during childbirth. To male surveyors,
however, such reliance on women and on older, non-scientific practices
reinforced an image of cultural backwardness that, in their view, demonstrated entrenched ignorance and necessitated modern reforms if
Aboriginal people were going to survive.[21]

In addition to noting different health practices, the surveyors further
reinforced a feeling of otherness towards Aboriginal people.[22] One surveyor reported: "The father also appeared to be very near the end from
[tuberculosis], but he reported that doctors in Edmonton three years ago
gave him only three months to live, and gloried in the fact that he was
still fooling them. Though he lives he is unable to do work of any sort,
all he can do is spit so he spits in whatever direction the face is pointing
when the necessity arises, in the corner, on the floor, in the doorway, and
once in a while in the can which he keeps for spitting into."[23] Several
such descriptions stressed the persistent elements of filth, poverty, and
adherence to "Indian medicine" or the circumventing of modern,
Western medical advice. Although the report does not explain what was
understood by "Indian medicine," it conveyed a set of activities grossly
inferior to Western medicine. Images of filth and disease permeate the
report, with family members described in a manner that deepened the
association between Aboriginality and illness.

The negative appraisal of indigenous medicine arose at times as ac-
cidental and at other moments as explicitly misguided on account of its
unscientific nature. One surveyor described a situation involving a Mr
Alphonse Gambler, who allegedly had "caused the smallpox scare" in
the Calling Lake District. Although Mr Gambler had been on a hunting
expedition when the opportunity for inoculation arose, "the natives
with very rare caution isolated him so that no one else took it,"[24] a passage that further emphasizes the presumed superiority of Western scientific medicine over indigenous healing practices, as the incident was
considered more an accident than a premeditated response, although it
extended no credit to the members of the community whose actions fell
into line with biomedical practices.

Behind such assumptions was the relationship between good health
and proximity to a modern hospital. In the first two decades of the twentieth century hospitals were built in urban areas as far north as Edmonton
and catered primarily to non-Aboriginal populations. Modern medicine, replete with its modern technological accoutrements, represented

progress. By contrast, unregulated health practices, including reliance on midwives and domestic healing techniques, represented, at least to provincial health surveyors, a less sophisticated health system and one that could be improved upon through the centralizing influence of a hospital or asylum.[25]

As the surveyors travelled farther north, health conditions worsened. Arriving on a reserve near Sandy Lake, one surveyor vaccinated twenty-one people and encountered "a child of twelve, female, in whom a rodent ulcer had taken away all soft parts of the face, save the eyes."[26] The surveyor also paid special attention to the status of people on reserve, recording them as treaty, simply native or Indian, or breed, terms that not only denoted differences in political jurisdictions or responsibility, but also, to this health official, seemed to provide clues about their degree of compliance with Western medicine, desire to work, likelihood to build houses, and to settle or engage in clean, moral habits. He claimed that the province had promised a hospital for the residents of Calling Lake in exchange for their labour on its construction. When residents refused to begin work until they had received a definite promise, provincial officials, rather than acknowledge this gesture as an astute negotiation tactic, regarded it as a lack of gratitude for the provincial initiative and proof of a negative attitude towards health and work.

Some surveyors distinguished between First Nations and Métis families, further demonstrating the way modern medicine had come to be understood as having a civilizing influence. Mixed blood, or "breeds," as the medical surveyor called them – he, like the people he surveyed, remained nameless in the report – allegedly were more willing to work than "Indians," and were described as more likely to be living in houses, rather than in tents. One entry stated: "we camped for the night in a breed's house, where I vaccinated eight breeds and two treaty Indians."[27] Again, these distinctions in labels seem to suggest not only different kinship connections but also different stages along a spectrum of assimilability that was tied in part to notions of intelligence, which was presumed to be higher as individuals embraced Western, Anglo-Saxon, and modern ideals, including living in fixed housing and subscribing to scientific medicine practised by licensed physicians. This notion of a spectrum also suggests that surveyors might have believed that assimilation was indeed occurring, and that direct intervention in these communities might not be warranted or financially feasible.

The reports more subtly described some of the tensions between Western and indigenous healing techniques by exposing an assumed ignorance about Western medicine: "One old medicine man, after openly proclaiming vaccination as false treatment and advising strongly against it, quietly slipped in by the back door and was vaccinated when no one else was around."[28] Whether or not this incident indicated a trend towards supporting vaccination and a growing acceptance of Western medicine, the surveyor recorded it as a triumph. Another case suggests that some people even regarded Western approaches as superior and perhaps all-encompassing. One woman, suffering from a series of ailments, including tertiary syphilis and grammata, reportedly sought medical intervention to restore her youth. The surveyor reported that "[o]ne eye was gone leaving a glaring ugly looking socket. The other eye was going. She wanted me to make her young and well, and was angry when I told her that no medicine could cure her."[29] In another instance, "[o]ne old man, a local muskakeweno or medicine man came to me covered with running sores and wanted to be cured ... I told him the only thing he needed was a bath and go home and wash with soap and water till he was clean."[30]

The medical inspector summed up his report with a set of recommendations and observations about the nature and problems of Aboriginals: "[T]he first and primary trouble with all these people is laziness. The children are allowed to do what they please at all times. There is no discipline; only girls are made to do any work, whatever."[31] The surveyor claimed that a "large cause of trouble is a propensity for gambling, and an absolute inability to value money. Added to this is a love for any sort of slop-wash which may produce a drunk."[32] But the most significant problem, he suggested, was the lack of discipline and authority overseeing this segment of the population, the result of which was unsanitary conditions and unsavoury relations that ended in venereal disease, polygamy, or illicit relationships, with multigenerational families living in single shacks or unmarried couples cohabitating in unhygienic conditions. The surveyor recommended that the province dispatch at least two young police officers to instil some moral discipline in the community, and that the medical community must follow, as "the death rate among children must be more than fifty per cent. Another generation will likely see the last of the Indians; two generations will see them all gone."[33] With such attitudes flowing south into the halls of power in Edmonton, neither the provincial government nor the Eugenics Board had a clear mandate to proceed with sexual sterilizations among the Aboriginal population as these communities appeared already to be disappearing on their own.

Reports about childbirth among the Aboriginal and Métis population helped to reinforce this conceptualization of race degeneration, suggesting that few members of these communities were in a position to benefit from the introduction of modern medicine in any case, owing to cultural or biological differences. In the early 1930s physician Mary Percy Jackson provided obstetrical care in the Métis village of Keg River, in the Peace River district of northwestern Alberta. In her report, published nearly twenty years later, she described the community as suffering from a lack of medical knowledge and clinging to unhealthy traditions. The language she used exhibits her disdain for the women she encountered in the community, writing, for example, that "most of the old squaws had had more than a dozen children and had often delivered themselves alone under a spruce tree somewhere."[34] She suggested, however, that, little by little, subsequent generations of Métis women were embracing more modern techniques, and many now delivered their children in a log house rather than outside, but few yet sought medical intervention.

Percy Jackson's depiction of childbirth in northern Alberta underscores the fundamental distinction she saw between white, modern Western, hygienic approaches to childbirth and the rustic, traditional, dirty, haphazard practices of the women in this Métis community. She recalled how the women regarded her with disdain, and suggested that "my gown, mask and gloves are accepted as a harmless eccentricity; they know that all that is really required is a pair of scissors and a piece of string."[35] She nonetheless acknowledged that her acceptance in the community rose when she provided chloroform to ease the pain of labour.

Percy Jackson concluded her report with reflections on her thirty years of service in the north and her optimism about the slow northward reach of modernity. She observed a change in the local diet resulting from increased roadways into the region, but ultimately she continued to regard these communities as "primitive" and in need of further guidance from the urban, white south: "It will be interesting to see what happens in the future," she wondered, "as Northern Alberta is opened up and the full force of changing conditions hits these primitive people."[36]

Set against this colonial backdrop, Alberta's eugenics program did not see fit to expend resources on Aboriginal communities. Successive reports confirmed this position as communities remained in abject poverty or suffered under poor conditions. Armed with theories of social Darwinism, reformers and policy makers could take comfort in the evidence that their promotion of an ideal society – one that included provisions for aggressive population control and social planning – were beginning to bear fruit. In this case, the natural experiment derived from the consequences of colonialism rather than the direct intervention of an official eugenics policy.

Making Eugenics Law

In 1928 Alberta passed Canada's first Sexual Sterilization Act. Race, however, did not emerge as a specific criterion for the program, and initial reports from the Eugenics Board did not suggest that racial considerations, whether Aboriginal or immigrant, were explicitly part of the motivating factors behind decisions to sterilize individuals. Intelligence and mental and physical fitness remained the key ingredients in the eugenics law. Debates at the high level of politics, within the medical community, and among middle-class reformers continued to centre on the theme of progress, and framed the eugenics discourse as a rational and sympathetic solution to the burdens of poverty and hereditary defects. Race, class, and gendered perceptions of intelligence and ability folded into these debates in more subtle ways.

Newspaper accounts of debates in the provincial legislature indicate that concerns about the bill did not include opposition to the policy itself, but rather focused on the manner in which the governing party introduced it.[37] The UFA, with its majority in the legislature, already had reached a consensus on the terms of the proposed legislation at its party conventions, with significant support from its women's wing.[38] Only one member, Lionel Joly, MLA for St Paul, broke party ranks, vehemently opposing the bill on the grounds that it was unfair, "as it would not reach all mentally diseased people; that it will open the door to abuse; that it will not accomplish that for which it was intended; that it gives too much power to the board which would be created; and finally that it offers mutilation as the price of liberty for the inmate of a mental hospital."[39] Joly's objections went unheeded during this round of discussions, although many of his concerns were later revisited. Conservative opposition leader C.Y. Weaver focused on Joly's last point, that of trading freedom from the institution for the potential to reproduce. He agreed that the cost-saving measures associated with a sexual sterilization bill were attractive to the government, but he worried that "the one obsession of persons in mental institutions was the desire to gain their freedom at any cost and surely it was a terrible alternative which this bill would place before them. They must agree to sterilization as the price of their freedom."[40] The People's League of Alberta, a short-lived communist group, complained that the proposed bill was unconstitutional, but without official representation in the legislature it was unable to generate sufficient local support, and its objections went nowhere.[41]

The legislation came into effect in January 1929, and involved the creation of a Eugenics Board headed by philosopher John M. MacEachern, who had trained in Leipzig, Germany, before taking up a position at the new University of Alberta in 1911.[42] The original group of Board members was small: in addition to MacEachern, it consisted of two surgeons, Edgerton Pope from the University of Alberta and E.G. Mason from Calgary, and recording secretary Mrs J.W. Field from Spurfield, Alberta. The deputy minister of health, Dr Malcolm Bow, also attended the early meetings.

At its inaugural meeting on 29 January, Board members focused on establishing the terms of legal obligation and liability associated with the program's activities. These kinds of discussions stretched over several meetings before any surgical operations were carried out, and primarily addressed issues of consent, jurisdiction, and the terms of institutional discharge in relation to sterilization. Several of these issues had been raised as points of opposition to the bill, but Board members moved to address them. First, they sought clarification on the kinds of institutions that would fall under the Board's jurisdiction, as regulated by the Mental Diseases Act. They unanimously decided that, in addition to cases for the provincial mental hospital at Ponoka, the Board should consider the cases of children brought to the Provincial Training School for Mental Defectives at Red Deer. Some of the children at that institution were wards of the state, having been orphaned at birth or taken away from their parents at a young age; still others had been brought in voluntarily by their parents. Restricting the legislation to those institutions and not allowing referrals from schools, residential or otherwise, meant that a concerted focus on mental and physical fitness, rather than other undesirable characteristics, guided this stage of the program. Next, the Board unanimously passed a motion outlining the standards for carrying out its decisions, including recording all deliberations in a case file; obtaining personal consent from patients where possible; appointing only certified surgeons to perform the operations; and hiring social workers to conduct follow-up studies with discharged patients.[43]

The second meeting, held two months later, involved further discussions about liability and more detailed recommendations on procedures.

In particular, Board members agreed that case histories for each patient should include a careful family history as well as confirmation of nationality, to help determine which jurisdiction would be financially responsible for pending operations. These discussions centred on laying the ground rules for carrying out operations, along with associated selection and discharge criteria. Deliberations also emphasized nationality as a key variable in identifying candidates for sterilization, but made no explicit mention of Aboriginal features or distinct racial characteristics of any kind.

The issue of consent raised further discussion. On this matter, the Board sought a ruling from the attorney general on how to proceed if a patient refused to grant consent or appeared incapable of providing it due to deteriorated or incapacitated health. The Board forwarded two scenarios to the attorney general for his consideration: "1. The husband being considered incapable of giving consent to his own sterilization, and the wife being able, and refusing to give her consent; 2. The husband being considered capable of giving consent, and doing so, and the wife refusing to give consent."[44] Board members agreed that they should wait for a response before proceeding with any cases that fell into these categories. Meanwhile, they decided that, before initiating any operations, they needed to conduct more research into how other eugenics programs assessed the "possible effect of the operation on the patient, physically, mentally and morally."[45] In the process of gathering such information, California arose as a model program. That state already had gained a reputation for its aggressive sterilization program, and boasted of the substantial savings that such an approach brought.

At the third meeting, on 12 April 1929, the Board considered its first patient. After debating the issue of surgeons' fees, which it concluded should be set in accordance with the standard College of Physicians and Surgeons' fee schedule for the province, the Board examined the case of a male patient from the mental hospital at Ponoka. The patient was approved for a vasectomy that same day, although the procedure ultimately was delayed until the Board received the attorney general's final approval of the overall consent criteria.[46] That approval materialized a month later, with further procedural guidance, and by October the man's case had moved along to the surgeon.[47]

The pace at which these events unfolded indicates a strong desire by Board members, as well as by the Alberta government, to move forward quickly with the sterilization program. Within ten months the terms and conditions had been set and surgeries begun. The meetings, now held monthly, rotated around the province from the mental hospital in Ponoka to the Edmonton Mental Health Guidance Clinic to the Provincial Training School in Red Deer, but the active participants remained constant. In fact, over the Board's forty-three-year mandate, with four or five members present at all times, only twenty-one individuals served on it, creating a strong institutional culture and allowing it to maintain its core values with only periodic input from new or infrequent members. Only one member ever had formal training in genetics.[48] The government was routinely updated and often consulted for legal and political advice, further underscoring the close connection between it and the Eugenics Board's activities.

Ten months after the first Board meeting, the first patient was scheduled for sterilization surgery and a second case was brought before it. A social worker had reported that the patient was a feeble-minded minor, incapable of providing consent, and that her parents lived outside the province.[49] The Board accordingly decided that the health minister should act as guardian and give consent for surgery, which was duly granted at the next meeting, a month later. The case prompted the Board to draft consent forms specifically for the health minister, who subsequently could act as guardian for similar cases where obtaining consent might prove problematic and where candidates reasonably might be considered wards of the government.

The first two patients, and most of the rest who followed, initially were identified as candidates for sterilization by virtue of their residence in government-run mental institutions. A social worker would approach them and inquire about their family and social history before referring them to the Board. After reviewing the social worker's report, the Board would interview each patient directly, and one of the two surgeons affiliated with the program would undertake a medical examination of the patient. Board publications indicate that patients were also assessed using psychometrics or IQ tests, but the results of such tests, beyond a tallied score, rarely appeared in the recorded deliberations. Once approved, the surgeries would be performed either at the University of Alberta Hospital or at the General Hospital in Calgary by one of the program's two surgeons. Finally, the Board would consider the matter of the patient's discharge from the institution following the surgery. Patients were expected to return home to their parents, husbands, or wives within a month or two of the operation, barring any further complications due to infection caused by the surgery.

With these procedural policies in place within the first year, the Board gained confidence that sexual sterilizations would reduce both the rate of reproduction among those considered a threat to the mental and moral stability of the province and consequently lead to substantial cost savings for society. The Board continued to believe that the primary targets of sterilization were people who had been institutionalized in a provincial mental hospital or related facility. Those people were not profiled by race, ethnicity, gender, or class; the language of the policy explicitly focused on intelligence and mental deficiency.

The cost associated with these surgeries was a matter that fell outside the normal practices of surgeons, and therefore prompted additional reflection. Initially surgeons received $150 for a salpingectomy, which involved the severing and removal of sections of the Fallopian tubes, and $60 for a vasectomy, requiring the surgical ligation of vas ducts. The Board, however, felt that these fees were too high, considering that these particular operations were a public expense and likely to increase over time. It suggested, therefore, that the appointed surgeons instead should collect a monthly honorarium of $300, that the fee for a vasectomy should be reduced to $25, and that the fee for a salpingectomy or tubal ligation should remain at $150 due to the more complicated nature of such operations. If the number of surgical operations exceeded one hundred in a year, the Board would consider increasing the amount of the honorarium.[50]

Within the first year of its activity, the Board also planned to expand its mandate, sensing that it would not reach its full potential if it remained limited to eugenics sterilizations only among institutionalized populations. Moreover, the process of obtaining consent for each case was becoming slow, tedious, and often complicated. The original legislation stipulated that the Board had the authority to select sterilization candidates from recognized provincial institutions covered under the Mental Diseases Act. By October 1929, less than a year after the program's establishment, the Board considered enlarging this pool by working with the medical profession, public health nurses, and the Committee for Social Hygiene to develop criteria for identifying potential candidates who had not yet been admitted to an institution. Their reasoning was that preventative measures, which included sterilizations, would help to reduce the costs associated with institutionalization. Working with these other organizations in the community meant that sterilization candidates could be identified before they became a burden on the government through institutionalization. In addition to broadening surveillance measures, the Board also considered extending its reach even further by encouraging voluntary sterilization and urging parents to present their children for sterilization upon request.

Pushing its role still further beyond the scope of the existing law within its first year, the Board pressured the provincial government to require couples to undergo a medical examination before being granted a marriage licence, a proposal that had been put forward earlier by the UFWA. The Board also suggested that the government revisit the law on contraception and relax restrictions on birth control.[51] In forwarding these recommendations to the attorney general, the Department of Psychology at the University of Alberta, and the National Committee for Mental Hygiene, Board chairman J.M. MacEachern "expressed the sincere desire of the University to cooperate to the fullest extent with the Department of Health in its effort to cope with one of the most serious problems of today."[52]

The Eugenics Board's efforts, first to streamline the identification process and then to extend the pool of candidates beyond its original mandate, met with considerable support from policy makers, reformers, and professionals alike, and a lack of political opposition in the legislature. The program thus got off to a strong start. The cases themselves provided the examples from which precedents formed around issues of consent, cost, and discharge. As more cases came to the Board's attention, more guidelines were established and, within a short time, the program was functioning relatively smoothly and without public criticism. Mental health professionals praised the program's effects on reducing the psychiatric population. By ostensibly eliminating the danger of transmitting mental diseases or deficiencies to progeny, hospital superintendents could discharge patients with confidence that they were reducing the rate of mental illness. Based on this logic, eugenicists believed that the distribution of mental illness within the population would decline or even be eliminated over the course of several generations.[53] Reports in the national medical literature commended the Alberta program for its foresight in developing such a successful program with broad-ranging potential for improving humanity. Local enthusiasts claimed that "there have been no criticisms of this work in Alberta and it is progressing steadily and smoothly." Supporters expressed their admiration for the "steadily growing faith in sterilization as an effective and reasonable method of bringing about at least a partial solution ... for the mentally subnormal," and stated that "[sexual sterilization] may be taken at least one step toward racial improvement."[54] Thus equating mental illness and racial degeneration, supporters heaped praise on eugenicists for managing to curb reproduction within specific subgroups of the population, with the idea that subsequent generations would reap the benefits. The same logic applied to First Nations communities, although their racial degeneration was expected to take place more naturally without direct medical or government interventions.

Despite the optimism about the alleged success of the program, however, it became evident within a few years that social planning through eugenic sterilization measures was not reducing the perceived financial burden on the government or the burden on society more generally. Medical officials began noticing that some discharged patients had difficulties with their post-sterilization lives. In one case a woman felt that the operation had robbed her of her "womanhood," and argued that the government therefore ought to support her, which ran exactly contrary to the intended spirit of the program. A social worker observed that several of the female patients who had undergone sterilization had a tendency to "gain in weight and in a general feeling of well being."[55] At the same time, however, among married patients, sterilization brought a sense of relief and protection from further pregnancies. These mixed results, from frustration and malaise to empowerment and relief, brought unanticipated responses and stymied the Board and eugenicists in their attempts to interpret the social implications of these post-sterilization attitudes.

Most of the cases the Board approved for sterilization were those of individuals who had been diagnosed as mentally defective – that is, whose IQ fell below 70.[56] Psychotic, manic-depressive, and schizophrenic patients represented 42.7 per cent of cases and the bulk of the remaining individuals slated for sterilization. Many of these patients, however, expressed resistance to the operation and refused to provide consent, with men resisting more often than women.[57] Many female candidates for sterilization were married with children, and might have welcomed the opportunity to control their fertility legally, while others might have felt uncomfortable challenging a doctor's orders. By contrast, the majority of male candidates were single,[58] and their more frequent resistance to sterilization might have been prompted by concerns about their masculinity and virility (for more discussion on gendered differences, see Chapters 3 and 4).

This discrepancy also suggests that a numerical analysis provides only part of the story behind the history of sterilization. Men and women during the first decade of the program were often presented in relatively equal proportions, although men more often and more successfully resisted the operation and refused to provide consent. The same scenario emerged among Aboriginal candidates. Although it is difficult to get a clear idea of the strategies or tactics used to display such resistance, it is instructive that sufficient numbers of individuals opposed the operation. Rather than conclude that the early phase of the program targeted women or specific ethnic or racial groups, as a crude statistical analysis might suggest, it is evident that many individuals escaped sterilization using the legal channels available to them. People considered mentally defective, or subgroups already under the authority of the state, including First Nations communities, had fewer resources with which to mount their resistance. In this way, intelligence and perceptions of intelligence arose as important indicators of mental fitness and increasingly influenced the activities of the Board.

The University of Alberta also played an important role in supporting the eugenics program, and added grist to the mill by reinforcing the connection between intelligence and fitness in a manner that assumed a veneer of class dynamics. The university's president, R.C. Wallace, addressing the Canadian Medical Association in 1934, urged physicians to support research into eugenic causes. He claimed that "we are being satisfied with a mediocrity of quality, both physically and mentally, and this reflects itself in our imperfect ideals and limited progress. Science has done very much to raise the quality of the stock in the domesticated animals which man has reared for his service; it has done virtually nothing to raise the quality of the human stock."[59] Wallace suggested that science had yet to unlock the mysteries of human behaviour or the mechanisms of the mind. Pointing out that medical progress had been applied unevenly to the population, Wallace said that "nature's weeding-out process has not been permitted to proceed in the earlier years, and the types that survive until forty are not all hardy."[60] He went on to emphasize the importance of being well born and the danger of ignoring mental attributes, including intelligibility and the risk of degeneration. Speaking from his podium as university president, he added that "the fact remains that children of the professional classes make a higher contribution through intellectual ability than those of the classes inferior in intellectual training."[61]

Wallace thus combined class and race concerns with a direct plea to the medical community not only to support eugenics efforts, but also to acknowledge the class degeneration at work in their own families. He suggested that upper-class or more intelligent families gained access to birth-control measures for selfish reasons, while families of less means had neither the inclination to use birth control nor access to it. Although he did not discuss the legality of contraception, he clearly viewed the problem as one of different class values. In the midst of an unprecedented economic depression, coupled with environmental devastation, particularly in southern Alberta, Wallace complained that the unchecked fertility of the lower classes threatened to overwhelm the more intelligent families and create an untenable burden on government, which provided support in the form of prisons, hospitals, and asylums. To him, eugenics was a progressive solution to a dire economic problem infused with fears of class degeneration or Anglo race suicide.

Wallace's sentiments also resonated with members of the mental health community in Alberta who regarded eugenics as a plausible solution to the province's purportedly growing population of mental defectives. Some proponents felt that sexual sterilization offered an opportunity to discharge patients from institutions quickly and confidently, given that the surgery removed the risk of progeny.[62] Such an attitude, however, also indicated a lack of regard for the social realities faced by individuals who were subsequently discharged into communities: although these patients were rendered incapable of reproduction, sterilization had no effect on their psychiatric or intellectual disability.

The intensity of the Depression profoundly influenced public attitudes towards charity, welfare, and entitlement. Large, government-funded institutions, including mental hospitals, stood as a reminder to voters that, although the province gave very little financial support to under- and unemployed people or hard-luck farmers, it remained willing to cover the expenses of patients who were considered incapable of working. Eugenic sterilization thus gained renewed support during this period for its promise to reduce the number of people in government-run mental health facilities. The Depression also helped to forge another connection in the public's mind – that of equating poverty with lowered intelligence.

Amending Consent

Although medical experimentation and therapy usually involved some basic consideration of a patient's consent well before the Second World War,[63] the concept of informed consent became routine only as a result of the trials of Nazi war criminals at Nuremberg and the investigation of the scientific experiments the Nazis had conducted on humans during the war. At the culmination of the international tribunal on medical experimentation in 1947, a declaration on medical ethics, known as the Nuremberg Code, provided the ethical basis for future experimentation, although the Code itself contained no provisions for its enforcement. Informed consent seized upon the notion that patients first had to be given information about the consequences and side effects of treatment as well as those anticipated if the patient chose not to undergo treatment.

In Alberta the Eugenics Board had long wrestled with the logistical challenges of obtaining permission or consent from patients or their next of kin, as the original law required and as was consistent with trends throughout North America, both in eugenics programs and in medicine more generally. As Nancy Campbell and other scholars have shown, however, obtaining consent from members of institutionalized populations poses particular challenges and issues of concern.[64] In the case of patients in Alberta, discharge from the institution was often at stake. As well, access to medical services was sometimes tied to consent, as was access to experimental therapies or specialists, which could be particularly significant for individuals living in marginalized circumstances where access to health care was at a premium, including in First Nations communities.[65] These circumstances produced coercive situations that manipulated the concept of free and informed consent.

The number of individuals approved for sterilization in the province steadily increased throughout the 1930s, but the need for consent had periodically slowed down the process and frustrated Board members. For instance, a young woman living at the Provincial Training School for Mental Defectives in Red Deer was under observation for sterilization when the Board received news that the girl's mother was eager to consent to the operation so that her daughter could return home. The mother's intervention sped up the process, and the young woman was immediately approved for sterilization.[66] It is unclear how much the mother knew or understood about her daughter's circumstances, but according to provincial law her daughter could not be released until the Eugenics Board had reviewed her file. In this way the Board played an important role in monitoring the discharge of patients, and it was extremely rare for the Board to agree to a discharge order unless the patient had been approved for sterilization.

Other cases demonstrated, however, that, even when consent was granted, family members who disagreed sometimes intervened to delay or alter the Board's decision. One young woman was approved for sterilization after her father consented to the operation, but her brother strongly opposed the measure and the operation was postponed until a more consensual decision was reached in the family.[67] Other deferrals of Board-approved surgeries occurred when family members could not be reached or failed to return the consent forms in a timely fashion; often, such cases involved individuals whose parents lived outside the province or country. These cases gradually fell under the jurisdiction of the minister of health, who then personally assessed whether the province should authorize the operation or send the individual to another jurisdiction.

In cases of married patients, the Board required consent from the spouse before proceeding with the surgery, but this sometimes proved difficult to obtain. Women whose husbands refused to grant consent remained institutionalized.[68] In one case a child was taken into custody by the Child Welfare Department while the Board waited for the proper consent to proceed with her mother's sterilization.[69] When her case was revisited, the woman claimed that she "wished to have the operation performed without implying any conditions as to the care of her child," and the woman signed the consent form voluntarily. The woman's own lawyer objected to the surgery, however, claiming that her "voluntary" consent had been linked to the assumption that the child would be returned to her afterward. The Board ruled that, since the woman was not a minor, her lawyer had no authority in the case. After consulting with the attorney general, the Board approved her case and she received the surgery.[70] The reports do not indicate if she resumed custody of her child.

By spring 1937 the Eugenics Board had approved the sterilization of 1,008 individuals, divided nearly equally between men and women,[71] but only 492 individuals had actually been sterilized. The discrepancy hinged upon consent. The superintendent at the Provincial Mental Hospital in Ponoka and the psychiatric social worker assigned to the Eugenics Board reported that nearly one-third of the males were discharged from their respective institutions without undergoing sterilization because the Board had not received consent, and only 36 per cent of men approved for sterilization actually underwent the procedure. In contrast, it proved easier to obtain consent for females, 66 per cent of whom were sterilized.[72] The superintendent at Ponoka and the Board's social worker did not elaborate on the gender-related complications of obtaining consent from approved patients, concluding that "the work of sterilization in the province of Alberta has been carried on very quietly and efficiently and the results have been pre-eminently satisfactory."[73] Nonetheless the issue seriously impeded the Board's work.

In light of the many idiosyncratic circumstances that complicated efforts to obtain consent, the Board eventually recommended amending the legislation to simplify the process. On 14 April 1937 the Social Credit government, which had inherited the Sexual Sterilization Act when it took power in 1935 and which wanted to reassure voters at the height of the Depression that government funds were being used effectively to ensure long-term solutions to chronic health and welfare expenses, removed the Board's need to obtain consent from a patient in cases where individuals were found to be mentally defective. The revised Act stated:

> If, upon examination of any mentally defective person, the Board is unanimously of the opinion that the exercise of the power of procreation would result in the transmission to such person's progeny of any mental disability or deficiency, or that the exercise of the power of procreation by any such mentally defective person involves the risk of mental injury either to such person or to his progeny, the Board may direct, in writing, such surgical operation for the sexual sterilization of such mentally defective person as may be specified in the written direction.[74]

With respect to individuals diagnosed as psychotic, however, the revised Act still required that consent be obtained, stating that "[sexual sterilization] shall not be performed unless such person being in the opinion of the Board a person who is capable of giving consent, has consented thereto, or when the Board is of the opinion that such person is not capable of giving such consent, if such person has a husband or wife, or being unmarried has a parent or guardian, resident within the Province, the husband, wife, parent or guardian of such person has consented thereto."[75]

To solidify the government's authority to make unilateral sterilization decisions regarding individuals deemed mentally defective, the amendment included a clause that gave blanket protection to the surgeon, anesthetist, or any person who assisted with sexual sterilization operations: "No person shall be liable in any civil action or proceeding for any thing done by him in good faith in purported pursuance of this Act."[76] Following the amendment, the Board began increasing the rate at which it authorized sterilizations and the average age of sterilization patients began to decrease. Previously the term "passed" had been used following the patient's physical and mental assessment but its use did not imply that consent had been obtained. Now, many patients considered mentally deficient were assigned a "passed clear" notation that fast-tracked the process leading to surgery; the Board rarely recorded additional or protracted deliberations of such cases.

A 1942 report praised this new approach as progressive because of the financial savings it offered the provincial government. By 1942 the Board had approved over 1,600 individuals for sterilization, and 315 males and 490 females had received operations, saving, a contemporary study claimed, $93,810 in costs as a result of the subsequent discharge of these patients from institutions.[77] The study also reminded readers that many of the families targeted under the scheme had not been born in Canada, while its comparative silence on Aboriginal families suggests that they were not on the program's radar during these first decades of the eugenics program.

The shift in consent procedures coincided with a growing silence about eugenics both in local medical journals and the newspapers. Previously the Board had regularly published its statistics as annual reports to the province, which were routinely copied in the *Alberta Medical Review* and sometimes in international medical journals. As the number of surgeries increased and the need for consent declined, these reports became perfunctory and, by the end of the war, disappeared from view altogether.

George Pierre

In the meantime complications began to arise with respect to Aboriginal patients. The first case appears in the Eugenics Board's minutes for 1932, when an Aboriginal woman's surgery was approved subject to the consent of both her husband and her Indian agent,[78] the inclusion of the latter moving the program into federal territory. Then, in 1937, one month after the amendment to the Sexual Sterilization Act was passed, George Pierre's case came to the attention of the Board. The extended correspondence on that file reveals some of the complexities that brought federal authorities and discordant perspectives into the discussions in a more direct manner.

The recent change in legislation meant that the Board did not require George Pierre's consent to go ahead with the surgery, but members nonetheless opted to contact his Indian agent, with the medical superintendent for the Provincial Mental Hospital in Ponoka explaining that "[i]t is now no longer necessary to obtain the consent of the parents or the patients for the sterilization of mental defectives. As this case has been passed by the Eugenics Board and is otherwise ready to undergo the operation for sexual sterilization, before taking any action in the case I should like to hear from your Department as to whether or not you have any objections to our proceeding in the usual manner."[79]

The Indian agent seemed unsure how to respond, and referred the file to his superiors in Ottawa. The joint response from the federal minister and local agent stated:

> The Department has no power to authorize the sterilization of an insane Indian. It has no objections to the operation and would regard it with approval if carried out in accordance with the laws and regulations of the Province. It cannot, however, agree that any Indian should be sterilized without the consent of his relatives, and of himself as well, if he is mentally competent to understand the results of the operation. It is not beyond the realm of possibility that Indians might get the impression that there was a conspiracy for the elimination of the race by this means.[80]

In a subsequent letter the Indian agent stressed that the operation should be deferred until the Board had obtained consent from the patient's family. Despite the provincial law that authorized the Board to proceed without consent, the Indian agent feared that a dangerous precedent could be set if it did so.[81] The provincial authorities responded, however, with some degree of disdain, claiming that "the patient is not willing to be sterilized but, according to the present Alberta Sterilization Act, his consent would not be necessary. Notwithstanding this latter fact it has not been our policy to operate where there are extenuating circumstances, which, in this case, would be the fact that he is an Indian."[82]

This response is striking, as the medical superintendent explicitly explains that "extenuating circumstances" that might guard against proceeding with a case include "the fact that he is an Indian." The passage further underscores the degree to which Alberta's eugenics program appeared to concentrate on other segments of the population during its first few decades and in fact might have avoided Aboriginal patients due to these acknowledged complications. Ultimately the medical superintendent agreed to defer the case until the family consented to the operation.

The Board's notes on the George Pierre case end at this entry. It is unclear if the surgeon eventually performed the desired vasectomy, if his family refused to provide consent, as had George Pierre, or if he remained in the institution indefinitely. Two and a half years later, however, another case concerning an Aboriginal man deemed mentally defective appeared before the Board. Although the Board approved the man, Bobby Warrior, for a vasectomy, it referred to the earlier correspondence concerning George Pierre and, yielding to the Indian agent's concerns about perceived genocidal conspiracies, agreed to delay the surgery until obtaining consent from the Warrior family.

At a time when the Board was rapidly increasing the approval rate for surgeries, in part due to the changes in the law that allowed it to sidestep the issue of consent, its deliberation in these cases is noteworthy, if short lived. By the early 1940s more such cases had come before the Board, which once again indicated that it required a more efficient way of handling them. Once again the Board contacted Ottawa, seeking blanket support for proceeding with Aboriginal cases. In a letter to the Department of Indian Affairs, the medical superintendent for the Provincial Mental Hospital in Ponoka complained that "it is regrettable, however, that the Department ... has never seen fit to approve of the sterilization of Treaty Indians for obvious reasons."[83] He went on to describe the details of a particular case that required specific attention, ultimately concluding with a request for consent to sterilize a male Aboriginal patient.

By this time officials at both the federal and provincial levels of government appeared to have grown more receptive to the idea of applying Alberta's eugenics program to First Nations communities, and, initially at least, its main targets were male. Perhaps, as other historians have suggested, the notion of the dying race was already being replaced by a growing recognition of Aboriginal resilience. Quite likely, the loose classification of mental defective also encompassed elements of race, as it had come to assume class and foreign dimensions. Rather than challenge the provincial approach, Indian Affairs in Ottawa responded with a definitive statement that indicated a new attitude: "*this Department has no objections to the laws of the province being carried out and any action taken in accordance with Provincial law will not meet disapproval* [emphasis in original]."[84]

In January 1943, at its 113th meeting, the Eugenics Board discussed the contents and implications of this correspondence, and confirmed Ottawa's shift in perspective "concerning cases of Treaty Indians, who might from time to time be presented to the Board."[85] By the late 1960s the sterilization rate among Aboriginal people surpassed that among all other racial or ethnic categories,[86] but the Board, having secured its desired outcome with respect to consent during the discussions of the 1940s, did not see fit to revisit the issue for the duration of the eugenics program.

In 1969 psychologist Dr William Blair chaired a report on the state of mental health in Alberta, drawing specific attention to the dramatic increase in Aboriginal sterilizations. The Blair Report acknowledged that the eugenics program had received some critical attention, but maintained that the policy rested on sound scientific principles.[87] It explained that the justification for sexual sterilization had expanded in recent years to include social or socio-cultural as well as biological factors. In some cases, for example, the Eugenics Board now recognized as suitable sterilization candidates children who might be genetically normal but who "would have virtually no opportunity for viable nature within the context of the biological family,"[88] thus effectively expanding the Board's purview to include eugenic considerations for children who might be raised in an impoverished social environment.

The Blair Report exposed a number of areas where Board members had rushed cases or collected insufficient evidence before proceeding with a recommendation for sterilization. In particular, the report cast doubt on the linkage between low intelligence ratings and the resulting sterilization decision based on "emotional or delinquency or subcultural (e.g. Métis) factors [sic]."[89] Although these changes in procedure had not appeared in the Board's minutes or recorded discussions, the report's comment suggests that, by this time, the Board viewed simply being Métis a sufficient reason to garner a low intelligence rating and consequently warrant a recommendation for sexual sterilization.

By the 1970s, as the formal eugenics program came to an end, First Nations activism blossomed. Allegations of abuse circulated in the popular press and implicated the legacy of colonialism, a by-product of which appeared to be coerced sterilizations.[90] Although Alberta's eugenics program had not targeted Aboriginal communities explicitly at its inception or in the language of its recorded activities, colonial elements of degeneration, inferiority, and assimilation remained deeply embedded in its practices. As the concept of a dying race was replaced by an image of a more resilient culture, eugenicists quietly adjusted their approach in concert with government authorities to extend sterilization practices into these communities such that, by the end of the institutionalized eugenics program, Aboriginal women had become its chief targets.

Chapter Three

Sterilization Redefined: Violet and Irene

Hallelujah to Hysterectomy
(Let's Stop Talking about Sex and Do Something about It!)
Speak to me not of birds and bees
Of the passion of flowers keep mum
About the amorous habits
Of snakes and rabbits
I prefer from now on to stay dumb.
In my day I have functioned with no little success
As a human producer ad nauseam
But my last trump is played
I was recently spayed
Of the vital organs which causeam.
In future, my thoughts will be mostly concerned with
Things – spiritual, social, intellectual
Three cheers! Jubilation!
I'm past pollination
With a brand new outlook sexual.
I can plan strenuous trips any time of the month
I can tweak my husband at random
To that Doc with a knife
Who has so changed my life,
A magnum of brandy, I'll hand 'm!
And all I can say to my gal friends is this…
Hysterectomy's the one bed of roses
For gals over forty
Who, tho still feelin' sporty
Loathe the contraptions of Bessie Moses!
                    – a patient of Dr Edward H. Richardson, Jr[1]

One of the leading feminist reformers on the prairies was Saskatchewan's Violet McNaughton, instrumental in establishing wings of the
United Farm Women in Alberta, Saskatchewan, Manitoba, and Ontario,
and the voice behind the women's pages of the *Western Producer*, an
agrarian-based newspaper widely read by farm families in the region.
An ardent feminist and agrarian socialist, McNaughton's influence on
women's issues across the prairies was significant.[2] Her perspective,
however, differed from that of some of her contemporaries who connected eugenics and contraception with lower-class and mentally deficient people. For McNaughton, contraception was a matter of health for
all women. Its use, she suggested, helped to reduce the incidence of
maternal and infant mortality and generally improved the well-being of
a family by allowing couples to choose when to have children and how
many. Redefining sterilization along these lines exposed differences
within the feminist movement, but also revealed some of the paradoxical rhetoric espoused by supporters of eugenics.

Sterilization of healthy mothers required direct compliance by physicians and relied upon women's convincing their doctors that having
more children presented health risks. Some members of the birth-control
movement recognized the need to include physicians in their campaigns
directly, in an effort to forge links between women and the health care
profession. In preparing for a convention of the United Farm Women of
Canada, one concerned farm woman suggested they get the medical
and nursing associations on board because, although they could be the
most powerful opponents of a more liberal birth-control law, they were
also its strongest advocates.[3] A California woman wrote McNaughton
that "[m]y doctor said [the diaphragm is] the best and easiest way she
knew of, and it's the method they are fighting to get thru for the birth
control."[4] She explained the class imperative and eugenic justifications
for her doctor's role: "They have clinics etc., here and they show you
how to use them, those that is mostly for the poor that the Welfare and
country have to take care of. It's supposed to be only legal for the doctors
to tell those who already have 5 living children."[5] The writer spelled out
the economics of birth control, and in doing so revealed an issue that lay
at the heart of the class-based medical system:

> I know of one [doctor] in LA who charges $40, and one who charges $50 if
> married and $75 if single, and another who charges $125. These are all in
> LA. It's a common subject now-a-days and everyone seems to have their
> own ones. Its like my Dr. says (Dr. White) (She's a real woman) when the
> birth control information becomes legal it will knock a good deal off the

doctor's business, especially the ones who do the illegal operations. I asked her if she didn't think it would hurt her practice. She's an obstetric specialist. She said when she had to make her living off poor people who couldn't feed the ones they had, she'd quit doctoring. She charges according to your income and circumstances. She tells all her patients who want to know. As she says, there's no money in the poor cases. They very often can't pay at all; but she doesn't turn them down. She says she feels right sorry for them. She says there's enough rich folk to make up ... One day I was in her office and she had a call come in to rush to such an hospital in Hollywood ... They were millionaires and she said it would cost them $1000, if all went well and more for extra. I told her that would be a fortune for me, and she said "say, if I charged them what I charge you they wouldn't let me in the door."[6]

Whether inadvertently or intentionally the letter writer had tapped into another current in the changing context of birth control – that of the gender dynamics in the profession. As Angus McLaren argues, "although many eugenicists opposed birth control because they feared it would limit the fertility of the 'fit,' a number of McNaughton's supporters clearly believed eugenics provided a rationale for birth control."[7] In addition to conveying birth-control information to the recipient of the letter, this advice helped other women on the prairies by spreading it to McNaughton and into the women's column of the *Western Producer*.

Feminists in the birth-control movement maintained that modern women, by controlling their fertility, made better, more loving mothers because they could devote their energy and finances to the children they chose. Voluntary motherhood, they espoused, offered a more appealing approach to the modern family than the alternative, so-called Vatican roulette, which resulted from the *coitus interruptus* method.[8] In addition to placing control in the hands of women, birth control and its decriminalization promised to help reduce the incidence of maternal and infant mortality, particularly those that arose from botched abortions. McLaren found a claim by a Member of Parliament in 1947 that, in contrast to the 47,000 Canadian soldiers who died in the Second World War, as many as 21,000 women had perished in childbirth since 1926 and that 4,000 of these deaths were related to complications arising from abortions.[9]

Like her feminist reformers in Alberta, McNaughton had strong views on the topic of birth control and, like some of them, she also had a personal stake in the campaign. After developing a pelvic tumour, in

1911 McNaughton had had a hysterectomy.[10] Yet, although she remained firm in her convictions regarding birth control and women's political rights, and although her own hysterectomy undoubtedly influenced some of her beliefs concerning motherhood and family values, she was, according to historian Georgina Taylor, "reticent about the specific details of the operation and careful about the people with whom she discussed her resulting childlessness."[11] Indeed, when her close friend and political ally Irene Parlby, president of the United Farm Women of Alberta from 1916 to 1919, underwent a hysterectomy in 1918, McNaughton did not confess to having had a similar operation. Parlby, by comparison, described her ordeal in detail to McNaughton:

> Here is damnable luck. I had a hemmorage – can't spell it – but got through Girls Conference and then thought I had better see a doctor and get patched up as had to speak at University service today, when he saw me he insisted on getting another man and putting me under chloroform to have a proper exam – they found 3 tumours in my womb, and say they must remove the whole thing, and I shall have to be on my back for 6 weeks and not able to do anything for months. I am cussing just as I thought we were going to have such a splendid year and accomplish so much.[12]

In reply McNaughton offered Parlby general condolences but stopped short of sharing the details of her own experience. Parlby wrote again from her hospital room: "Many thanks for your two letters received since I came into hospital and also for your sympathy." She went on to recommend the surgery to McNaughton, stating: "Now about yourself – if you have to have this same job done do not put it off – it makes it all the harder on you as your general condition is getting worse all the time. My womb was just full of tumors big and little and doctor says if I had put off – most probably I would have had to spend 2 or 3 months in hospital … What a nuisance ones internal organs are to be sure."[13]

Neither woman openly spoke or wrote about her hysterectomy or appeared to publicly reflect on her own surgery in relation to her advocacy of eugenic sterilizations, women's health, or the sanctity of motherhood. McNaughton, in fact, did not discuss her surgery even with any of her colleagues or feminist friends. Parlby, meanwhile, seemed frustrated that her surgery had taxed her body and forced her to retire from political office before she felt ready. Months after her operation she explained her distress to McNaughton: "the doctor who operated on me before in Lacombe [Alberta] came out and gave an ultimatum that I must 'quit all public work for a year, or become a chronic invalid' so there was nothing for it but to send in my resignation – I doubt if having got out of it I shall ever have the courage to tackle it again."[14]

Like McNaughton, Parlby's sterilization did not seem to affect her views on motherhood or eugenics, although she continued to praise the science of eugenics for its benefits to society. In an address six years after her operation, Parlby explained: "curious, is it not, that we cull our flocks and herds, allowing only the finest and most physically perfect to breed, and yet when it comes to the human race we allow the mating of the most diseased and imperfect both mentally and physically."[15] She reminded her fellow feminists that they were indeed "mothers of the race," and perhaps she included herself in that category as one concerned with the well-being of society, despite her own inability to bear children.[16]

Unlike Parlby and McNaughton, their contemporaries Emily Murphy and Nellie McClung represented a more typical image of traditional womanhood in the sense that they were mothers of four and five, respectively. Murphy and McClung shared many of the feminist principles held by their fellow agrarian feminists, but their perspectives on reproductive rights and motherhood exposed some of the more delicate fissures within the women's movement, even when these women did not openly reflect on their personal experiences in public or private correspondence. Unlike the avowed principles of so-called second-wave feminist reformers – particularly those who, after the Second World War, would claim that the "personal is political"[17] – these feminists chose to conceal their personal experiences in their political expressions.[18]

The internal dynamics of the maternal feminist movement shifted in the 1930s as the Depression took hold. Several prominent feminist reformers left the scene: Henrietta Muir Edwards and Louise Crummy McKinney died in 1931 (McKinney's grave stone reads simply "mother"), and Emily Murphy followed in 1933, leaving McClung, McNaughton, and Parlby in considerable positions of power in the women's movement. As well, historian Linda Revie suggests that low grain prices and drought placed additional severe hardships on prairie families and influenced attitudes towards birth control as economic considerations slowly chipped away at moral arguments against contraception.[19] For some families, sterilization emerged as a viable option to control fertility, not so much for reasons of eugenics as a safe, permanent solution to family planning. Letters in the women's pages of newspapers and sent to political parties pointed to the availability of information about contraception, including sterilization; the issue was also discussed in articles in medical journals and papers presented to medical conferences. In Alberta, surgeons and obstetricians faced a conundrum when presented with married women who appeared healthy but who sought a sterilization operation. Physicians sought guidance from their legal and professional bodies regarding the ethics of sterilization not performed for eugenics purposes, a debate that then exploded as medical authorities across Canada considered the ethical and legal implications of sterilizing healthy married women.

At the time, under Canadian federal law, contraception, abortion, and infanticide were strictly illegal.[20] The 1892 Criminal Code stipulated that anyone who "sell[s], advertise[s], publishes an advertisement or has for sale or disposal any means or instructions or any medicine, drug or article intended or represented as a means of preventing conception or of causing abortion or miscarriage" was guilty of a criminal offence.[21] The law remained unchanged until 1969, when the government of Prime Minister Pierre Trudeau decriminalized contraception, abortion, infanticide, and a number of previously prohibited sexual acts, including homosexuality.[22] In the nearly eight decades between these two landmark pieces of legislation, significant changes at the economic, feminist, religious, and medical levels altered the way in which sterilization was understood. In particular, the aggressive genocidal application of sterilization by Hitler's Germany sent ripples of fear through Europe and North America, especially in areas where eugenics and sterilization already existed as controversial issues.

The notion of voluntary sterilization therefore needs to be considered in this broader historical context, bookended in Canada by two pieces of legislation that swung the door open for the legal use of sterilization as a form of birth control. US scholars have shown how some women – married ones especially – sought sterilization as a form of fertility control at a time when contraceptives were illegal.[23] Rebecca Kluchin finds that, with 7.9 million procedures by 1975, sterilization had become the most popular method of contraception used by married couples in the United States.[24] Historians Gunnar Broberg and Mattias Tydén show that, in Sweden, where one of the most aggressive eugenics programs took root, sterilization policies initially targeted mental defectives, but by the 1940s married women increasingly sought access to surgical sterilization as a way to limit family size. Women in Sweden, as elsewhere, tried to convince the medical and political authorities that large families imperilled their physical, mental, and social health. Sweden's laws changed in 1941 to reflect this demand from middle-class women, and included new provisions for "exhausted mothers" and "weak" women. Broberg and Tydén find that, in 1945, only 6 per cent of sterilizations in Sweden applied to women in this category, but by the 1950s the proportion had increased to more than 50 per cent.[25]

Canadian historians have yet to explore the shifting context and use of sterilization in the latter half of the twentieth century, as either a choice or an extension of eugenics programs aimed at reducing mental deficiency and raising more ideal families.[26] However, if one brings together elements of the birth-control movement and the history of sterilization, both eugenic and voluntary, and looks beyond the Second World War, it becomes clear that Canadian women promoted a sterilization agenda that was much more complicated than that explained through the eugenics program alone.

Married women in Canada were part of these broader international trends, and similarly participated in different parts of the feminist, birth-control, and eugenics movements, which at times knitted together and at other moments pulled apart into separate threads. The situation in Alberta grew increasingly complicated: the law provided for sexual sterilization for eugenics purposes, but raised questions on the part of women and their obstetricians who sought the legal sterilization of healthy women. Discussions at meetings of the Eugenics Board stressed the financial benefits of the sterilization of mental defectives, rather than offer services to so-called competent individuals – indeed, the Board considered charging healthy patients for these surgeries to offset the costs associated with the eugenics sterilization program. At a meeting in June 1931, for example, the Board refused to consider a case that it considered medical rather than an issue of eugenics, and that even though the Board believed it had the authority to grant such a procedure, it should not "be performed at the expense of the Government."[27] Although the Board's files contain no further comment on this case, it is indicative of the Board's desire to distinguish between cases of attempted voluntary sterilization for contraceptive purposes and operations on individuals at risk of spreading genetic disorders to their progeny.

Sterilization as a form of birth control or fertility regulation had some supporters in the birth-control movement in Canada, but surgery as contraception was often separate from other forms of fertility control. Contraceptive devices such as diaphragms, douches, pessaries, and tonics could be obtained discreetly and used privately, even without a husband's knowledge, let alone under the observational lights of the operating room in a hospital with a surgeon and staff standing by. Some physicians supported the birth-control movement and even risked legal charges for distributing contraceptive devices, but sterilization required full compliance with a surgeon, which invariably required hospital space as well. Hysterectomies, involving the full removal of the ovaries, and salpingectomies, or tubal ligations, which meant the removal or cutting of the Fallopian tubes, were invasive procedures that proved difficult to procure. Their effectiveness, however, appealed to families interested in curbing fertility on a permanent basis.

Historian Angus McLaren suggests that, during eugenics debates in British Columbia in the mid-1920s, the strongest proponents of sterilizing feeble-minded individuals were "such luminaries as Nellie McClung, Emily Murphy, Henrietta [Muir] Edwards, and Helen Gregory MacGill."[28] These women praised motherhood as a fundamental right of women and a sacrosanct contribution to the nation – provided the right kind of women produced the right kind of children. They feared that poor, immigrant, and feeble-minded women were reproducing at a faster rate than their Anglo-Saxon counterparts, and that eugenics measures, including birth control, should be aimed at such less desirable families. The converse of their argument, as their logic implied, was that women of their own status should produce more children. Other feminist reformers, however, took a slightly different perspective, situating sterilization along a birth-control spectrum that they viewed as a woman's right regardless of the class to which she belonged. McLaren reports that Violet McNaughton, "an active political progressive and feminist, was convinced that the health of women and children was influenced by family size and used her column [in the *Western Producer*] to elicit the support of her readers."[29]

Although some women dared to write openly about such taboo subjects as sterilizations and abortion, most did not submit their stories to local newspapers or publicize them in any fashion, particularly while birth control of any kind remained an indictable offence under the Criminal Code of Canada. Uncovering their experiences, then, requires piecing together fragments of gossip and rumour, in combination with women's writings that sometimes offered hidden clues or advice to other women.

Details concerning contraceptive advice had long appeared in coded forms in the women's pages of newspapers and journals and in letters to the editor. Violet McNaughton at the *Western Producer* received and distributed birth-control advice behind the scenes through her regular columns,[30] and her correspondence files reveal a veritable network of women involved in these activities. Catholic papers took a different position on the issue, but the pages of the Saskatchewan-based Catholic newspaper, the *Prairie Messenger*, suggest that local Catholics were concerned about birth control, sterilization, and eugenics for both Catholic and non-Catholic women. Throughout the 1920s, 1930s, and into the 1940s, articles in the *Prairie Messenger* expressed fixed ideas on the topics of birth control and abortion, but sterilization presented different challenges to Church doctrine. The early focus on eugenic sterilization and control of the allegedly mentally defective population convinced some writers that sterilization in specific cases helped to ease the financial burden on churches and states that invested in providing social services. Hitler's Catholic roots also stymied German Catholics in western Canada on this issue, as they initially tried to justify certain acts of sterilization while condemning others. Alberta physicians also recorded their concerns, both medical and legal, when asked to perform sterilizations, offering perhaps the most conclusive proof that sterilization operations occurred on the margins of the eugenics program in that province. Together these records indicate that married, middle-class women in Alberta, Catholic and Protestant alike, behaved in step with their counterparts throughout much of the United States and Europe in seeking surgical and permanent solutions to birth control.

The sexual sterilization of women considered mentally healthy, morally fit, and routinely of ideal stock raised different concerns about mental hygiene, race degeneration, and reproductive choice. Alberta's law seemed logical to reformers who considered the issue in the context of race degeneration. After the Second World War, however, as sterilizations among healthy, middle-class women increased, the issue began to be seen as more about reproduction and individual and family health, and less about race degeneration or social degradation. The gradual cultural shift from thinking about reproduction as an issue of the health of the nation to one more suitable to the confines of individual families re-engaged feminists, religious communities, politicians, physicians, and families in contentious debates about sexual sterilization, eugenic and otherwise.

As women increasing joined the ranks of physicians, many working in obstetrical practices, some began to challenge the wisdom of a legal and moral ban on contraception.[31] Feminism itself also changed over this period: early feminists such as Emily Murphy, who as a member of an urban professional class had been a vocal advocate for eugenics among the poor, no longer suited the model feminist of the second wave. Socialist feminists argued, for example, that birth control should not be hoarded by the elite members of society, but should be shared with their sisters in all classes – in particular, working mothers in the lower rungs of society – and not as a matter of force, but as a legitimate choice. Women were entering the workforce in record numbers, shaking up perceptions of the relationship between gender and class and challenging women to consider their reproductive futures differently. Across class and religious lines, women began demanding access to information and, ultimately, medical interventions to help wrestle control over their bodies away from their husbands and doctors.[32]

These fundamental cultural changes occurred very gradually and often under the public radar. As evidence of sterilizations among healthy women grew and attracted public attention, however, opponents responded with outrage. Religious leaders condemned such acts as selfish and materialistic, while the medical community tried to regain control over the situation, initiating a number of inquiries into the health parameters surrounding sterilization and abortion. The debates ultimately returned full circle to mental health as a barometer of morality. Women and men with psychiatric disorders – particularly those deemed mentally deficient or feeble minded – were susceptible to involuntary sterilization based on the hypothesis that they were both incapable of responsible parenthood and likely to pass on a biological defect to their progeny. Conversely, otherwise healthy women who sought sterilization operations in an attempt to control their fertility subsequently ran the risk of developing a psychiatric disorder due to the stress of the procedure, its permanence, and its implications for degrading natural womanhood. The complaint that sexual sterilization surgery fundamentally affected womanhood resonated with advocates and resisters alike, who argued, for example, that the "patient thought that she was no longer a real woman."[33]

Objections, however, applied unevenly across categories of involuntary and voluntary surgical candidates. Clinical reports, from Canada and elsewhere, demonstrated that healthy women who had undergone sexual sterilization surgeries, including tubal ligations or hysterectomies, developed psychiatric disorders.[34] There was no clear consensus within the medical community as to whether these psychiatric disorders represented an underlying problem or had been caused by the sterilization, but the debate once again revealed deep differences in the ways in which lower-class women were expected to behave compared with their middle-class sisters. A Liverpool study indicated, for instance, that "the results also show that members of the lower classes were more satisfied than upper social classes,"[35] whereas a Glasgow study found that over half of the requests for sterilization upon a Caesarean section delivery and within days of a vaginal delivery came from Roman Catholic women.[36]

On the Canadian prairies, class and religious differences framed the early debates about eugenic sterilization, but the Depression softened the edges of class conflict as many families were plunged into financial crisis. Gender seemed to trump religion when it came to sterilizations on the prairies, but Catholic hospital administrators and newspapers fought against this transgression. As in other jurisdictions, Catholic women on the prairies sought out contraception, including sterilization surgeries.

During the 1930s the economic strain on prairie families raised a number of serious health issues that spilled into concerns about large families. Middle-class women and vocal feminists began advocating for changes to birth-control laws, including better medically regulated access to contraceptive information and devices. Many of these women recognized the tremendous strain caused by multiple pregnancies, regardless of socio-economic status, and realized that the Depression was placing more and more families in financial peril.

Although for some women sterilization became an extension of birth control, for others it remained an act beyond the pale – an aggressive and unnatural measure to control fertility. As the debate in Alberta on contraception began to consider the use of these more invasive surgeries, the discourse shifted to one about women's rights. By the time that Hitler's genocidal application of sterilization laws appeared in Alberta newspapers in the mid- and late 1930s, sterilization had already become a more public topic of discussion. Women increasingly pitted themselves against a patriarchal legal system and a patronizing set of moral and religious arguments levelled at them from pulpits and platforms. The women's movement gradually responded to the broader political, economic, and cultural changes of which it was a part, and slowly began redefining itself. Already in the 1930s traces of a feminist movement defined by gender, and less divided by class, emerged on the Canadian prairies.

Birth Control, Feminism, and the Catholic Opposition

By the 1930s, as the issue of contraception gained momentum among women's groups, Violet McNaughton had become wholeheartedly in favour of birth control and deviated from some of her contemporaries in advocating for physician-assisted and regulated contraception for women across classes. Unlike Emily Murphy, who had supported birth control, including sterilization, for women of the lower classes and particularly for individuals and families considered feeble minded, McNaughton saw sterilization as part of a broader set of women's rights. Her views revealed a closer association with the agrarian socialist movement, and the letters she received from other farm women likewise reflected this difference within the birth-control movement. For example, one letter to McNaughton, as editor of the women's pages at the *Western Producer*, identified women in a more collective sense without dividing them into categories of class or intelligence. The writer described the birth-control debate as a struggle against powerful and irrational men who unflinchingly culled their livestock herds, but considered it unconscionable for women to seek reproductive control. She continued:

> I was so very disappointed to see that she [a woman who put forward a motion on legalizing birth control] so lacked the faith in her own convictions as to offer to withdraw her motion because some man had the nerve to criticise the motion and quote the Bible commands as he read them to her ... I have grown hardened to Bible Commands when quoted by men to cover their own selfish ends ... They use every care to see there isn't more horses raised than needed pigs according to their feed bins or cattle according to their pasture. But the most helpless little bits of all nature is "God's Will."[37]

The Catholic Church's condemnation of birth control and abortion stemmed from a fundamental belief in a traditional set of circumscribed roles for the sexes, including safeguarding women as subservient, but distinctly celebrated, mothers of the race. The Church regarded as blasphemous any medical or private interventions aimed at challenging this natural role, and levelled criticism at women and their increasingly secular doctors who believed otherwise. For instance, an article in the *Prairie Messenger* fulminated against "women who have been defrauded of their most glorious privilege," fearing that "the race ... is being robbed of its future in the name of medical science," and arguing that "physicians ... know that their sacred calling is to cure and not to kill."[38]

By 1938 the United Farm Women of Alberta (UFWA) had made a thorough inquiry of the birth-control issue in that province and had come out in support of relaxing the law restricting its use. Rather than openly criticize the Catholic viewpoint, however, the UFWA instead pointed to several Protestant and other religious groups – including the Federated Council of Churches in the United States, the Central Conference of Jewish Rabbis, the American Unitarian Association, and the Methodist Episcopal Church – that had embraced birth control as a matter that ultimately supported national health, rather than simply corroding it. The UFWA also noted the growing support for birth control from medical, nursing, and labour organizations, as well as from members of the professional classes, including economists, statesmen, doctors, and philanthropists. The UFWA argued that birth-control measures, contrary to earlier criticisms, did not in fact reduce the number of births in "desirable families."[39] Citing evidence from the Netherlands and New Zealand, both of which already had birth-control regulations in place, the UFWA noted that these countries had experienced a population increase and reduced their rates of maternal and infant mortality. The most vehement critics of birth control, the UFWA maintained, were those who clung to Catholic religious views or who believed that birth control appealed exclusively to a selfish, materialistic, and even secular middle class.

In a resolution presented by Myrtle Roper, the UFWA urged the "speedy removal of all barriers due to legal restrictions, tradition, prejudice or ignorance which now prevents parents from access to such scientific knowledge on this subject as is possessed by the medical profession."[40] The resolution also encouraged women to demystify the taboos surrounding birth control by talking more openly about the subject: "Have you been hesitating about mentioning such delicate personal matters as birth-control in your home? Have you been horrified at the boldness of some women who have broached such subjects in your club meetings? Well, if the Church of England and the Bishops of that church from their pulpits and in public meetings of every kind can urge consideration of these questions, surely we women talking among ourselves can afford to discuss them."[41]

The resolution thus reframed birth control as a women's issue and a family issue, and reproductive rights as collective rights that spanned class and geographic location. "All over the world today we see women in a great social revolution, struggling for emancipation, protesting against sex servitude and asserting their right to voluntary motherhood."[42] The claim that the lower classes and the feeble minded were out-producing the more desirable elements was countered by the suggestion that "these statistics do not tell of the overworked fathers, of the unceasing and increasing pain of over-burdened mothers, of the agony of children fighting their way against the handicaps of ill health, insufficient food, lack of education and toil that breaks the spirit."[43] Even if women were more suited for work in the home, "that doesn't necessarily mean that any woman shall have so large a family as to make a drudge of her for the rest of her life." The resolution pointed out that "our great women writers, teachers, painters, musicians, physicians, leaders of public thought, etc., are with very few exceptions all women with small families. If they had been compelled to put their spiritual and physical strength into the bearing and rearing of large families, we should never have heard of them."[44]

In speaking against the resolution, Emilie Briggs of Magrath, Alberta, cited religious arguments and population statistics that emphasized the dwindling numbers of children born to families in the middle and professional classes, echoing the concerns raised by University of Alberta president R.C. Wallace a decade earlier. She concluded by encouraging Alberta women to "be brave, clean, resolute, with a firm determination that we be not merely wives, with no loftier ambition than to tamper with the sacred issues of life, but rather than we be mothers in the true spirit of motherhood, with the untiring zeal to fill the full measure of our being here as instruments in the hands of God in peopling, Christianizing and redeeming the human family."[45] In returning to the arguments of religious opponents of birth control, Briggs thus emphasized the importance of family values as inseparable from Christian morals.

Canadian historians have debated the degree to which religion was in decline over the course of the Victorian era and into the twentieth century and how secular ideals and modernism stimulated cultural shifts in moral authority. Ramsay Cook, for example, in examining the concurrent and coordinated emergence of science, liberalism, and Darwinism as the roots of modernism, argues that, in the latter half of the nineteenth century, these features chipped away at religious doctrine and gave rise to a new language of equality through science. He suggests that Richard Maurice Bucke, the superintendent of the Asylum for the Insane in London, Ontario, recognized in science a new religion of equality, justice, and rational order poised to bolster social reform movements with renewed credibility that fused spirituality with social and life sciences.[46]

In the early part of the twentieth century the Social Gospel movement arose as an amalgam of biological and life science principles, socialism, and spirituality. The reinvention of spirituality, in combination with Darwinistic principles, provided an intellectual backbone for a new religious philosophy that promised to reform the working classes by recasting them within a new spiritual discourse, one wedded to science.[47] Scholars such as Mariana Valverde have argued that social reform movements in Victorian-era Canada reflected a complicated mixture of state, civil society, family, medical, and philanthropic impulses that, taken together, challenged religious interpretations of purity and replaced them with social and moral hygiene theories. In this context, cultural morality itself shifted from something designed chiefly out of religious pulpits to views increasingly engendered by the secular discourses of nation building, state regulation, and public health.[48] While historians such as Richard Allen argue that a new Christianity emerged during this period that ultimately instilled a new social conscience,[49] David Marshall argues that Christianity bowed to a more secular agenda dominated by materialism and leisure. Marshall tracks the decline in church membership following the world wars, and suggests that the emerging welfare state assumed many of the responsibilities once held by churches, while the atrocities of the world wars crumbled faith in Christian humanity.[50]

Michael Gavreau and Nancy Christie challenge this interpretation, instead arguing that the cultural shifts did not represent a rejection of Christian theology or spiritualism; rather, religion in Canada recalibrated in the first half of the twentieth century to embrace the challenges of modern social welfare in new ways, especially through a renewed institutional involvement in social work and health care.[51] These historiographical debates suggest that the religious and cultural context of the early to mid-twentieth century was changing, and much of that change affected religious participation and spilled into other areas of society, including health and medicine, and plausibly even more directly into areas of mental health and degeneration.

Within the context of birth control and eugenics, religion continued to influence discussions on the Canadian prairies. Among the loudest and most condemning voices of birth control within the religious landscape were those of Catholics, whose numbers climbed from 39 per cent of Canada's population in 1921 to 40 per cent in 1931 and to 42 per cent by 1941.[52] On the prairies, Catholics were more numerous in Saskatchewan and Manitoba than in Alberta until mid-century, when the numbers of Catholics became more evenly distributed among the three provinces.[53]

Confronted with questions of medical science, prairie-based Catholics fell between the explanations provided by the historians above. Although articles in local Catholic newspapers suggested that they positioned themselves against an increasingly secular scientific explanation for reproduction and contraception, they nonetheless reinserted themselves into these debates by providing services in the aid of mental health. Particularly beginning in the 1940s, the Catholic position from western Canada maintained that the Church had a vital role to play in supporting mental health initiatives in their communities. This shift in emphasis away from contraception specifically and into the more complicated territory of madness and alienation gave renewed purpose to Catholic outreach, and allowed the Church to maintain its social position as the battle over the morality of sterilization stretched into family values.

A key organ in this context was the *Prairie Messenger*, a weekly newspaper that connected prairie Catholics to world events, travelling lectures, papal encyclicals, and local current events from its base in Muenster, Saskatchewan. Benedictine monks of St Peter's Abbey had established Muenster at the turn of the twentieth century, and set up St Peter's College as an affiliate of the University of Saskatchewan in 1921. The college became a centre for Catholic education and boasted one of the largest libraries in the region. Located in an area with a high proportion of German Catholics, St Peter's College and its *Prairie Messenger* became an important institution for distributing Catholic literature throughout the prairies during this period.

On the issues of birth control, marriage, and reproduction, the *Prairie Messenger* exhibited firm views. Two clear lines of argument emerged in articles in the 1920s that matched those opposed by the women's organizations: first, that the liberal use of birth control among middle-class families contributed to a birth dearth in the most desirable segment of the population; and, second, that contraception corrupted marriage and ultimately destroyed Christian family values. In presenting these views, the paper often looked beyond Canada's borders to bring readers' attention to the ways in which other communities dealt with these concerns in an effort to connect with the global Catholic community. Reporting on a national congress of the Dutch Catholic League of Large Families, for example, the paper stated: "neo-Malthusianism was charged with undermining of family life and of the people's happiness, with the harming of woman's health, with injuring the nation's welfare and destroying religion."[54] In a similar vein, a Vancouver-based report suggested: "It is certainly important to improve the race, but it is still more important to perpetuate. The argument that small families mean better and happier children is unsound. Members of small families are apt to be selfish."[55]

The *Prairie Messenger* made a concerted attempt to combat the contemporary feminist movement with opposing perspectives from Catholic women who maintained more traditional views on femininity and family. At an address in Honolulu, Miss Alma Myers, an attorney and self-identified Catholic convert, stated: "The ones, however, who generally indulge in it and who seek to spread this vice are at the outset not in ill health and not suffering from poverty in any form except the poverty of ideals and moral standards. The reasons are indeed camouflaged, and the real reasons are selfishness, self-indulgence, and a lack of appreciation of the true values of life. They are indeed materialists, who worship ease, comfort and the sensual appetite."[56] Her pointed words struck at the heart of Catholic fears, not of contraception, but of the challenges modernism posed to Christian values.

Taking this position one step further, by the mid-1920s the paper began describing the dangers associated with birth control, and in particular how it wrenched away moral turpitude and even stimulated disease among women. In an effort to bolster its position, the paper featured an address by a medical professional who contended that "contraception is not in harmony with nature and is therefore wrong according to any standard of morality, indulgence with the aid of contraception, whether marital or extra-marital, is an unnatural sexual vice, because it gives sexual pleasure in a manner and for a purpose contrary to the biological aim of the act." The physician added: "Let it also be remembered that interference with the organs of reproduction will see an increase in female disease and consequent production of more unhealthy and deformed children. Contraceptive teaching is physiologically wrong."[57] Combining feminist and medical voices in the charge against contraception, the Catholic paper warned its prairie readers that, far from alleviating physical or mental complaints, contraceptive actions and thoughts produced ill health.

The Church first directed its condemnation of contraception at non-Catholic families, but over time its targets broadened to include health professionals who allegedly pedalled birth-control advice: "We are informed that under the cloak of science, doctors, clinics, hospitals, visiting nurses, social workers, economists are counseling the use of contraceptives as a scientific means of solving domestic and economic problems ... Doctors, hospitals, clinics furnishing such information should be avoided by all Catholics."[58] This criticism played into a broader challenge to medical authorities, as physicians gradually absorbed more professional territory that traditionally had been the jurisdiction of the Church.

On 6 January 1931 Pope Pius XI issued an encyclical on Christian marriage in which he spoke at length of the modern evils of divorce, birth control, and sterilization, condemning each act as crimes against marriage. The *Prairie Messenger* published his address in full, and provided helpful editorial comments to guide readers through his message: "In vigorous and lucid terms, the Holy Father condemns the far-reaching and deplorable evils of divorce, companionate marriage, birth control, abortion, sterilization and the distorted views propagated under the general name of 'emancipation' all of which, he warns, scorn and degrade the institution of marriage and imperil the welfare of the individual, the state and society, and cause the loss of souls."[59] The newspaper, which republished segments of the encyclical in subsequent years, hailed the pope's unwavering condemnation of these acts as one of the most significant statements of the twentieth century, and it emphasized the importance of resisting the temptations wrought by science that claimed to modernize the family and elevate the status of women by encouraging them to engage in unnatural acts. The pope firmly maintained the immorality of such acts, and acknowledged how even faithful Catholics had been persuaded by secular arguments: "the most pernicious errors and depraved morals have begun to spread even among the faithful and are gradually gaining ground." Redrawing the traditional boundaries of appropriate behaviour of the sexes, Pope Pius reiterated: "Let women be subject to their husbands as to the Lord, because the husband is the head of the wife, as Christ is the head of the Church."[60]

On the matter of contraception the pope acknowledged the birth-control movement, and reconfirmed his position on the issue: "Some wish it to be allowed and left to the will of the father or the mother; others say it is unlawful unless there are weighty reasons which they call by the name of medical, social, or eugenic 'indication' ... the destruction of the offspring begotten but unborn is forbidden."[61] He went on to declare a position of zero tolerance on abortion, even when the mother's health lay in jeopardy: "As to the 'medical and therapeutic indication' to which, using their own words, We have made reference, Venerable Brethen, however, much we may pity the mother whose health and even life is gravely imperiled in the performance of duty allotted to her by nature, nevertheless what could ever be a sufficient reason for excusing in any way the direct murder of the innocent?"[62]

The matter of sterilization particularly enraptured the pope, whose total condemnation was the first papal statement on the topic:

> Finally, that pernicious practice must be condemned which closely touch-es upon the natural right of man to enter matrimony, but affects also in a real way the welfare of the offspring. For there are some who, over solici-tous for the cause of eugenics, not only give salutary counsel for more certainly procuring the strength and health of the future child – which, indeed, is not contrary to right reason – but put eugenics before aims of a higher order, and by public authority wish to prevent from marrying all those who, even though naturally fit for marriage, they consider, accord-ing to the norms and conjectures of their investigations, would, through hereditary transmission, bring forth defective offspring, and more, they wish to legislate to deprive these of that natural faculty true marriage.[63]

Following the encyclical the *Prairie Messenger* seemed buoyed in its moral position on fertility. It published a spate of articles condemning laws and practices that loosened the bonds of marriage or that elevated the status of women through birth control. For example, a California bill proposed that parents could opt to undergo sterilization operations if they believed their children would become a burden on the public purse or would develop mental deficiencies, a proposal the paper lambasted as one to "prevent parenthood."[64] The blame often was aimed at physi-cians who helped to distribute information or perform operations that allegedly led to the decay of morals and the corruption of marriage.

The paper also published a number of articles highlighting the more enlightened approaches of even non-Catholic doctors who espoused anti-birth-control logic. For example, it proudly drew attention to a statement from the president of the American Medical Association, who "vehemently denounced the practice of birth control," despite his not being Catholic. In a similar vein, the paper added that "President Er. Wm. G. Morgan, who is not a Catholic, expressed himself as follows: 'the question of birth control is of vital importance to the future of our country, since it affects directly the survival of the white race and its dominance in world progress.'"[65] As further evidence of opposition to birth control by a non-Catholic medical authority, the paper reprinted an aggressive statement by Dr Howard Kelly, Professor Emeritus of Gynecology at Johns Hopkins University: "All meddling with sex relations to secure facultative sterility degrades the wife to the level of a prostitute. There is no right or decent way of controlling births but by total abstinence."[66] A final example came from a female physician, Dr Mary Sharlieb, who had expressed her views first in the *British Medical Journal*. She argued that "an experience of over forty years convinces me that artificial limitation of the family causes damages to a woman's nervous system."[67]

Drawing on such powerful statements from non-Catholics, the *Prairie Messenger* thus attempted to convince its readers that it was indeed gaining ground in the contest over contraception, and furthermore, that the Catholic Church had retained control of its status as a vital moral authority. The paper reminded readers that Catholics represented a critical perspective in defence of the family, and in Manitoba and Saskatchewan Catholics claimed credit for defeating legislative bills that would have provided for the sterilization of people deemed mentally defective.[68] This claim bolstered the suggestion that Catholic views represented the mainstream or majority perspective and that sterilization represented a form of misguided science and corrupt values. In Saskatchewan, as policy makers entertained a sterilization bill, the *Prairie Messenger* urged its readers to pressure their representatives, Catholic and non-Catholic alike, to oppose the bill: "We need not for a moment think that we as Catholics stand alone in opposition to the proposed measures of sterilizations, for we have plenty of supporters of other creeds, men of every profession and walk of life."[69]

Throughout the early 1930s the issues of sterilization and eugenics heated up as countries passed laws permitting these acts for both eugenic and non-eugenic reasons. Meanwhile, the *Prairie Messenger* maintained its firm position, castigating other regions and religions for foundering on these issues. Family values, however, even according to Catholic doctrine, did not extend to families with members considered mentally defective. When the Nazis introduced the Law for the Prevention of Hereditarily Diseased Offspring in 1933,[70] the German Catholic *Prairie Messenger* softened its approach slightly: "Let it be merely said that to prevent mental defectives of the lowest grade from marrying would not be unjust. They are of such low mental calibre that they cannot have an adequate concept of the nature of marriage and would prove only a burden to themselves and the State."[71] In holding this view the paper remained consistent with Catholic perspectives in Germany,[72] and in responding to this apparent paradox in Catholic doctrine the editors of the *Prairie Messenger* explained: "the position of Catholics is often misunderstood. It may surprise some non-Catholics to know that we admit that 'society has the right to protect itself adequately against the danger resulting from the presence and the increase of the mentally diseased ... And yet the Catholic Church cannot endorse the modern science of Eugenics in its entirety.'"[73]

As the eugenics program in Germany gathered momentum and the sterilization debate in North America grew more intense, the newspaper featured more articles on the topic. Concerning Hitler's sterilization law, the paper reported that the compulsory sterilization of individuals suffering from venereal disease, chronic alcoholism, inheritable diseases, or guilty of sex crimes was justified as "necessary to stave off a threatening degeneration of the nation."[74] As the Nazi campaign grew ever more aggressive, however, the Catholic Church resumed its former position of zero tolerance of sterilization,[75] and the *Prairie Messenger* once again began publishing the views of medical experts who were against sterilization at any cost, but now the emphasis shifted to encompass a wider set of dangers: "sterilization facilitates sexual promiscuity, which spreads social disease."[76] The paper argued that such cases justified the maintenance of long-stay custodial hospitals to contain individuals with low IQs and severe disabilities who, if sterilized, could become promiscuous with the risk of pregnancy removed. Subsequently, articles appeared that focused on mental health and reinserted the Catholic Church into the equation, suggesting that, "wherever a temple is destroyed a sanitarium has to be erected."[77] The current cultural climate, the paper argued, had led to collective madness in which insanity replaced religious adherence, and secularization and modernization contributed to immoral and indecent acts. In this cultural moment, the Catholic Church identified an opportunity to extend its reach into salvation through mental health.

By 1935 the *Prairie Messenger*'s tone had shifted considerably away from a tolerance of sterilization, even of people deemed mentally defective. Instead the paper began to focus on lobbying efforts at local and international levels to overturn existing sterilization laws and stop proposed ones. Redoubling its efforts to condemn any form of birth control, the paper reminded readers of the slippery slope from private birth-control methods to surgical sterilization and abortion: "the birth control movement is a deadly cancer on the body social and the world over."[78] The solution, the paper argued, was simple: "there is positively only one way of solving the birth control problem and that is bringing Christ closer to the hearts of men."[79]

The relationship between an alleged epidemic of insanity and secularization offered a compelling argument for Catholics, but it also appealed more broadly. Governor General Lord Tweedsmuir claimed that "one of the reasons for the recent alarmingly rapid increase in mental patients is the decline of religion."[80] Religion, it seemed, could reinvest itself in the service of humanity by addressing the issue of mental illness, particularly since such disturbances emerged from the insanity of secular living.

Seeking Sterilization

Despite Catholic opposition to birth control, including sexual sterilization operations, men and women in the twentieth century had long searched for methods to control their fertility, a quest in which Catholics and Protestants alike participated. Sterilization offered an attractive option for families who wanted to limit the number of births indefinitely, and a relatively safe and effective procedure performed by medical professionals was preferable to alternative methods such as tonics or home-made devices, which had a lower rate of success and a higher rate of variability. By mid-century evidence surfaced in a variety of arenas, primarily in medical publications, that women and men were using sterilization as a form a birth control.

A study conducted by the Iowa Medical School, for example, stated that, "until the perfect contraceptive is discovered, tubal ligation will be a common procedure. A 1955 study of 2,713 white married women showed that in 9 per cent of the couples between 18 and 30 years of age, one of the spouses had been sterilized, usually the woman."[81] The reliability and convenience factors arose as two key reasons married couples would choose this route over other birth-control measures. Opposition to such operations, according to the Iowa study, came chiefly from Catholic physicians. "Protestant and Jewish physicians concur," the study explained, "in that over 98 per cent of them believe that sterilization is justified in at least some circumstances, whereas only 48 per cent of Catholic physicians agreed."[82]

Nonetheless, during the 1940s and 1950s, as healthy women negotiated with their doctors at the margins of the law, opponents of sterilization inspired claims that the procedure would lead to promiscuity, regret, and serious mental illness. Despite such claims, the voluntary sterilization of married women began to capture medical and legal attention, although much of it remained out of the public view. Members of the medical profession had to deal with a growing demand for voluntary sterilization by patients who were not suited to the eugenics program and for whom contraception and sexual sterilization remained illegal. Despite Alberta's eugenics legislation, individuals considered healthy were restricted from receiving the operation on the grounds that it was immoral. Women nonetheless demanded that their physicians, many of whom had long been involved in underground networks of contraceptive distribution, provide sexual sterilization surgeries.

These women did not leave behind a trail of records of their attempts to secure such operations, so it is difficult to determine how often they occurred, but physicians' records point to the increased frequency of requests after the Second World War. The identification of any such attempts encourages us to reconsider the roles families, the medical profession, and the state played in family planning and population control exercises. Put differently, Alberta's eugenics legislation might not simply have been another example of social control by the medical profession, but might indicate that some Albertans astutely used the law to gain access to legal contraception.[83]

The realization that healthy individuals were attempting to take advantage of the sterilization law raised concerns among medical officials. An article in the *Alberta Medical Review* in 1949, reprinted from the *Canadian Medical Association Journal* (*CMAJ*), claimed that sexual sterilization was "being done, as well, for healthy individuals who request it, usually for insufficient reasons of a temporary nature. There is not a month but what the [Canadian Medical] Association has to inform some enquiring doctors that they may not accede to requests from healthy persons for sterilization – that such a procedure must be considered illegal till shown to be otherwise."[84] The tone of the article was one of concern, particularly for the "casual attitude adopted by doctors towards the sterilization of patients and over the consequent increase in the number of sterilizations being done."[85] The article went on to describe a case from 1947 where a married woman with children had asked her family doctor whether she could be sterilized. The physician agreed that such a procedure could be done if her husband agreed. During his clinical observation, however, the physician discovered a cyst on one of the woman's ovaries, which necessitated its removal. He then asked her if she would like her other ovary removed as well. She agreed, and was effectively sterilized without her husband having been consulted.

It is difficult to determine how many cases like this might have presented themselves to family physicians, perhaps even in the privacy of that relationship, where the husband was not present to object or even to gain knowledge of the procedure. Although the removal of the first ovary would have been permissible under the law given that it constituted a threat to the woman's life, the second procedure transgressed the legal parameters and ultimately brought the physician to the attention of the Canadian Medical Protective Association. The article occasioned further discussion of voluntary sterilization, and closed with a strong statement distinguishing between healthy and unhealthy, or illegal and legal, sterilization cases: "Voluntary sterilization of the healthy is a wholly separate and different problem. Excluding from the discussion those cases covered by one or two provincial acts allowing sterilization under specific conditions, voluntary sterilization of the healthy must be considered wholly illegal … Requests from healthy individuals, man or woman, for sterilization must be refused, promptly and finally."[86] The article concluded unequivocally: "voluntary sterilization of the healthy should never be done."[87]

Two years later, in 1951, another article appeared in the *Alberta Medical Review* describing the case of a woman who had given birth by Caesarean section, during which the surgeon had identified a number of cancerous fibres on her Fallopian tubes. Determining that these fibres were likely a risk to her life, he had removed her ovaries immediately following the C-section. When the woman learned that she had been sterilized, she sued the surgeon, who was forced to admit that the fibres in fact had not been an immediate danger to her life, and was fined for not providing her with an adequate opportunity to consent to or resist the procedure.[88]

Caesarean sections thus provided timely opportunities for sterilization operations. The 1951 article in the *Alberta Medical Review* indicated that, of twenty-seven C-sections conducted in Lethbridge over six months, seven had also involved sexual sterilization.[89] By this time, women, especially middle-class married women, increasingly were giving birth in hospitals, rather than at home or outside the institutional walls of a medical centre as had earlier been common.[90] Historian Wendy Mitchinson, in a study of birthing in Ontario, finds that one doctor in the 1940s "was willing to do a C-section for no other reason than to sterilize a woman at the same time."[91] In one hospital between 1925 and 1939, over 40 per cent of the C-section deliveries were followed by sterilization. Although it is unclear how many of these operations were undertaken to prevent future health risks, their regular occurrence suggests that they were available to women with children who negotiated them with their physicians.[92]

Surgeons also played a heavy-handed role in deciding whether to sterilize a woman immediately following a C-section delivery. Several health risks increased as a result of this method of delivery, including an elevated risk of bursting the uterine walls in subsequent pregnancies. In other cases, however, C-sections gave surgeons a rare glimpse inside a woman, enough to at times detect abnormalities, including tumours and cancerous fibres. Nonetheless, Mitchinson's work in Ontario and the Alberta records suggest that women exhibited more authority in these situations than is often assumed. Women increasingly requested this surgery of their obstetricians and, as Mitchinson indicates, "the solution for non-Catholic physicians was to sterilize the woman at the same time as performing a C-section."[93] Moreover, she argues, despite appearances, women often exercised a degree of control and agency in these decisions.[94]

A year after the Lethbridge case was published, an article in the *Alberta Medical Review* responded to allegations of a near-epidemic of ovarian cancer in southern Alberta necessitating sexual sterilization operations. In a subsequent study the Alberta Medical Foundation learned of at least forty-eight cases of married women with children where the clinical notes mentioned only complaints about menstruation or prolapse, and although cancer could not be confirmed in these cases, the women had been sterilized for therapeutic reasons.[95]

While C-section deliveries, cancer, and even the threat of cancer widened the approved options for sexual sterilization for married women, physicians also noted the health consequences associated with socioeconomic stress, which was further exacerbated by repeated pregnancies. This consideration not only broadened eugenics-based justifications for sexual sterilization but also opened up the issue to include male sterilizations. A 1947 editorial in the *CMAJ* claimed: "The happiness of a large family can be beyond estimation, but economic changes have inexorably made large families impossible in all but exceptional cases, and the physical and mental effects of rapidly repeated pregnancies lead to an intolerable strain, which birth control properly used can prevent."[96] Such circumstances, the editorial suggested, could be used to justify sterilizing the husband: "It had been stated that the operation was illegal, but it might be asked for by the man himself under certain circumstances. Experience had shown however that whilst such sterilization might be desired at a given time, it might be regretted later on."[97] Indeed, the vasectomy created its own moral and medical challenges, as I discuss in Chapter 4.

At the end of the 1950s the *Alberta Medical Review* featured a lengthy article on sterilization, and again reminded readers that the topic regularly appeared in letters and inquiries from Canadian physicians. The secretary-treasurer of the national association, Thomas Fisher, asked, "why are so many requests for sterilization being made by patients: Are they spontaneous? Do they originate with the patients? Or are they the result of suggestions made by the doctor?" He then reiterated that sterilization was strictly illegal unless it was absolutely necessary for the preservation of health.[98] He also recognized, however, the increasingly elastic definition of health, especially when it involved the potential for sexual sterilization. For example, he described a circumstance laid out in a letter he had received from a concerned physician who had attended a woman pregnant with her fifth child. The family doctor wrote that "it will be all her health can stand to raise her five children. She became pregnant in spite of careful contraceptive measures. Because of the trauma involved in sterilizing her, would it be legally possible to sterilize her husband instead?"[99] This scenario elicited significant debate over whether the health concerns were specific to the woman or might encompass a married couple or even an entire family. Ultimately Fisher deferred to the legality of such an act, and recommended that sterilizing the husband in this case would be illegal unless the family resided in Alberta or British Columbia, where eugenics programs were in place and where, at least from the medico-legal position, such a procedure might be procured.

Sexual sterilization for married couples remained contested through the 1950s and 1960s. By the 1970s, however, as the federal laws on birth control and abortion changed, sterilization became one of the most popular forms of birth control for married couples. Indeed, by 1970 it was estimated that one in ten US married couples had volunteered for sterilization surgeries,[100] as disenchantment with oral contraceptives following a spate of life-threatening side effects from the birth-control pill raised the profile of surgical sterilization as a safer, albeit permanent, form of birth control.[101] Also by then Britain had added vasectomies to the list of operations covered under the National Health Service. Prior to this change, a British survey of sterilized men from 1967 to 1970 found that 98 per cent were "completely satisfied and so were their wives."[102]

These findings generated a wave of interest among Canadian medical authorities, particularly as they considered extending voluntary sterilization surgeries to men.[103] The executive director of the Royal Alexandra Hospital in Edmonton indicated that "sexual sterilization has become an unexpected popular form of birth control and [is] being requested by an increasingly large segment of the population and is recommended by an equally increasing proportion of the medical profession. The adverse publicity that has been so prevalent against the 'pill' is making this swing to sexual sterilization all the more evident."[104] Indeed, with the changes to the Criminal Code of Canada, the resulting increase in voluntary sterilizations was overwhelming Alberta hospitals. As the Royal Alexandra's executive director noted, "[i]n 1966 twenty six female sterilizations were performed but in 1969 there were four hundred and fifty five female sterilizations done. In the first six months of 1970 there have already been four hundred and four performed."[105] Edmonton hospital administrators feared that the rising demand for sexual sterilization operations would create an untenable strain on hospital resources. Furthermore, since Catholic hospitals refused to provide sterilizations, other hospitals had to take on the extra demand,[106] even though "twenty seven percent of the patients sterilized were Roman Catholic."[107]

In spring 1970 Rockyview General Hospital in Calgary developed criteria for approving sterilization cases, and "became the first accredited hospital in the city" openly to provide sterilization surgeries for married women. Rockyview granted women sterilizations if they met one of the following four criteria: 1) if a woman had five or more children at any age; 2) if a woman had four or more children and was over twenty-five years of age; 3) if a woman had three or more children and was over thirty years of age; or 4) if a woman was over thirty-five years of age. These criteria, however, left no room at all for single women who sought sterilization surgeries.[108]

Throughout the inter-war and post-war period the mythology surrounding sexual sterilization changed considerably. Women such as Violet McNaughton and Irene Parlby espoused radical views on birth control during the early part of the century, but appeared too ashamed or reluctant to discuss their personal experiences with sterilization. Although married women in western Canada increasingly gave birth in hospitals after the Second World War, over time they began to request that their physicians provide them with contraceptive solutions, including sterilization. The fact that sterilization remained illegal, was opposed on moral-religious grounds, and required compliance from a number of actors, including hospital staff and surgeons, suggests that the desire for the operation remained firm. Yet the spectre of mental illness continued to cast a shadow over family planning strategies as the debate went on about who allegedly should not reproduce and whether it was acceptable to cater to those who dared tamper with healthy reproduction.

Chapter Four

Vasectomy, Masculinity, and Hyperactivity: Ken Nelson

In 1998 Ken Nelson stood in the Legislative Assembly of Alberta to watch Premier Ralph Klein respond to public demands to compensate the men and women who had suffered under the eugenics program. Ken had been sterilized in 1960 when he was a boy living at the Provincial Training School for Mental Defectives in Red Deer.[1] As the *Edmonton Journal* reported, "'I stood in the legislature gallery today and watched the premier of Alberta take the rights away from 700 people,' said Nelson, his voice straining with emotion, after the Conservatives tabled legislation to limit the rights of people sterilized in government-run institutions from 1928 to 1972 to sue for compensation."[2] The premier attempted to invoke the notwithstanding clause of the Constitution after "he noted the sterilizations, part of a government-run eugenics program, occurred before many of today's taxpayers were born. 'We think it will be in the best interests of the people to limit the liability for something we were not responsible for many, many years ago.'"[3]

Ken Nelson's comments drew public attention to the history of male sterilization and the legacy of long-stay institutionalization. Men's perspectives and actions in this debate had long been silenced, partly owing to cultural conventions that expected them to act with unrestricted sexual expression, while women were conversely expected to bear the burden of heterosexual sexuality and its consequences. The pathologization of boys and men as potentially more aggressive and sexual not only affected their participation and credibility in the sterilization debate, but also influenced their experiences in psychiatric institutions throughout the twentieth century. While women bore the burden of sexual sterilization, the combination of eugenics discourse and experimental psychiatry after the First World War saw institutionalized boys

and men bearing the brunt of invasive treatments aimed at curbing behaviours considered aggressive.

According to a 1996 National Film Board of Canada documentary,
"The Sterilization of Leilani Muir," Ken was eight years old when he
was transferred to the Provincial Training School at Red Deer. Before
then he had lived as a ward of the province at a Protestant Home for
Boys. He characterized his time at the Provincial Training School as one
that was profoundly confusing, first due to the lack of information surrounding his transfer and later due to Alberta's coercive sterilization
policy. He claimed that "we were never convicted of any crimes, but
you almost felt as though you were a prisoner. That you had no rights.
Those rights were taken away from you." Ken described how he felt put
upon by Training School officials. At one point he was brought before a
group of people and asked a series of questions regarding his stay at the
institution, including how much he liked the place. He later remarked
that you "wouldn't dare say no [or contradict these people]. Little did I
know, but this was the Eugenics Board. These were the people that were
going to decide our fate." After a short interview and with no information about the consequences of the conversation, Ken was referred for a
vasectomy. "All of a sudden I was told by the ward charge," he remembered decades later, "that I would be going in for an operation."[4] After
leaving the institution Ken eventually married and became a stepfather
to his daughter, Crystal. His first-hand experiences as a husband and
father further challenged the wisdom of a policy that restricted fertility
and invasively altered the options for raising a family among children
who had been institutionalized.

Sexual sterilizations of boys and men within the purview of Alberta's
eugenics program operated on some of the same principles that applied
to institutionalized women – namely, the desire that they not be able to
pass on their supposed mental deficiency to another generation. The
discharge of sterilized men from the institution initially raised alarm
that they might engage in riskier sexual behaviour or that deviant sexual activities were proof of their mental disorders in the first place.
After the Second World War, however, such fears gradually shifted
from connecting eugenic vasectomies and male sexuality towards a
better understanding of the relationship between male hormones and
masculinity. Alberta studies in this vein increasingly focused attention
on boys and young men in the Provincial Training School, and brought
attention to concerns such as hyperactivity and learning disabilities. As
a result, these individuals increasingly became susceptible to psycho-

pharmaceutical experimentation alongside their sustained involvement in the sterilization program.

Men's involvement as patients in this history has often been overlooked, both historically and historiographically, relative to females, and male subjects have more often remained quiet. Men who came through Alberta's eugenics program rarely attracted significant public attention or became part of precedent-setting cases warranting full disclosure. Men did not form support groups or work together using collective action to campaign for better access to vasectomies. When they looked for vasectomy services, they did so quietly within their peer groups, sometimes shepherding their friends into doctors' offices after being regaled with testimonials about the positive results of so-and-so's recent vasectomy. There was no male champion of men's rights in the wake of eugenics legislation to point out the ways in which men had been treated badly or denied their reproductive rights. Even in the context of voluntary vasectomies, men as subjects seemed to take a backseat in the discussions.

Male Eugenics

Despite this lack of interest in their experiences, men represented 42 per cent of the total number of sterilization operations performed as part of Alberta's eugenics program between 1929 and 1966, at which point the annual reports stopped recording the male-to-female ratio. The proportion of men among those who underwent sexual sterilization surgery reached a low of 34 per cent in 1949 and rose to a peak of 57 per cent in 1953.[5] In total, 1,926 men were recommended for sterilization between 1929 and 1966 and 1,041 underwent the procedure (the corresponding numbers for women were 2,146 and 1,410), indicating that the male body did not escape the scrutiny of medical reformers interested in reducing institutionalized populations, particularly among people deemed mentally defective.[6] Indeed, before the end of the Second World War, more men than women (992 versus 946) were recommended for sterilization. In all but two years between 1934 and 1943, men were consistently recommended for sterilizations more often than women,[7] although women subsequently outnumbered men on the sterilization rolls for all but one year for the remainder of the program.[8] These numbers suggest not only that gendered considerations for sterilization changed over time, but also that the peak in male sterilizations corresponded with the worst of the Depression and the outbreak of the Second World War.[9]

Most eugenics programs, in fact, sterilized women more often than men.[10] In North America, policies emphasized the relationship between eugenics and women, and historians typically have considered the toll that eugenics programs took on feminism and women,[11] or examined the critical roles that women in general and feminists in particular played in promoting an enduring discourse on eugenics tied to birth control.[12] In Alberta, as Jana Grekul notes, women were more likely than men to be recommended for sterilization,[13] a discrepancy that partly reflects an understanding of the impact of the operation on masculinity: for men, "the operation would be a blow to [their] pride or vanity."[14] Ultimately, 64 per cent of women who were recommended for sterilization underwent the operation, compared with 54 per cent of men.[15] Men thus seemed better able or more likely to resist the operation, either by refusing to grant consent or by stalling. Part of the gender discrepancy, Grekul suggests, is tied to notions of power and consent, but as examined earlier, women were also more likely to volunteer for sterilization rather than simply accept their fate as passive victims of a coercive policy.[16]

Gendered analysis of sterilization recommendations, surgeries, and consent involves competing expectations of women and femininity and men and masculinity. These features become more complicated when one looks beyond middle-class mores and communities. For some individuals, ideals of femininity and masculinity had already played a part in determining their committal to a mental health institution.[17] Concerns about promiscuity, aggressive sexual activity, and homosexuality emerged in this context and applied unevenly across the sexes. Interpretations of pathological male behaviour, fear of rampant or deviant male sexuality, and concerns about men's intelligence and capacity for responsible parenting differed from expectations placed on women in these areas. Just as Grekul analyses some of the double standards and feminine ideals placed on women in the mental health system, the masculine alternative is worth exploring in greater detail.

As noted, men have largely escaped scrutiny as subjects of Alberta's eugenics programs and the corresponding assault on masculinity. The *Prairie Messenger* published lengthy and regular columns dedicated to the health of families, mental health, birth control, and sterilization, but very rarely included considerations of ordinary men. Similarly, medical professionals wrote about their experiences with the eugenics program or requests for birth control from married couples, but almost invariably concentrated on the plight of their female patients. Men, when discussed at all, were most often considered with reference to their wives or as appendages to a series of problems that were conceptualized as women's issues, rather than issues that might be important to men or to the family unit. At the policy-making level, the fate of men and their reproductive rights also escaped judgment – indeed, they were not singled out in the Criminal Code regarding birth control. As a result, the laws regarding vasectomies raised new challenges to legal, medical, and political actors trying to assess the potential threat posed by voluntary male sterilizations in the second half of the twentieth century.[18]

Court cases in Alberta in the 1990s stemming from the backlash against the Sexual Sterilization Act also bear out this characterization of the eugenics program as one aimed at women. In preparing for the Leilani Muir trial, one of her lawyers' approaches had relied on a feminist interpretation: "The theory here is the most basic of feminine concerns – a woman should not be stripped of her right to reproduce simply to meet the convenience of others, her parents and the managers of the mental hospital."[19] The argument and supporting evidence continued to stress this point, with an Alberta government official maintaining that, "while Alberta's legislation allowed sterilization of both sexes, the Government now admits that virtually only women were sterilized,"[20] a statement that simply was not true.

The silence about male sterilizations in the media, religious quarters, and political channels did not mean, however, that contemporary Albertan politicians and lawmakers were unaware of the program's effects on men. In 1943 Ernest Manning assumed the premiership following the death of his predecessor, William Aberhart. Manning had two sons, William Keith and Ernest Preston, both called by their middle names. The premier's biographer relates that "Keith suffered oxygen deprivation at birth, which destroyed a part of his brain, leaving him prone to epileptic seizures, coordination problems, and arrested mental development."[21] Keith spent several years in a residential school in New York and later lived in the Provincial Training School in Red Deer, at great expense to the family. Keith's disability exposed the Mannings directly to the realities of the mental health system and to the financial and emotional strain that comprehensive care put on families. Preston later recalled feeling somewhat ashamed of his older brother, worrying that he would have a seizure while they were out together in public. When reporters questioned Ernest Manning's wife Muriel in 1996 about whether her son had been sterilized at the Provincial Training School, she avoided the issue,[22] although she admitted that some parents had sought this operation for their disabled children out of fear that the care of future grandchildren would fall to the aging grandparents.

Before becoming premier, Ernest Manning had suggested that medical professionals ought to have the authority to decide the reproductive futures of children and adults who could not make rational decisions for themselves. He explained, "you've got these tragic cases of people that are sometimes little more than vegetables ... how far can you argue that they should have the right to function as what we would refer to as normal human [beings] when, tragically they were not normal human beings?"[23] For Manning this issue was not abstract, and his response represented his combined experiences as a father of a child with disabilities and a political leader capable of putting his ideas into action. Yet the issue did not amount to a line in the provincial budget; the eugenics program was merely one more obligation Manning had inherited from his predecessor. By then the program had already undergone two amendments to widen the scope of its purview and to remove the need for informed consent. Manning was personally and professionally aware of these changes, and maintained the program without further adaptations until his term as premier ended in 1968.

Keith Manning entered the Provincial Training School in 1962, in which year the Eugenics Board recommended sterilizations for forty-eight men, thirty-three of whom eventually underwent the surgery; many would not have been asked for their consent if their diagnoses confirmed that they were mentally defective.[24] Despite the historical legacy of eugenics as part of a grand scheme of race betterment or ethnic cleansing, Alberta's program did not fit that description entirely. Rather, Depression-era politics on the prairies gave rise to a set of more humanitarian attitudes associated with eugenics out of concern for the plight of families struggling to deal with disability and mental health, even among high-profile politically connected families.[25]

Sterilization Operations

Men facing sterilization surgery received one of two orders: vasectomy or orchidectomy. A vasectomy involves severing and usually removing a section of the two vas, or tubes, running from the testicles behind and under the bladder and entering the penis, to ensure that they can no longer deliver sperm during ejaculation.[26] The operation does not produce immediate effects, but after a few months sperm are cleared from the active system and the man should be rendered sterile. Vasectomies represented the vast majority of the operations recommended for males by the Eugenics Board.

Orchidectomy, or castration, involves the full removal of the testicles and thus the body's ability to produce sperm and regulate hormones in the testes. This operation is considerably more invasive and has the combined effect of altering sexual function and desire by involving the endocrine system. Its application was reserved for special cases where an adjustment in hormones was considered advantageous for improving behavioural outcomes.

By the time Alberta implemented the Sexual Sterilization Act in 1929, programs had been in effect in the United States for several years. That year, the *Journal of the American Medical Association* published a study based on voluminous data from California, which boasted it was "where more elective sterilization has been done than in all the rest of the world together."[27] The California eugenics program had begun in 1909, and by the end of 1928 the state had sterilized 3,232 men and 2,588 women, more than Alberta sterilized through the duration of its program. California, like Alberta, drew subjects from institutionalized populations and targeted individuals deemed mentally defective, although it also considered eugenic sterilization for a range of mental disorders, including psychotic, depressive, and manic.[28]

In these cases most patients were put under a general anaesthetic "because they are dealing with the insane and feebleminded," as Robert L. Dickinson, a California physician, asserted.[29] Based on experiences in both California and Indiana, states with long-standing eugenics policies, researchers found no change in sexual desire for males who underwent vasectomies. Physicians were primarily concerned with the risk of increased sexual desire on the part of sterilized boys, but discovered that, even among adolescent boys whose hormones were still changing, the vasectomy operation did not rouse additional aggressive or excitable behaviour.[30] Based on his experiences in California, Dickinson recommended that "sterilization, not castration, should be done," explaining that "sterilization does not cause castration, nor does it unsex either sex. The operation of sterilization is not dangerous to health of life."[31]

As the history of Alberta's eugenics program came to light in the mid-1990s due to lawsuits by former patients, both male and female, who demanded retribution and apologies, more information emerged about the operations that had been performed on men. In the Leilani Muir case, for example, Gerald Robertson, a law professor at the University of Alberta and author of a book about mental disability and the law, offered an interpretation of cases in which sterilization had been recommended for sexual misconduct, citing "a number of cases where the individual who was recommended and approved for sterilization was noted to have engaged in consensual homosexual activity, bestiality, or homosexual activity with young boys."[32] The examining lawyer, Jon Faulds, followed up by asking how the categories of "sex reactions," "sexual irregularities," and "promiscuity" had changed over time or influenced the decisions of the Board in determining sterilization candidates. Robertson responded that "there was no record either in the minutes or in the documentation on file as to the reasons for sterilization ... The one exception to that was cases of orchidectomy or in the case of women oophorectomy [removal of the ovaries] or hysterectomy."[33] As examples, Robertson cited file number 2549 from 1949, where the Board had recommended castration or orchidectomy "because of [the patient's] sexual aggressiveness,"[34] and file 2675 from 1950 for an orchidectomy for the same reason. In file 4602, from 1970, a younger boy had received a recommendation for an orchidectomy "in view of this boy's apparent overt sexual assaultiveness [sic] towards female staff and the possibility of exacerbation as he gets older and stronger."[35] Under cross-examination, Robertson explained an instance of a man he observed in the records who had received a second operation. Initially the male patient had undergone a vasectomy to render him sterile, but upon his release into the community he was convicted of raping a thirteen-year-old girl. His case elicited discussion among Eugenics Board members as to whether an individual could be recommended for a more invasive surgery in situations where the subject expressed aggressive sexual behaviour.[36] In preparing for his testimony, Robertson had reviewed the 20 per cent of the original case files still extant, and had gauged the Board's practices in a random sample of those files. These cases therefore offer glimpses into the Board's activities and their prevalence, but they do not show the whole picture.

The first scheduled orchidectomy in the Eugenics Board's minutes appears in 1937. The case occurred before the change in the consent law and therefore still required permission from the boy's parents. The file indicates that the Board recommended a full castration, but in the event that the parents would not consent to that more invasive operation, a vasectomy would suffice.[37] The following year only a few orchidectomies warranted noting in the minutes, including one for a patient diagnosed with psychopathic personality disorder, though not mentally deficient, and another who was simply described as "Eskimo."[38] A case in 1944 was downgraded to vasectomy, although Board members felt that, due to the patient's "history of exhibitionism," an orchidectomy was preferable. This patient, however, was illiterate, and an accurate IQ rating proved difficult to obtain; in the absence of the legal authority to proceed without consent, the Board accepted the vasectomy as a viable alternative to which parents usually consented.[39]

The absence of a full set of patient records now prohibits a retrospective analysis of male patients and corresponding recommendations, but contemporary reports and publications offer further insights into the reasons behind some of the decisions regarding male sterilization operations. For example, in a medical article on experiences in the Provincial Training School, physician James Russell Grant reported that the nature of the patient population in that institution, as elsewhere, reflected gender differences in the reasons for committal. Of those patients who fell into the moron category and were the likely subjects of eugenics efforts, the males "appear as psychopathic personalities and criminal offenders," whereas the females in this category "are more likely to seek help and advice from welfare workers and guidance clinics, or by reapplication to the Training School, chiefly on account of personality disorders or neurotic symptoms."[40] Grant hinted at the degree to which male disorders and abnormalities often related to expressions of aggression, whereas disordered females tended to be more withdrawn. Whether or not Grant's distinction in this instance was overdrawn, gendered characterizations influenced diagnoses at the point of admission, which subsequently affected the likelihood of individuals' coming before the Eugenics Board at all.

Prior to arriving in Alberta Grant had worked as the registrar of the Maudsley Hospital in London, England, which was then shifting towards more emphasis on children's mental health after serving during the Second World War as a military institution. The Maudsley gained a reputation for developing better criteria for understanding the particular behavioural and psychological features of adolescents.[41] Staff at the Provincial Training School in Red Deer soon adopted a similar focus on adolescents and, consequently, in the post-war period the Eugenics Board increasingly began approving sterilization surgeries for such patients.[42]

Grant further described the Provincial Training School as the institution best suited for children who were unruly or who had become a burden on their families due to low levels of intelligence or physical and mental impairments. Of those in the moron category, which represented individuals with an IQ below 80 and considered chronically mentally deficient, he insisted that "low-grade morons are patently aware of their defect," suggesting that these individuals were easier to manage given the widespread acknowledgment of severe disability.[43] By contrast, he felt that individuals in the high-grade moron category were more apt to deny their "disability and are never made fully aware of their limitations, perhaps through the constant encouragement they are given in institutional life ... thereby they come to meet the world on equal terms, which they cannot in fact do."[44] Such distinctions between "high-" and "low-grade" morons, in fact, guided the Eugenics Board's decisions.

The moron category of patients, according to Grant, represented a serious challenge to administrators seeking to deinstitutionalize children or send them home to families, because upon discharge they were liable to be taken advantage of, both socially and sexually. For boys and young men, this challenge might be manifest in aggressive sexual liaisons, whereas girls and young women were more likely to become victims of sexual assault. In either scenario, disabling their reproductive functions was a prophylactic measure against pregnancies, but the simpler procedures did not protect them from sexual activity.

Character disorders represented another category in the Provincial Training School population. As Grant explained, "character disorder has been taken to mean persistent misconduct trying the patience of society, or such that the parents themselves have declared the child beyond their control." He went on to specify that "it does not include masturbation, isolated minor sexual offences, or isolated instances of theft or aggressive behaviour. It does, however, include extreme single instances, such as murder." Within this category the gendered dimensions became more evident, as patients were committed and examined on the basis of small crimes and legal transgressions, including theft, assault, promiscuity, prolonged unruly behaviour, and rowdyism.[45] Grant claimed that, prior to admission to the institution, none of the male patients had been "charged with rape or attempted rape, or been involved in a heterosexual offence," whereas "a large proportion of females have been concerned in illegitimate births and promiscuity." Here, too, Grant's interpretation of this difference lay in the way other members of society interacted with youths diagnosed with character disorders. The young women, he believed, were at greater risk of becoming "easy prey for the wiles and depredations of 'normal' society, at a time when their character has been insufficiently fashioned to compensate the limitations of their intellect."[46] Young men, on the contrary, showed no previous predilection towards sexual offences prior to committal. Fearing that they might develop such habits, however, it became imperative to examine them at a young age before they developed a sexual appetite. Curbing their sexual interests was critical for their future release into the community, and the eugenics program had been premised on this ideal.[47]

In the United States the medical literature vacillated on the relationship between sterilization and sexual acts.[48] Some states, including Indiana and California, initially targeted boys and men for sterilization in a concerted effort to reduce aggressive sexual activity, homosexuality, and masturbation. Over time, however, those attitudes shifted to include a greater emphasis on criminality and heredity, while concerns over sexuality disappeared behind these broader discussions. In a 1950 study of vasectomized patients from mental health and penal institutions, the topic resurfaced with a slightly different interpretation. Researchers found that patients reported a great deal of satisfaction after being sterilized. Few men claimed to experience an increase in their libido, and the numbers of institutionalized men now requesting vasectomies seemed to be on the rise. Indeed, the authors noted that "many boys, learning that the procedure was often a step on the road toward parole, had stopped [Dr Butler at the Sonoma State Home in Eldridge, California] as he passed to ask, 'Doctor, isn't it about time for my operation?'"[49] These insights are a poignant reminder of the institutionalized context in which sterilization decisions took place and the consequences attached to these decisions regarding a lifetime of confinement or release into the community.[50] The differing interpretations surrounding male sexuality and sterilization also suggest that there was no scientific consensus on the issue.

Discharge and Deviance

In post-war Alberta the three imperatives of fiscal conservatism, psychiatric experimentation, and eugenics came together in a manner that justified the continuation of the eugenics program as a way to broaden the scope of psychiatric research and treatment.[51] Periodically the superintendent of the Provincial Mental Hospital in Ponoka, Randall MacLean, had pleaded with his medical colleagues to pay closer attention to the realities and shortcomings of the mental health system. In 1942 he had written: "Mental Hospitals are very expensive of construction and primarily are not designed nor staffed nor in a position to house and care for seniles, epileptics, mental defectives or incurable, physically incapacitated individuals. These types actually militate against obtaining best results in the handling of the mentally ill. They constitute very undesirable influences in any active treatment Mental Hospital." Although admissions in these categories represented a minority of cases, MacLean repeatedly lamented that such incurable patients should be cared for at home or in designated institutions, and not be mixed with patients suffering from acute psychoses, who, he argued, could be rehabilitated: "Mental Defectives likewise are likely to be upsetting to the mentally ill, as they are frequently unstable, mischievous, cruel, scheming and crafty in their behaviour."[52]

MacLean's comments reflected a number of cross-cutting currents within contemporary psychiatry. Mental hospitals were grossly overcrowded, and despite efforts to organize patients according to disease, rather than class and gender, the complexity of co-morbid conditions combined with a lack of understanding of disease etiology forced hospital staff to rely on crude observations. It is partly due to these conditions that, as historians such as Joel Braslow, Jack Pressman, and Edward Shorter have pointed out, the period between the 1930s and into the 1950s represented an important turning point in psychiatry.[53] Shorter describes it this way: "In the first half of the twentieth century, psychiatry was caught in a dilemma. On the one hand, psychiatrists could warehouse their patients in vast bins in the hopes that they might recover spontaneously. On the other, they had psychoanalysis, a therapy suitable for the needs of wealthy people desiring self-insight, but not for real psychiatric illness. Caught between these unappealing choices, psychiatrists sought alternatives."[54] During this period psychiatry embraced a number of radical therapies, bodily interventions such as insulin shock therapy, malaria therapy, electroshock or electroconvulsive therapy, lobotomies, and, by the 1950s, a host of pharmacological interventions. Although in hindsight these therapeutic innovations have been described as barbaric, malaria therapy and lobotomies earned their innovators Nobel Prizes for path-breaking research.[55] Teaming up with neurologists and emphasizing a physical and increasingly scientific approach to mental health, psychiatry, at least according to Shorter, realigned itself with its biological roots after a brief flirtation with Freudian psychoanalysis.[56]

The development of these physical interventions, however, grew out of a culture of experimentation in psychiatry that was fuelled by a sense of desperation, overcrowded institutions, and increasing disillusionment among psychiatrists about their inability to cure and rehabilitate patients deemed mentally ill. This desolate situation affected patients facing a lifetime in an institution or alienation in a community; it also affected psychiatrists whose reputation as a medical sub-specialty remained in jeopardy as the discipline languished in an area that seemed separate from the triumphs and progress felt in other fields of medicine. These features of psychiatry helped to pave the way for experimentation in search of rehabilitation in mental hospitals as well as more sophisticated explanations for disorders, drawing especially upon recent developments in biochemistry, neurology, and endocrinology.

Within this culture of enthusiasm for experimental psychiatry and physical treatments, psychiatrists and staff working with patients confined under the Sexual Sterilization law felt relatively free to extend this approach as they explored therapeutic objectives in their institutions. Indeed, under the dual pressures from the provincial government to reduce the number of people living in the institution and from the medical community to devise more sophisticated etiological and prognostic studies, Alberta psychiatrists were under pressure to experiment. By the 1950s the testing of psychopharmacological agents amplified these pressures, and experiments increased in the institutions under the mandate of the Eugenics Board.

For instance, the superintendent of the Provincial Training School, Dr Leonard J. Le Vann, gauged the reactions of children in the institution to treatments for schizophrenia, and developed a hypothesis that low-grade mental defectives, or morons, were in fact exhibiting a kind of proto-schizophrenia. Combining elements of psychodynamic or Freudian theories and older notions of schizophrenia as a disease of adolescence, Le Vann suggested that mental deficiency was actually a remnant of an earlier evolutionary species. The implications of this research for the eugenics program were significant: if Le Vann could establish a clinical relationship between psychotic disorders and mental deficiency, a diagnosis of mental deficiency would mean that a patient's consent no longer would be necessary before proceeding with a sterilization operation. It would also mean that psychotics, who represented the largest group of institutionalized patients, could be sterilized without consent and ultimately discharged.

Le Vann had arrived in Alberta in 1949 after graduating from medical school in Edinburgh in 1943. He had had a short stint as the staff psychiatrist at the Manitoba Mental Hospital in Brandon before moving to the Provincial Training School in Red Deer. At that time, the University of Alberta also appointed him as an adjunct lecturer in the Department of Psychiatry.[57] The College of Physicians and Surgeons of Alberta, recognizing his expertise in psychiatry, granted him a licence to practise and ultimately appointed him superintendent of the Provincial Training School, from which position he oversaw all operations and activities related to its institutionalized children.

During the court proceedings in the 1990s it became clear that, despite his considerable experience in psychiatry, Le Vann in fact did not have specialist training in the field. Correspondence from the 1970s with provincial health officials indicates that they understood this gap in his training, but paid him as a specialist as an acknowledgment of his expertise, although they did not extend the title of specialist to him because he had not completed the requisite academic training.[58] Upon further investigation of his qualifications, it was discovered that he had obtained the British equivalent of a Licentiate of the Medical Council of Canada, or a medical degree. He nonetheless had often signed his letters using the initials LRFPS, which was not a recognized qualification and the subsequent legal committee could not discern its meaning. He had also claimed to be a fellow of the Royal Society within the London College of Medicine, a designation that had no correlation in Alberta and did not convey any additional specialization in psychiatry. Despite his lack of qualifications as a psychiatrist, he conducted psychiatric experiments on children at the Provincial Training School and, during the early 1950s when he worked at the Red Deer Guidance Clinic, even signed his letters for a time as "the clinical psychiatrist." In 1960 he became the superintendent of the Provincial Training School, which gave him unprecedented access to the entire institutional population, although he still failed to meet the formal requirements for practising psychiatry in the province.[59] Nevertheless, during the 1950s and 1960s, Le Vann gained distinction for his research and leadership in the field of children's mental health in the province. He was one of the few staff members who regularly conducted research and published his results in medical journals. His publications showcase Le Vann's interest in somatic or bodily therapies – physical interventions as key to curing mental ailments. His support of sexual sterilization stemmed from this broader fascination with physical therapies.

Le Vann was not alone in recognizing the relationship between boys and aggressive – even pathologically aggressive – behaviour. Several scholars have identified the ways in which gender historically has shaped admissions and diagnoses, particularly among the psychiatric population.[60] By the post-war period some of the gendered understandings of hyperactivity were even assigned to children. Ilina Singh shows that, during the 1950s and 1960s, drug advertisements for hyperactivity concentrated exclusively on boys, noting that, "between 1955 and 1998 all children pictured in advertising campaigns for minor tranquilizers and stimulant drugs are boys." Singh further reports that, in the post-war period, "a new generation of experts in boys' psychology have argued that we are 'medicalizing boyhood' with stimulant drugs in a contemporary setting which is so fast paced and competitive that boys are forced to live up to a 'culture of masculinity' much before their time."[61]

Although Singh's study focuses on otherwise normal boys, she helps to demonstrate the contemporary relationship between medicalized hyperactivity and boys. Matthew Smith's historical study of the medicalization of hyperactivity suggests that the increasing focus on hyperactivity as a learning problem itself stemmed from conditions set during the Cold War – in particular, the rising emphasis on education and intelligence, which were tied to notions of Western superiority in the ideological conflict with communism and which had captivated pediatricians, child psychologists, teachers, and politicians, who increasingly supported research and observations regarding children in institutional learning environments.[62] Although Le Vann's subjects were not expected to become middle-class professionals, he nonetheless worked within this cultural context in assessing children deemed mentally deficient. His concentration on hyperactivity and learning abilities shifted his focus towards boys in the institution and made them more likely subjects of his psychiatric experiments, while the boys' bodies functioned as the instruments for the pharmaceutical trials.

Le Vann also kept in close contact with the Eugenics Board. In 1949, when he joined the staff at the Provincial Training School, he was welcomed by the Board's chairman and encouraged to take note of the procedures so that he could assist them in detecting potential candidates for sterilization from his new post.[63] From that point onward, he became a regular attendee of the Board's meetings, although he was never formally a member. Le Vann's activities first appeared in the Board's records two years later, for helping to arrange for consent from a parent and for urging the Board to hold off on sterilizing children until they had reached adolescence, feeling "that the sexual tendencies of those [children] presented may be better evaluated at that time."[64] If a trainee was up for parole, however, the Board would intervene and review the case regardless of the child's age.

In an early article based on his work in Alberta, Le Vann considered the presence of hallucinations in patients diagnosed with manic depression, and recommended electro-convulsive shock therapies for controlling such symptoms.[65] Although this practice was gaining currency in psychiatry, the cases he described reveal his detection of co-mingling symptoms. One case was that of Anne P., a twenty-nine-year-old single girl who had religious hallucinations involving the presence of the Virgin Mary and Jesus Christ. Her parents did not speak English and the "girl," as she was described, had masturbated since the age of thirteen. Le Vann recommended two shock treatments every two days. He thereafter found that Anne's mood had changed positively and that she recognized the "silliness" of listening to these voices, although she still had auditory hallucinations.[66] Another case involved Colin I., a fifty-five-year-old married man who also had auditory hallucinations, although his were more paranoid in nature than Anne's in that he believed officials were conspiring to harm him. Colin had admitted to "severe drinking bouts," which Le Vann felt exacerbated the presence of voices in his head. After two rounds of electric shocks, the intruding voices disappeared and Colin claimed that he wanted to return to work as a bricklayer.[67] Le Vann's clinical case notes in this article reveal his interest in the social and moral or environmental triggers underlying severe psychiatric problems. In Anne's case, her masturbation and possibly her unmarried and non-English status contributed to her condition, whereas Colin's drinking clearly emerged as a poor influence in his life, which might have led to his delusions. In both cases, electric shocks appeared to provide relief.[68]

These two cases helped to set in motion a number of studies in which Le Vann elaborated on his suggestion that, despite the shift in mental health circles towards emphasizing environmental influences on behaviour, genetics and biology remained a firm factor.[69] Le Vann claimed that "indeed the picture of comparison between the normal child and the idiot might almost be a comparison between two separate species. On the one hand the graceful, intelligently curious, active young homo sapiens, and on the other the gross, retarded, animalistic, early primate type individual." On this basis he did not agree with his contemporaries that schizophrenia represented a deterioration of the mind, but instead represented a "prototypical homo sapien[s]," which Le Vann called a "congenital schizophrenic."[70] The implications of his theory bolstered the genetic argument that mental illness was in fact inheritable, and therefore individuals with mental illnesses, even of the psychotic type, were subject to sterilization.

Some of his colleagues supported the assertion that schizophrenia might be related to mental deficiency and more broadly connected with theories of degeneration, and thus was present in children before the typical onset of psychotic symptoms characteristic of schizophrenia in the adolescent years. James Russell Grant, for instance, explored the dual existence of symptoms of deficiency and schizophrenia as a syndrome called "propfschizophrenia," a term coined by US colleagues Bromberg and Schilder.[71] In his study Grant relied on an untested theory to prove the existence of schizophrenia among the population of low-grade mental defectives,[72] but, with the permission of the then director of mental health for the province, Randall MacLean, and the support of colleague Le Vann, had the local ward nurses administer the tests on one hundred institutionalized children and young adults who had been classified as having a high- to low-grade IQ. The youngest children, ages five and six, became flushed and tended to fall asleep within a few hours. Some of the older children and young adults complained of visual disturbances and dry mouth.[73] Grant concluded that an overwhelming majority of the cases tested showed signs of underlying schizophrenia, and recommended further studies on children to understand better the hereditary underpinnings of degenerative mental deficiencies.

By the mid-1950s, as antipsychotic drugs increasingly became available for controlling symptoms associated with schizophrenia, Le Vann began administering them to the children living at the Provincial Training School, effectively treating them for symptoms he believed would develop into schizophrenia. He maintained that this approach was critical because most of the children had been admitted to hospital with limited communication and social skills and had come to the residential school on account of their "abnormal or hyperactive behaviour" at home.[74] The newly available tranquillizing drugs allowed for substantial changes in the institutional setting, including the freedom to "abolish restraints, to open ward doors and to institute educational and training procedures" for all but the "hard core of mentally defective children who have not responded successfully to therapy with chlorpromazine" or other tranquillizing agents.[75] In a study of thirty-three patients ranging in age from five to forty, Le Vann concluded that the use of tranquillizing antipsychotic drugs "does make considerably easier the care of the hyperactive mentally deficient children."[76] Where previously these cases had been difficult to manage and had posed administrative challenges, the application of tranquillizers improved the capacity for nursing care. In addition to the improved conditions for staff, the results also encouraged Le Vann to continue exploring the relationship between mental deficiency and schizophrenia.

Le Vann believed he was on the cusp of making a significant contribution to psychiatry through his focus on childhood disorders. In 1960 he published an article boldly placing his own work alongside that of Eugen Bleuler, who had coined the term schizophrenia in 1908,[77] and that of the Maudsley Hospital in London. Le Vann felt that the Provincial Training School, with its rather closed staff and patient population and extensive resources for vocational, occupational, and recreational training, offered a suitable location for contributing to this growing field of study.[78] Moreover, his relatively free access to institutionalized children, many of them wards of the province, opened the possibility of engaging in a variety of experiments on a vulnerable population. Under Alberta law Le Vann did not require additional consent from the children or their guardians to conduct these studies.

Le Vann's later studies further demonstrate his attempts to find links among hyperactive behaviour, learning disabilities, schizophrenia, and mental deficiency. He continued to administer new antipsychotic and tranquillizing substances to his young patients, surmising that a typical response corresponded to a specific disease category. Given the range of disorders that Le Vann identified within this spectrum of mental deterioration, his subjects were mostly boys, since they were more often diagnosed in these categories. Indeed, in his first study there were twelve boys and only four girls, and the diagnoses included one girl and two boys with juvenile schizophrenia, two boys with autism, one boy with epilepsy and obsessive-compulsive disorder, one impulsive and emotionally unstable girl, one anxious and withdrawn girl, one boy with behavioural explosivity, and one abnormally small boy treated as an outpatient for anxiety-related concerns.[79]

After examining the children's physiological responses, Le Vann argued that changes in behaviour due to the use of psycho-sedatives helped to prove his claim that the etiology of mental retardation and deficiency was in fact related to schizophrenia. In 1961 he proudly claimed: "to the mental hospitals and residential schools for retarded children these drugs have revolutionized psychiatric care by the realization of the 'open door' policy and also by diminishing the need for the more hazardous type of physical therapies such as electro-shock and insulin-shock."[80] He also began administering anticonvulsant drugs to epileptic children, claiming that the drugs helped to prove the existence of underlying mental disease and that they controlled emotional outbursts, helping patients return to the community.

By the mid-1960s the Provincial Training School housed over eight hundred children in the category of mental retardation and maintained a waiting list of another one thousand children whose families sought their accommodation.[81] In one retrospective review of the sexual sterilization program, a former member of the Eugenics Board recalled that the "justification for sterilization was sometimes offered to ease off grounds supervision and off-grounds visits."[82] The conditions for mental health care in Alberta, as elsewhere, remained overcrowded, under-resourced, and neglected. As a result, Le Vann's experimental theory that tranquillizing drugs could reduce the number of patients requiring custodial care generated widespread interest from political authorities interested in reducing the overall psychiatric population.

Indeed, the overall goal of Le Vann, Provincial Training School staff, and the provincial health minister remained returning the children to the community. Most of them in fact would not return to their families, but instead would be released as adults with some modest training and skills intended to help them find employment. Le Vann held steadfastly to his belief that tranquillizing medications aided in the management of mentally deficient children, which was critical for their social training. He suggested that "the cardinal symptoms in the children must be relieved and, because their education must continue, the children must remain alert."[83]

In 1969 Le Vann published the results of his research using haloperidol, an experimental drug made by McNeil Laboratories, to determine if it improved mental alertness in children with attention and hyperactivity disorders. Here again, there was an emphasis on boys, the study group consisting of sixty-one boys and thirty-nine girls, approximately half of whom were under twelve years of age, the other half described as "adolescents."[84] Le Vann found that haloperidol did in fact help to reduce levels of hyperactivity, assaultive behaviour, and self-injury, but, like other major tranquillizers, the drug's side effects included tremors and muscular rigidity. He nonetheless felt that the improved capacity for remaining calm and mentally alert overwhelmed these relatively minor concerns.[85]

In a follow-up study, Le Vann reported that, by comparing reactions to haloperidol and chlorpromazine – the latter having already enjoyed commercial and therapeutic success as an antipsychotic medication – haloperidol performed more successfully to address problems of aggression,

hostility, and impulsivity.[86] Another of Le Vann's studies, using ana-
bolic compounds, relied on a patient group of seventy-four boys and
twenty-six girls ranging from four to six years of age.[87] In a study of
neuleptil, described as "a new phenothiazine," Le Vann examined the
drug's effect on sociopathic behaviours, including aggression and self-
destructive behaviour; in this case the patient group consisted of nineteen boys and eleven girls.[88]

Le Vann's research and interest in sexual sterilization came together
in one detailed case in the eugenics program. In 1963 the Eugenics Board
evaluated a young man described as having a borderline IQ and a schiz-
oid personality. Because the man's diagnosis did not include mental deficiency, the Board said that "sterilization cannot be recommended ... ,
but if epilepsy or simple schizophrenia can be entertained, then the operation subject to the consent of parent would be possible."[89] As in other
cases, the Board recommended re-evaluating the patient to see if his diagnosis or IQ might change to accommodate a waiver of consent.

Although boys and men fared better than women in the final breakdown of involuntary sexual sterilization surgeries, Le Vann's attempts
to draw a link between hyperactivity, schizophrenia, and mental
deficiency ultimately failed. He had tried to prove that pathological
behaviour more commonly associated with boys in the institution
was evidence of an underlying mental deficiency, which consequently
triggered a sexual sterilization operation. Although his theory ultimately failed to convince the medical community, males living at the
Provincial Training School bore the burden of his eugenically motivated
experiments.

Voluntary Vasectomies

Even as Alberta boys in institutional settings received vasectomies,
sometimes without their consent, men on the outside tended to stay
silent or subdued in discussions about birth control, men's rights, and
the relationship between voluntary vasectomies and modern masculinity. Vocal wives and women's groups meanwhile were proclaiming
that, as a fifteen-minute outpatient procedure, a vasectomy was a far
more attractive form of birth control than a hospital-based surgery for
women to have their tubes tied or enduring the long-term consequences of consuming a hormone-changing oral contraceptive.

Although the recollections of individual vasectomy patients or perspectives from fathers are muted in the records, their participation as

subjects filled an important role in shaping cultural attitudes towards male sterilization and birth control. Not only did men participate, willingly and unwillingly, but their bodies also bore the scars of medical experiments aimed at understanding the linkages between masculinity and sex, and later between schizophrenia and mental deficiency. Framed in the context of the post–Second World War reconstruction period, and dwarfed by the looming legacy of feminism that altered the language of reproductive rights, the politics of male reproduction underwent a significant cultural change. With it came a shift in the perception of masculinity from one associated with unbridled sexuality and hyperactive behaviour to one that denoted a more restrained or even contained image of responsibility.

Historians have tended to focus on the ways in which eugenics programs targeted women, particularly in the early phases of the movement, when the "mothers of the race" were both the prime motivators behind eugenics programs but also as motherhood itself came under intense scrutiny from social reformers.[90] The preoccupation of medical historians with motherhood in this period has helped to show how ideals of femininity became a product of social, moral, political, and medical thinking,[91] and has demonstrated how motherhood and femininity became constructed concepts, which ultimately shaped responses to reproduction and reproductive rights. Masculinity and fatherhood, however, have not attracted the same level of attention from historians in considering how intertwining notions of sexuality, class, intelligence, masculinity, and health combined to generate an evaluation of men in their roles as fathers.[92]

American historian Judy Walzer Leavitt, examining the medicalization of childbirth over the twentieth century, demonstrates that it had a profound impact on changing conceptualizations of masculinity and fatherhood, particularly among the middle class. She suggests that, by mid-century, "fatherhood became a focus of substantial public comment."[93] As opposed to the rugged manliness and bravery expressed during the world wars, the post-war period, she argues, demanded a more disciplined and constrained manhood – at the bedside of wives in labour, men were now expected to be gentle, tender, and even nervous.[94]

In another US study of health-related influences on twentieth-century ideals of masculinity, David Herzberg examines the proliferation of anti-anxiety and depression medications, and argues that mid-century commercial advertisements zeroed in on middle-class men who were battling to constrain their allegedly more natural manly impulses. The resulting conflict produced a crisis in masculinity.[95] According to the pharmaceutical ads, modern urban culture was producing pathological anxiety in men who had become shackled to office jobs and lived a sub-urban existence that forced them to control their impulses. The rhythms of contemporary life limited men who would otherwise be free, unen-cumbered, and even potentially wild. Civilization had evolved in a manner that had adjusted male roles and tamed biological expressions of manhood by replacing the wilderness with concrete jungles and the expectation that men would control their inner base instincts to fit into suits and navigate a more domesticated world. In short, Cold War men had to conform to modern expectations of psychological and emotional strength, and were expected to cultivate new, and potentially unnatu-ral, ideals of masculinity that centred on self-discipline. When male be-haviour failed to meet these revised standards of normality, it was open to being pathologized.[96]

In Canada, in contrast, there has been far less analysis of changing ideals of masculinity in the twentieth century. Christopher Dummitt has explored the relationship between modernity, men, and risk in post-war Vancouver, and argues that masculinity involved a reinsertion and redefinition of patriarchy in the more domestic political and cultural setting that emerged after the tumultuous and anxiety-producing Depression and war. The "manly modern," according to Dummitt, combined an emerging faith in experts with urban and suburban pat-terns of life that muted and in some cases directly challenged traditional masculine expressions. Men came to be regarded as "modernity's vic-tims, stretched out upon the altar of progress, baring their chests for the mechanical sacrificial knife."[97] When it came to modern men and birth control, however, they bore more than their chests.

By the 1950s expectations of men in the context of birth control began changing. The medical literature on vasectomies at this time often seemed to straddle the issue of contraception when it came to men. Several articles avoided the issue altogether by focusing on the ana-tomical or physiological effects of the operation without making explic-it comments about the patient population. Others openly acknowledged that vasectomies appealed to men across a wide social and socio-economic spectrum.

A US study from 1950, for example, identified a group of sixty-two men who had received voluntary vasectomies in North Carolina and followed their cases to get a better understanding of the men who sought this operation. Five of the men were African American and forty-five were white, and their average age was thirty-nine. Their educational backgrounds varied from having less than high school to being medical doctors, of whom there were ten. The vast majority were married with children, and most had sought surgery as a form of birth control. A minority complained of mental or physical discomfort following the procedure.[98] When questioned about the effects of the operation on their libidos, most of the men claimed that the changes, if any, were minimal and short lived, while "[f]ive patients attributed their increase in libido to the lack of necessity for contraceptive procedures and greater cooperation and response by the wife due to the removal of the fear of pregnancy." This finding led the researchers to conclude that a vasectomy had no discernible impact on the sexual performance or desire of men. There were also "no changes in external appearance or in sexual characteristics, such as pitch of voice or distribution of hair." As to the men's general satisfaction, "an automobile dealer volunteered the information that four other men had been sterilized on his recommendation ... [and] a real estate agent 'wouldn't take a million dollars for mine'... A Negro farmer with twelve children regretted that the operation had not been performed 'years ago.'"[99]

Unlike the concerns about intelligent parenthood for women, vasectomies for males, whether for eugenic or family planning reasons, avoided the issue of responsible fatherhood as a moral criterion. As Rebecca Kluchin shows in her study of sterilizations in the United States, "the increasing use of vasectomy signaled both a new trend in contraceptive decision making between couples and the medicalization of male contraception."[100] The increasingly accessible and relatively simple vasectomy had significant consequences for attitudes towards family planning that reached far beyond the clinic.

Canadians were part of these discussions, but some continued to frame the subject in eugenic and moral terms. A 1946 editorial in the *Canadian Medical Association Journal (CMAJ)*, in considering the effects on hereditary science, concluded: "it is clear that hereditary units or genes are so widely scattered that eugenic measures regarding these [vasectomies] are impracticable." Moreover, the editorial suggested, the topic of birth control raised a host of moral, religious, social, and political anxieties that usually overwhelmed considerations of the mental or physical effects on the patient. Contrary to the legal advice proffered through the Canadian Medical Protective Association (CMPA), the editorial argued that "contraception was one of the few subjects on which a general practitioner could speak with authority."[101]

Canadian officials remained more cautious than their American colleagues in their approach to voluntary male sterilization, and early discussions hinged on its legality. In an address to the CMPA, the dean of the Manitoba Law School, G.P.R. Tallin, suggested that "[a] man might be sterilized in the justifiable belief that it would be highly undesirable to have children by a wife of a certain type, but she might later be replaced and he might then regret his premature decision." Lingering regrets attributable to the sterilized male, he said, had led surgeons to abandon the operation.[102] Tallin reinforced the scientific wisdom bestowed on the medical doctor, who needed to remain firm in his principled practices. For Tallin the issue was simple: sterilization should be applied only as directed by law – that is, only when a woman's life or health was at stake. Sterilizing men was preposterous, since the health risks surrounding pregnancy for men were non-existent. Tallin's colleague, Thomas Fisher, secretary-treasurer of the Canadian Medical Protective Association, further explained that, if doctors performing these operations later had to face the court, "it is likely that none of the tear-jerking reasons that were presented to them [by their patients] will be remembered."[103] Regarding men he explained, "the situation is peculiar and anomalous and even paradoxical in that requests for sterilization come more from men than from women and most men survive pregnancy with little lasting harm. In all probability most requests from males for sexual sterilization can be answered promptly and unequivocally: no benefit will be conferred on the male and therefore the doctor should refuse to sterilize him."[104]

Despite Tallin's and Fisher's unequivocal stance, physicians and husbands continued to press authorities for a more satisfying position on male vasectomies. The crux of the issue for members of the CMPA rested on the health of the individual: "Patients often ask for sterilization because they say they dislike contraceptives. Doctors should recognize the patients' statements that they do not like contraceptive methods, that they want something else, constitute no reason why doctors should do something potentially harmful, and permanently so, to attain a result that patients, if they wish strongly enough, can attain by themselves doing something relatively harmless and which has, in addition, the advantage of impermanence."[105] According to this interpretation, doctors were directed to leave patients to their own contraceptive devices without running the risk of transgressing the law. In other words, physicians should turn a blind eye to underground contraceptive practices, but should not offer to provide medical services for male contraceptives.

Nonetheless the pressure from men for vasectomies continued. An inquiry into five Ontario hospitals in 1967 revealed that elective sterilization surgeries on males had been taking place, and produced thorny legal challenges. The Ontario physicians argued that, if patients provided informed consent, the surgery should be considered legal. Since male patients sought the operation for contraceptive purposes, however, it raised other Criminal Code issues about the use of birth control. Although the 1892 Code prohibited the use of any contraceptive devices, it made no explicit mention of male contraception per se. Yet surgeons worried that they could be charged with assault under this outdated law, regardless of consent.

Legal experts weighed into the debate too. Referring to a precedent-setting case in English law, Canadian lawyers suggested: "The decision would probably be favourable, if it be shown that the object was to preserve the life or health of the patient, or there were well founded eugenic grounds." This perspective seemed consistent with the medical protection interpretation, but the authors added: "There is no doubt that the courts would condemn any operation for sterilization which was done solely for the personal convenience of the patient ... It would be unlawful to sterilize a man so that 'he could have the pleasure of sexual intercourse without shouldering the responsibilities attached to it."[106] Moreover, some officials felt that well-adjusted and emotionally stable men would not choose any such operation, since it fundamentally undermined masculinity.

Despite such fears about a vasectomy's effects upon manhood, reports from the United States confirmed that married middle- and upper-class men, like their women counterparts, sought sterilization as a form of birth control. One study from California indicated that the "socio-economic status of these subjects is appreciably higher than the national average ... [O]ne-third of the men were at least college graduates. Over one-fifth were in managerial or professional positions. None was an unskilled laborer."[107] Other studies corroborated such findings, and still others found that working-class men were also beginning to demand the operation.[108] In another California study the rise in demands for vasectomies was directly attributable to men's discussing the surgery with their friends: "In every case the husband had at least one close personal friend who had undergone the vasectomy and was satisfied with it. In all cases but one the husband was accompanied by one or more friends who had either had this operation previously or who would also do so at that time."[109]

The growing demand for voluntary vasectomies from well-adjusted men suggests that the desire for an effective contraceptive trumped fears about its capacity to undermine masculinity. Moreover, it indicates that the conceptualization of modern masculinity was changing to suit a more responsible image that combined sex and a check on fertility. As with access to birth control for women, middle-class men proved to have the resources to facilitate their access to these surgeries, whether through word-of-mouth information from their peers, higher levels of education, or financial means, and working-class fathers were quick to follow. Lingering eugenic arguments about a birth dearth in the upper rungs of society did not appear to dampen the growing enthusiasm for voluntary male vasectomies.

British studies confirmed the rise in popularity of the vasectomy for birth control in that country, where, after 1966, more than 20,000 men were undergoing the surgery annually. L.N. Jackson, the director of the Simon Population Trust Voluntary Sterilization Project, which provided facilities and counsel for these operations, reassured men that the surgery was safe, effective, and, most important, kept a patient's masculinity intact: "After a vasectomy a man is no less a man than he was before. He remains completely masculine, his desire and capacity to perform the sexual act are quite unimpaired. Indeed, in many cases they are enhanced."[110] Jackson argued that a vasectomy was preferred over other forms of contraception, many of which had complications such as "long-term effects of the pill," allergies to rubber, or "pre-coital preparation which destroys the spontaneity of the sexual act."[111] He explained:

> With all these methods – except the pill, provided she doesn't forget to take it – a woman may be haunted and nagged by fear of a possible unwanted pregnancy. Such a woman can be sterilized if she can find a gynaecologist willing to sterilize her. Even then, unless she can afford to have the operation done privately, she will have to wait for a bed ... By contrast, the operation on the male is much simpler. It does not involve an abdominal operation, and can be done under a local anaesthetic. Many men suffer so little post-operative discomfort that they are back at work the next day.[112]

In a study of men who had received vasectomies through the British project, 1,012 men were asked about their satisfaction based on a series of questions, including its effects on their marriage and sex life and if they had any regrets and recommendations. The study found that "99% of the respondents would recommend the operation to others. In more than half of the cases there was no change in health or sex life; but where there were changes, they were for the better about 50 times more often than for the worse."[113] Far from a vasectomy's curbing sexual activity, these studies repeatedly implied that it offered a new level of sexual liberation for men.

Canadian doctors responded to such reports with trepidation, as they were anxious that the vasectomy not be used to foster promiscuity. A 1966 editorial in the *CMAJ* noted that, in Britain, voluntary sterilizations for men or women were legal, with written consent from both spouses, that they could be done for reasons other than physical or mental health risks, and that, since 1965, vasectomies were considered legal and permissible for any of the following reasons: eugenic, therapeutic, socio-economic, and convenience. The *CMAJ* argued that "[d]octors should not recommend for vasectomy men of any age who ask for it expecting to be rejuvenated. Applications from unmarried people should seldom be supported." It continued: "it seems among women at least 75% are entirely satisfied with [their husband's vasectomy] and only 5% express definite regret."[114] Canadians officials, however, continued to rely on health measures as the arbiter of access to birth control, in which case men and the vasectomy did not apply.

Vasectomy and the Pill

As men and their male physicians contemplated the legality of the vasectomy, a public health crisis emerged. The birth-control pill, which had been widely hailed as a feat of modern medical science and technology and praised (and condemned) for ushering in a new era of sexual liberalism, began to exhibit unwanted and severe side effects. As US historian Liz Watkins explains, "from the very beginning, scientists and laymen expressed concern that the use of oral contraceptives might be hazardous to a woman's health. Early clinical trials had revealed that women who took the pill experienced a variety of side effects, most commonly nausea, gastrointestinal disturbances, breast tenderness, weight gain, and breakthrough bleeding."[115] Physicians, it seemed, had not taken patients' concerns seriously when they complained about side effects. Healthy women of child-bearing age were not expected to develop serious, life-threatening symptoms, but they did: women who took the pill began developing cancer and blood clots, which caused strokes.

By 1969 women in the United States were being encouraged to think critically about their preferred choice of birth control. Barbara Seaman, a journalist and popular writer for women's magazines, published a book called *The Doctor's Case Against the Pill*, in which she condemned the use of the hormonal oral contraceptive and the medical-pharmaceutical complex that developed it.[116] Seaman's book struck a chord with feminists, especially those who had already begun organizing around women's health issues, and provided ample ammunition with which to challenge the medical establishment for more reproductive autonomy without hazardous consequences. In January 1970 an angry crowd of feminist protestors interrupted the hearings of a Senate committee, demanding that the US government address their concerns about the pill. Although the women were removed, Washington eventually pressured the medical and pharmaceutical establishments to provide more information about the oral contraceptive in the form of package inserts.[117] Throughout these debates American couples began demanding more information about birth control and its risks, and the Association for Voluntary Sterilization gained momentum as it received letters from couples inquiring about male vasectomies.[118]

In Canada the Thalidomide crisis, which caused approximately one hundred women to have miscarriages or give birth to children with congenital birth defects, had already caused women to become concerned about pills and pregnancies. Canadian physicians responded by cautiously advertising oral contraceptives to their female patients. Editorials in the *CMAJ* between 1966 and 1968 began discussing the negative side effects associated with the pill – including headaches, premature menopause, arterial emboli, asthmogenic effects, and thromboebolic disease[119] – and by the late 1960s Canadian women began challenging political and medical authorities to provide a better, safer pill. As historian Heather Molyneaux recounts, federal health minister John Munro was pressured to amend the Food and Drug Act in response to the dangers associated with the pill, likely fuelled in part by activities south of the border. In a 1969 article in *Chatelaine* magazine, the author "noted that even though [the pill] was considered safer than having a baby, many Canadian women were pressured to give [it] up … as a result of the reported side effects."[120]

The growing complaints and scepticism concerning the oral contraceptive for women redirected pressure for contraception towards men. A wave of vasectomy confessions appeared in newspapers and magazines on the heels of the pill controversy, illustrating the ease with which married men could safely and completely solve the problem of voluntary birth control in marriage. In spring 1970 the *Calgary Herald* began running a series of articles aimed at demystifying the vasectomy. These articles targeted married men, just as the pill advertisements had concentrated on married women.[121] For example, the newspaper intro- duced "Peter Keller, 40, ... a company president and the father of two children, aged 16 and seven. He is also one of the increasing number of men undergoing a vasectomy operation." The article explained that the operation cost between $70 and $100 and took a total of fifteen minutes. It estimated that, by 1961, 1,300 vasectomies had already taken place in Canada, and reminded readers that these operations had a track record with which to gauge their safety. It further noted that "[a] spokesman for [Planned Parenthood of Toronto] said that both men and women have called expressing concern about the pill. The men say they want to have a vasectomy so that they can get their wives off the pill."[122] In a similar vein an article in Good Housekeeping featured a New England minister boasting about his vasectomy: "I just felt it was my turn. There is one way a man can sort of balance out what the woman has done in bearing children. It's a husband's gift to his wife."[123]

While officials at the national level clung to the legal position on vasectomies, individual surgeons and hospital administrators began taking the matter into their own hands. Some, like Calgary hospital ad- ministrator J.C. Johnston, twisted the meaning of health to include con- siderations of socio-economic circumstances, psychological stress, or emotional stability related to the fear of producing more children. Johnston acknowledged that "a new wave of interest is developing amongst the medical profession, as well as male patients," but remained concerned about the legal interpretation: "The position would probably be favourable, if it be shown that the object was to preserve the life or health of the patient, or there were well founded eugenic grounds."[124]

Adding fuel to the fire, in 1970 Donald J. Dodds, former president of Planned Parenthood of Toronto and a general practitioner who had served in Toronto, Montreal, Boston, Halifax, and Curling, Newfound- land, published a small booklet describing his experiences with male sterilization, including his own.[125] He had performed vasectomies since 1959, and had grown frustrated with the difficulties he experienced in securing them. Like many others, he attributed the rise in their popu- larity to the publicity surrounding the birth-control pill. Dodds directly addressed the issue of masculinity in his booklet, stating that "a not insignificant proportion of the male population are firmly convinced that if they were rendered incapable of making women pregnant they would no longer be men ... Persuading such a man to undergo a sterilization operation could lead to him suffering from feelings of in- adequacy."[126] He went on to explain that this was a natural instinct and that losing the ability to reproduce might generate bad feelings, but that the intelligent man also might recognize that, in losing the ability to reproduce, he had gained a greater ability to control his life. Dodds added that "some women are convinced that sterilization would cause them a loss of femininity, and, as with men, sterilization in such instances would not be in their best interests."[127]

Dodds's comments tapped into changing ideals of masculinity. On the one hand, the vasectomy, by rendering them sterile, was seen literally and metaphorically to emasculate men. Yet sterility offered new degrees of sexual freedom, and in marriage this condition espoused a more modern image of restraint when it came to limiting family size. This conceptualization of modern masculinity, however, tapped into the changing nature of control, discipline, and perhaps even a new version of courageous manhood. Much like Judy Leavitt's gentle fathers who accompanied their wives into the delivery room during the birth of their children, the vasectomy arose as a rational, economical, even manly operation that dared the modern family to explore uncharted territory. Dodds, perhaps unwittingly, played into that sentiment and gave couples a checklist of questions and considerations before deciding to proceed with sterilization surgeries. The explicit target group, for Dodds, was married couples that had finished having children: "Husbands often seem less concerned than their wives that they might want more children if they ever re-married. Perhaps this is because by the time a man decides he would like to be sterilized, he has reached an age when he is becoming increasingly less tolerant of small children."[128]

After describing in detail the anatomy and physiology involved in the vasectomy, Dodds reassured his readers that the procedure, unlike castration surgery that removes the testes, "does not cause a man to put on weight, become weak, lose his beard, develop breasts or speak with a high-pitched voice, or to become effeminate in any way." He reassured anxious inquisitors that vasectomized men continued "to have the same sexual desires and feelings, to perform sexually as before, and to ejaculate semen fluid as before the operation. In other words, there is no difference in appearance, sensation or behaviour." Moreover, he explained, "more than three quarters of the men who have had vasectomies, and an even greater number of their wives, enjoy intercourse more."[129] Dodds's statements indicate that sex free from the fear of pregnancy, or a more liberated sexual expression, might indeed better suit modern attitudes towards sexuality, albeit within the confines of a married heterosexual relationship.

In the last section of his booklet Dodds considered sterilization for non-married, usually younger males. Here he did not suggest that the operation should be prohibited, but instead recommended steady counsel for those seeking a vasectomy. Dodds explained that such cases might appear radical or rash, and that doctors and counsellors should be prepared to question motive to ensure that the man understood the implications of his decision since, although reversing the operation was possible in some cases, it was not routine. In the end, though, Dodds felt that the emphasis on male contraception should mirror that applied to women: it should be reserved for married couples that had already reproduced.

Men in Alberta, like their counterparts elsewhere, responded to the increased flow of information about the vasectomy by demanding the operation from their physicians. In April 1970 the *Calgary Herald* reported that approximately 3 per cent of Calgary men between twenty-five and sixty years of age had received a vasectomy. One implicated physician, Dr E.S. Livingstone, claimed to have performed 2,500 vasectomies in Calgary since the late 1950s. The newspaper added that "[i]f a 10 per cent rate of vasectomies is achieved among Calgary men in the most common years of fatherhood, the ratio of couples using this method of birth control would be 'the highest in Canada,' the physician commented." Livingstone estimated that approximately four Calgary men sought vasectomy operations each day. Anticipating some of the fears and anxieties that had emerged in US studies, Livingstone reiterated that sexual function remained "intact. As the newspaper reported, "[i]n one sample of 100 Calgary men, 21 reported their virility (sexual urge) had increased after the surgery. Forty also said their frequency of intercourse had been augmented, and 62 said they were more satisfied by the act," and in follow-up interviews, "none of the patients said he was 'dissatisfied' with the overall result of his vasectomy." The newspaper said that Livingstone likened the vasectomy procedure to having a tooth extracted: "Vasectomy leaves the sexual organs otherwise unaltered, permitting intercourse and sustaining the patient's masculine body characteristics." He added that "[t]here is no typical man who applies for a vasectomy. They come from every walk of life."[130] Livingstone's more cavalier approach to the moralized views of vasectomies opened the door even further, implying that any man could request this surgery; moreover, he reiterated the increasingly common refrain that the vasectomy had no bearing on masculinity. In fact, the vasectomy was gradually evolving into an operation that improved or enhanced masculinity.

In the same year, the topic reached new audiences with a full spread in *Life* magazine. The popular article introduced vasectomy to its readers by depicting the life of Walter and Betty Brainerd in Tanafly, New Jersey. Walter was thirty-three years old and worked as a mathematician. His wife Betty was a thirty-one-year-old housewife. They had grown increasingly concerned about population control and feared that "young, successful, educated" people like themselves were "producing more children than any other group."[131] The Brainerds had decided that, although they were both healthy and able to conceive on their own, they would adopt children. They adopted Lisa, then shortly after conceived a baby, Pam. After Pam's birth, they went to New York for Walter to get a vasectomy. The article went on to explain that, in 1970, "75,000 American males will choose to undergo the same sterilizing operation as Walter Brainerd did. They may do so for altruistic or selfish or financial reasons, but in almost every case they will find the procedure a quick, simple and relatively painless way of making them infertile." Reorienting it as a male issue, *Life* explained: "In a sense, vasectomy may constitute birth control by overkill. But most researchers believe that its target – the male reproductive system – is the right one. It is simpler than that of the female."[132]

Chapter Five

From Sterilization to Patient Activism:
Doreen Ella Befus

"You'll never make it out in the world, Doreen. You'll never be able to learn enough to live like a normal person." I heard this over and over as I was growing up in an institution for the handicapped in Red Deer, Alberta. I wanted to learn how to sew and read better, but I was labeled as being too "retarded."[1]

These sentences introduced Alberta's *Decision* magazine's readers to Doreen Befus's arduous life journey. Doreen had had an auspicious start as an orphaned twin daughter of immigrant parents, who shortly after birth was placed under the custody of the provincial government. She spent her childhood and teenage years in the Provincial Training School for Mental Defectives in Red Deer. In Doreen's case, she qualified for institutional care after having been diagnosed with an intelligence quotient (IQ) of 55, placing her in the category of moron and making her a candidate for sexual sterilization. Ultimately, Doreen spent forty-two years in public institutions before being encouraged to take up residence in the community.

Beginning with accommodations with roommates in a sheltered Red Deer housing unit, Doreen was forty-nine when she struck out on her own in 1976 for the first time, moving to a one-bedroom apartment and supported through a combination of provincial and federal programs for adults with disabilities. She began searching for her biological family and connecting with her community, although this time on her own terms. For the rest of her life Doreen kept careful track of her activities in a journal, wrote countless letters of thanks to the various officials and service representatives she encountered, and became a tireless advocate for individuals who required additional assistance, be that physical, financial, or emotional. In 1988 Red Deer officially recognized Doreen's humanitarian efforts and presented her with the Air Canada Heart of Gold Award.

Perhaps one of the most notable features of Doreen's story is its endurance. She donated her copious letters, newspaper clippings, photographs, and a diary of her own thoughts to the Red Deer and District Archives and made copies for the local public library, making her collection a rare example of a patient-centred and former-patient-and-activist-centred collection of materials related to intellectual disability, institutionalization, and care in the community. Her foresight in this regard is commendable and further testimony to her unwavering mission to combat the stigma surrounding people with disabilities. Moreover, her records and family history challenge some of the fundamental assumptions concerning the contemporary validity of Alberta's sterilization program. Far from simply suggesting that the program was no longer suited to the rigours of modern society, Doreen's story offers sufficient evidence to raise questions about its original objectives and the lack of conclusive information surrounding genetic defects or the capacity of individuals with low IQ to care for others, including raising children.

Doreen's Biography

Doreen was born in 1926 to Russian immigrants Dave and Mary Befus, who farmed in southern Alberta. Mary had given birth to twin boys a few years earlier, but both sons died in infancy. She then had a daughter who survived and remained with the family. Dave and Mary had separated periodically, but in early 1926 they reunited and Mary delivered twin girls, Ella Glanda and Edna Marie, on 28 December. Ella was born with two extra toes, but Dr Gershaw, the attending physician, removed them within a few days. Ella also seemed weak, and the doctors recommended that she remain in the hospital for further observation. The family had no funds to pay for the extra care, however, and required government assistance to cover the expenses. From birth, then, Ella became entangled in the provincial welfare system.

Nearly two weeks after their arrival, the twin girls went home with their mother. Edna had been healthy throughout this period, but Ella continued to require extra attention. Over the next year, Mary and Dave once again separated, and eventually they divorced. At some point Dave remarried, and the girls were sent periodically to live with their maternal grandmother. Overwhelmed by the burden of three daughters and meagre resources after Dave's departure, Mary ultimately decided to put the twins up for adoption.[2] According to another version of the story provided by a former neighbour of the Befuses, Dave disappeared, and Mary claimed to be a widow who was then "forced to surrender both girls to the Department of the Lethbridge Courts."[3] Regardless of the truth behind the marital separation, Ella's future remained in jeopardy while her mother struggled to make ends meet in the absence of a supportive husband and surrounding family. There was no further mention of the maternal grandmother once the girls were put up for adoption.

A Norwegian family living in Iron Springs, Alberta, adopted Edna at the age of twenty-two months. Ella, however, remained unhealthy, and was put under the care of the Alberta government as part of the Children's Protection Act. She lived in a number of foster care homes, her last operated by a couple who were reportedly drunk and abusive. Under these circumstances the Department of Public Health once again moved Ella to another setting. At age seven, she was admitted to the Provincial Training School, where she would live for the next twelve years. At the point of admission, the medical superintendent claimed that "Ella was too much of a grown up name for a little girl" and changed her first name to Doreen.

Despite the lack of a family setting, "Doreen" recalled her time at the Provincial Training School as a positive one. "I was not unhappy," she claimed in a 1990s magazine article. "Reports by the staff described me always laughing and singing, I was well-liked by both staff and residents. I was never ill-treated. In fact, the nurses were loving and understanding."[4] Compared with her experiences at home and in foster home settings, the Provincial Training School offered Doreen a stable, structured environment where she was surrounded by other girls her age, many of whom had come from similar circumstances. In many ways life in the institution offered an improvement over her previous accommodations.

At age eighteen Doreen was brought before the Eugenics Board and recommended for sterilization. "No one told Doreen Befus what sterilization meant when she had a tubal ligation," claimed *Maclean's* magazine when it interviewed her in 1981 about this period in her life. Like other patients who had come before the Board in the 1940s, Doreen had not been asked for her consent, nor had the operation been explained to her. Many patients were told that they were having their appendixes removed. When interviewed for the magazine article, she explained that now "I'm fighting for the rights of mentally handicapped not to be sterilized ... Why can't they leave our bodies alone?"[5]

A 1956 report indicated that 69 per cent of the individuals discharged from the Provincial Training School had undergone sterilization under the eugenics legislation before leaving the institution. "The remainder comprise[d] a group consisting of extremes in subnormal IQ, patients discharged before the Sterilization Act was passed, and patients discharged, for various reasons, before sterilization procedure." The report also found that 23 per cent of discharged patients had married, and 94 per cent of those who married were women whose IQ ranged between 42 and 85 (the normal range was between 85 and 115). Many of these women had attempted to have their Fallopian tubes repaired surgically or to adopt, although the report was unclear as to how many of them realized they had been sterilized upon discharge. Only one woman reported that she had successfully adopted a child.[6]

Doreen was clearly not alone in her situation, although she differed from many of her peers in her reaction to the news of her clandestine sterilization. Many chose to conceal their past when they entered the community, some out of shame and others out of fear that identifying themselves as victims of the provincial eugenics program would expose them as former mental patients or as individuals labelled as mentally retarded. Doreen, however, took a different approach, and engaged in a moral crusade against what she saw as human rights abuses at the Provincial Training School on unsuspecting and often abandoned children. Only after she had been forced out of the institutional environment that, in essence, had raised her did Doreen embrace the opportunity to challenge some of the popular assumptions about people with disabilities.

Deinstitutionalization

In 1947 Doreen began providing domestic help for rural families in the Red Deer district while still a resident of the Provincial Training School. Later she lived at Deerhome, a provincial facility established in 1958 for adults with disabilities. Working closely with families piqued her interest in learning more about her own family, and from that point forward Doreen made a concerted effort to learn more about her mother and her older and twin sisters. She nonetheless continued to have strong ties to the institution that had been her main home throughout her adolescence, regularly returning to the Provincial Training School for medical attention, to visit friends, and to enjoy the comfort of familiar surroundings.

In the late 1960s large-scale institutions in all provinces came under pressure to reduce their patient populations. Some provinces, such as Saskatchewan, moved quickly, but Alberta adopted a more gradual

approach. Nevertheless, between 1975 and 1980, 62 per cent of the dis-
charges associated with this strategy took place across Canada.[7] Doreen's
formal discharge coincided with this trend: in the mid-1970s the
Provincial Training School, renamed the Michener Centre, was home to
2,300 residents, but by 1977 the number had dropped to 1,800.[8] Some
patients, especially the young and middle aged, went to new facilities,
including Deerhome, or were released permanently into the surrounding
communities, including Red Deer. Many elderly patients, however, were
transferred to old age homes, continuing a life of institutionalization.

Deinstitutionalization in the most literal sense involved the massive
depopulation of psychiatric institutions across the country. Downsizing
and eventually closing mental hospitals, however, had a rippling effect
on the economy, the workforce, public health and education, human
rights, and, most obviously, mental health care treatment and facilities.
The context for this trend involved a multilayered set of ideological and
cultural precedents. The end of the Second World War saw governments take on the task of reconstruction, which often involved an internal focus on infrastructure and the development of the so-called welfare
state.[9] But in the 1980s, the era of Reaganomics in the United States and
Thatcherism in Britain, the government of Brian Mulroney opened the
Canadian border to freer trade and weakened the social services infrastructure that previous governments had developed. Whether as a by-
product of the Cold War or the victim of the emergence of fiscal
conservatism, the post-war welfare state began to crumble under this
ideological shift. Child welfare, disability support, and provincial programs for social services, education, and health care – including most of
the hospitals concerned with psychiatric care – were all affected severely by such public policy.[10] The ideological shift created significant challenges for the more vulnerable members of society and for those who
cared for them in institutional settings.[11]

Despite these changes, an emphasis on an individual's value in the
workforce continued to frame discourses on ability and disability, as
they had during the rise of the asylum system in the nineteenth century.
In the age of the asylum and institutional care, work had functioned as
an essential component of therapy, allegedly teaching the moral virtues
of industriousness, discipline, responsibility, and skills. At the same
time, patient labour helped to ensure that large-scale psychiatric institutions were relatively self-sufficient as patients worked the gardens, ran
the laundries, and performed maintenance and cleaning on hospital
grounds. Some scholars, however, have pointed to the folly of assigning

value to work simply as therapeutic, but not providing remuneration for work conducted by institutionalized individuals. Labels such as ability and disability have come to be considered too simplistic, especially for evaluating human value, worth, and dignity,[12] and more sophisticated studies of disability move well beyond these rather utilitarian black-and-white categories.[13]

In a post-asylum world, work became a means for survival, but too much work threatened to undermine social services provisions. The emergence of sheltered workshops filled the role of asylum-based work therapy in a quasi-remunerative environment, sheltered at times from direct labour competition, but subject to economic markets. The rise of these new working regimes often rested upon the efforts of volunteers as well as subsidies from a variety of government and non-profit organizations. Although the institutional nature of work changed, the valuation of patient and former patient labour remained underappreciated and the relationship between therapy or rehabilitation and employment continued to exist in murky territory.

The structural changes brought on by the closure of long-stay hospitals and the physical impact of such closures on the landscape and economic outlook of many communities did not necessarily bring about significant differences in the experiences of alienation or vulnerability faced by many individuals who interacted with the mental health care system. Deinstitutionalization might have signalled the end of the age of the asylum and the dawn of an entirely new system of mental health accommodation, but it did not coincide with a decline in the numbers of individuals and families seeking assistance. Quite the opposite occurred. Although the asylum ostensibly had provided a set of services, however problematic, under one roof, the post-asylum world involved a complicated matrix of services that did not belong to a single government department or even fit neatly into a constitutional federalist framework. Medical services alongside housing and employment needs in combination with financial and family support services often involved a delicate degree of bureaucratic coordination in a Kafkaesque world of red tape.

But not everyone lamented the downsizing of these institutions. Some embraced, and even demanded, an end to the incarceration of individuals deemed mentally disordered or labelled intellectually disabled. This sentiment stemmed from a number of cultural movements that had gathered momentum in the midst of rights-based campaigns. Building on the strengths of civil, feminist, and gay and lesbian rights

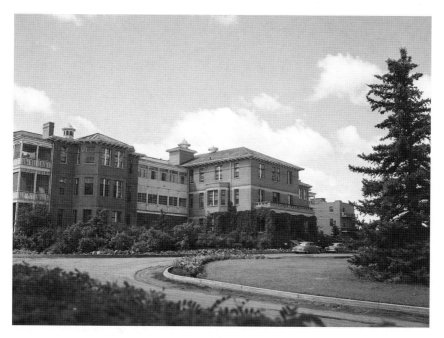

Provincial Mental Hospital, Ponoka. Provincial Archives of Alberta, PA1637

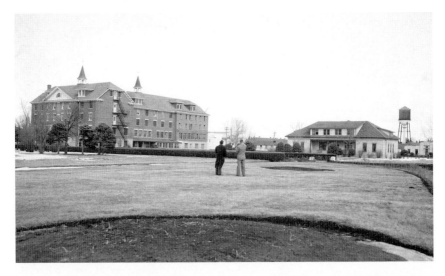

Provincial Training School for Mental Defectives, Red Deer. Provincial Archives
of Alberta, PA767

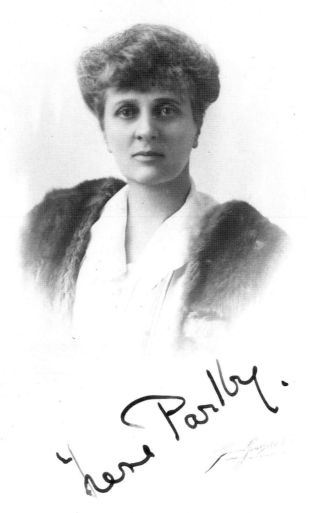

Irene Parlby. Provincial Archives of Alberta, A3353

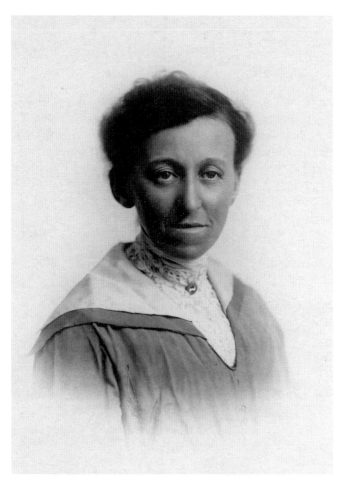

Violet McNaughton, circa 1920. Saskatchewan Archives
Board, S-B2043

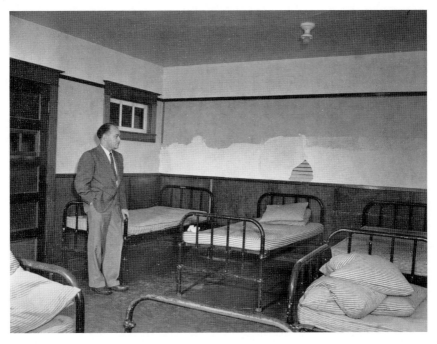

Dr Le Vann in an empty ward at the Provincial Training School for Mental Defectives. Provincial Archives of Alberta, PA767.6

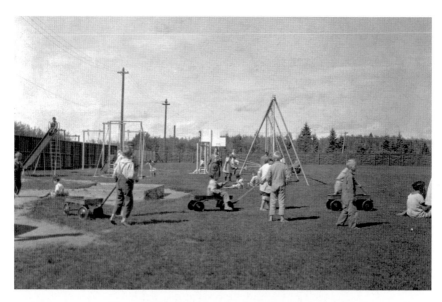
Children in the playground at the Provincial Training School. Provincial Archives of Alberta, photo: A10256

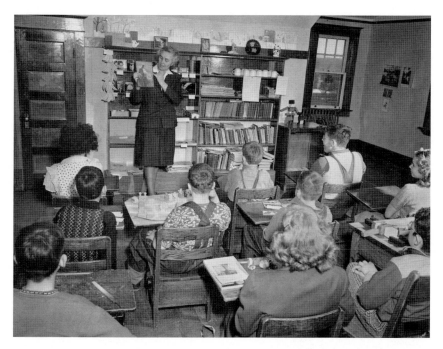

Children in a classroom at the Provincial Training School. Provincial Archives of Alberta, photo: PA767.7

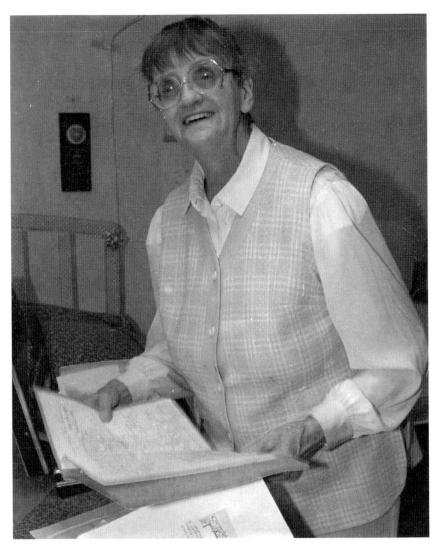

Doreen Befus in the 1990s. Courtesy of the *Red Deer Advocate*

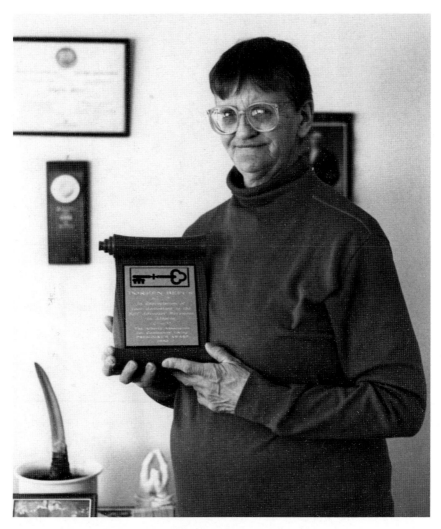

Doreen Befus receiving an award in the 1990s. Courtesy of the *Red Deer Advocate*

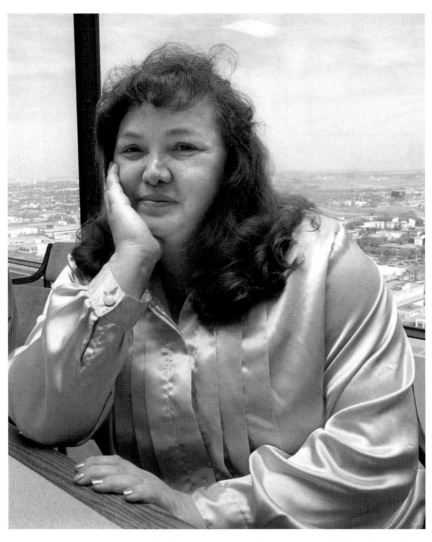

Leilani Muir, 1995, during her suit against the Alberta government for sterilizing her. Courtesy of the *Edmonton Journal*

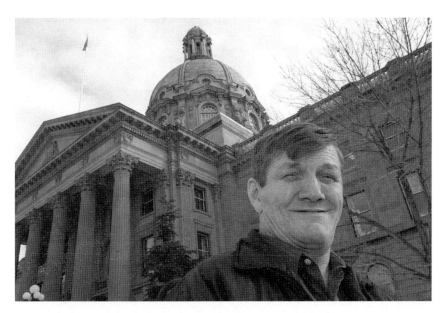

Ken Nelson in front of the Alberta Legislative Building after receiving a private apology from Premier Ralph Klein for having been sterilized as a child. Courtesy of the *Edmonton Journal*

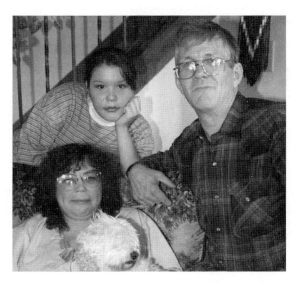

Ken Nelson with his wife Percy and her daughter Crystal, 1996. Courtesy of the *Edmonton Journal*

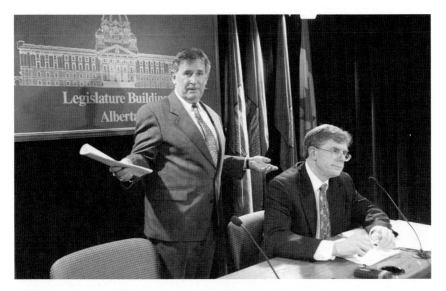

Premier Ralph Klein and Justice Minister Jon Havelock address the media, 1998, amid rising legal action by 700 sterilization victims. Courtesy of the *Edmonton Journal*

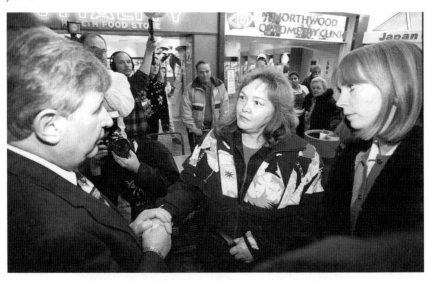

Leilani Muir receives a personal apology from Premier Ralph Klein while a BBC film crew observes, 1997. Courtesy of the *Edmonton Journal*

movements, patients began campaigning for their place in the human rights discourse. Disability rights activists engaged in aggressive campaigns for better access to services,[14] while psychiatric patients and their families began lobbying for anti-stigma campaigns, alongside demands for adequate housing, basic health services, voting rights, and access to safe employment. Some of these campaigns were fuelled by and gave inspiration to a set of intellectual critiques that questioned the way mental disorders were understood and treated.

Some intellectuals, including Thomas Szasz, a California-based psychiatrist, went so far as to pronounce that "mental illness was a myth" that had no basis in scientific or medical reasoning.[15] Michel Foucault began his career with a trenchant critique of the significant power psychiatrists wielded to determine what was and what was not acceptable social conduct.[16] In a world where free will was leached away by modern aspirations of productivity, capital accumulation, and moral authority, Foucault seemed to lament the opportunities that such a worldview created for individuals to police normality and to discipline members of society, including through the use of institutions. The evolution of an anti-psychiatry perspective, sometimes cross-fertilized with post-modernism, provided fodder for critiques of institutions.

But well beyond the highbrow critiques of institutional power or the medicalization of human behaviour, family members and former patients began mounting their own criticisms of deinstitutionalization. Their campaigns assumed a different edge, but became a critical aspect of the "people first" campaign and anti-stigma lobbies that grew in response to the rise of care in the community. Their lobbying efforts exposed the new face of mental health as one that was sorely underfunded, underresourced, and overpopulated.

Life after the Institution

Doreen's life became part of this trend, both as a deinstitutionalized individual and as someone who then championed the rights of people with disabilities in the community. She was released into Red Deer, where she lived semi-independently at first with the help of social services, including regular contact with a social worker, and a variety of public supports. Although she had been working outside the institution since the early 1960s, the labels, public surveillance, and social criticism associated with an institutionalized identity followed Doreen into the community. Beyond the walls of the hospital Doreen became an active member of her community, providing child care support for local mothers and helping her fellow deinstitutionalized friends and acquaintances face a new set of life challenges as they tried to negotiate the contours of outpatient care, social services, bus routes, bill payments, and the rhythms of an independent life.

For the first few months after Doreen left the institution for good and moved into a group home in Red Deer, she remained in regular contact with her doctor at Deerhome while she underwent an operation for phlebitis. Her move out of Deerhome triggered a dramatic set of changes in her life, not the least of which were living on her own, paying her own bills, becoming an active member of her church, securing appropriate employment, maintaining social services appointments, cooking, cleaning, and assuming a host of responsibilities. She was familiar with some of these activities, having cooked and cleaned as a trainee in provincial institutions. Managing money, however, had only ever been an exercise within the protective walls of the institution, while taking public transit and making appointments with social workers, doctors, psychiatrists, and others had never been part of the closely monitored functions of the institution. Life on the outside was very different, and people like Doreen, who had spent their entire lives in a carefully structured and supervised environment, carried many of their institutionalized habits into the community.

Furthermore, Red Deer, in common with many communities that once hosted large-scale institutions, is relatively modest in size. Former patients who might have exhibited characteristics of an institutionalized existence or who required extra time at the grocery till or needed help figuring out the bus schedule were not necessarily easily absorbed into the community. The combined social stigmas of disability and institutionalization that followed people out of provincial facilities into such communities created a new set of challenges for them as they faced a host of practical and psychological obstacles to overcome, whether their new-found independence was sought or thrust upon them. The public programs developed to ease this transition from full-scale institutional living to an autonomous existence were often ill-equipped to address these finer points of acceptance in the community.

Doreen's candid reflections on these qualitative features of deinstitutionalization provide an intimate, and undoubtedly unique, set of insights into the realities of life beyond the asylum. Although in many ways she represents a successful case, her encounters with friends and fellow deinstitutionalized men and women cast doubt on the assumption of unadulterated freedoms associated with so-called independent living. Her own actions suggest that deinstitutionalization reinforced feelings of injustice and anger towards a paternalistic state that had once sterilized people who did not meet an intellectual standard and that later had pushed those same people into a community without altering its perceptions of them as citizens. Doreen and others, however, did not blindly accept this fate; instead, they used the tools of the state to challenge an unjust conceptualization of ability and disability and to carve out a different path for citizens with disabilities.

On her own Doreen embraced a new phase of life, one marked by social activism and advocacy for individuals with disabilities. Generating strength from her religious convictions, Doreen spent the next twelve years writing letters to editors, dignitaries, and even the Queen, promoting the rights of individuals with handicaps and working closely with deinstitutionalized people to help them realize their capabilities. She stated, "when I speak, I hope to change people's attitudes toward the handicapped from believing in their own abilities. Handicapped people are like everyone else."[17] Doreen became involved with a variety of organizations, including the Alberta Association for the Mentally Retarded, the Epilepsy Association, the Brain Injury Society, the Hearing Impaired Society, and People First, in her efforts to help combat stigma and promote an abilities agenda. Her own journey into activism reveals her tenacious spirit and her sincere belief in the good of all people. These elements are clear through her actions, but a closer look at her more intimate and immediate responses shows that her activism was not inevitable but rather evolved out of her experiences in the community.

Doreen's Diary

On 1 September 1976 Doreen marks in her diary the occasion of her first stay in the group home: "I was transferred from ASH [Alberta School Hospital] Deerhome to the New Group Home in West Park. As I will have to be on social assistance, welfare is paying my board and room plus meals. I shall also get spending money. I shall receive some rehabilitation pay."[18] From this point forward regular entries describe the social workers with whom she comes into contact, the meals she eats at the group home, and the various tasks she performs to help both the staff and the residents at the home, including preparing meals and cleaning the house. The entries continue daily as Doreen meticulously catalogues her activities, almost as though she is filling in a chart.

Within a week Doreen seems to grow restless, missing friends who remain institutionalized, and on 8 September she returns to Deerhome to have coffee with some of them. She also accompanies the social worker to the Social Welfare office, where she picks up her next cheque. She seems to slip into a routine of returning to the institution while trying to find her way in the community. For the next few weeks she continues to record her daily activities as she settles into a pattern of cooking, cleaning, attending doctors' appointments, and returning to the Social Welfare office either to pick up cheques or to connect with her social worker. Throughout this busy schedule Doreen often finds time to visit friends at the nearby institution and to help out around the group home, including helping other residents meet their schedules.

At the end of September, in a manner that she would later embrace with regularity, Doreen writes to the editor of the *Red Deer Advocate*, hoping that the newspaper will publish her insights on trying to integrate into the community. She opens by boldly stating: "I would like to say how pleased I am that the government had decided to open up the new group homes out in the community."[19] She praises both the provincial government and the community for creating opportunities for people with handicaps and disabilities to live relatively normal lives, rather than being shut away in hospitals or long-stay institutions. In the community "they are given the chance to learn to take on responsibility for themselves like learning to do things in a normal way: taking the city bus to work, go shopping and ... also learn to cook."[20] Doreen attributes her love of writing to the new freedoms associated with life in the community, which allow her to participate in events at the public library and to practise her writing with help from the group home staff and other members of the community. Moreover, she feels that this form of expression is something she was not encouraged or inspired to do when she lived in the institution.

In addition to her self-discoveries, she feels strongly that life in the community allows former residents to gain self-confidence as they realize they are not "helpless" or "hopeless," but in fact have talents that are of value in the broader community.[21] In a plea for social compassion, she writes that she had been "helping these residents in mental hospitals [who now have] hope. These patients can learn. All it needs is the love and understanding and promise of the government for allowing these group homes ... [so that] residents are not feeling neglected and shut out from the world, they are given a chance to live a normal life within the community with other people, which is the best thing that ever happened."[22] She emphasizes in particular the merits of attending school in the community, an environment she associates with building confidence and acceptance. As she reflects, "years ago there was nothing and residents were put out at institutions and never given a chance to go back to school or given any guidance to what they could learn."[23] The group homes situated in the community offered a variety of learning opportunities, both formal and informal. Perhaps most important for Doreen, those opportunities existed alongside other so-called normal activities, which went a long way towards demonstrating acceptance and normality for individuals with different kinds of abilities.

After a month Doreen's daily diary entries shorten to a single line, now assuming a staccato-like rhythm with short jot notes recording only highlights: "Oct. 2 stayed home did diary work ... Oct. 7 out to supper with Hamers ... Oct. 16 to church dinner ... Oct. 23 stayed home did baking."[24] Although she continues meticulously to keep track of each day's activities, she rarely records personal details, instead concentrating on outings or activities.

Then, on 1 November, the two-month anniversary of her stay at the group home, Doreen devotes over three pages of her diary to a thorough set of reflections. For the first time since starting her diary, Doreen expresses feelings towards life in the group home and her identity as a disabled individual. She begins by thanking the people she lived and worked with – a move that would become a signature feature of her writings in years to come – and within a few lines she expresses her gratitude for living with other "handicapped people": "it is so nice to have someone to talk with openly, the handicapped and the others who are working with us."[25] She goes on to explain the pressing need for staff and residents to get along and to talk more openly. She seems to imply that she and some residents had tried to help other residents but that the staff felt this was inappropriate interaction. She ends the entry on a positive tone, grateful for her experiences and reminding herself to thank the staff for all the "good work[;] you are all doing a wonderful job."[26]

Doreen's entry hints at a symptom of the transition from institutional living to semi-institutional or group home accommodations. At the Michener Centre and Deerhome, institutions she had lived in for nearly fifty years, residents were required to clean the facilities and had regular tasks assigned to them, both as part of their therapy, rehabilitation, and training, and also to promote the smooth functioning and self-sufficiency, where possible, of the institution. Group homes, however, functioned differently. Residents paid for their room and board, even when that payment came directly from Social Services as part of their welfare provisions. The role of the residents consequently shifted from patients to consumers or clients, and from wards of an institution who were expected to contribute to its daily maintenance to semi-independent residents whose additional work might encroach upon the role of paid staff or run counter to the needs of the facility. If Doreen's case was typical, however, she was not adequately prepared for this transition. Although her notes reveal a litany of details regarding her daily tasks, they make no mention of social workers discussing how she might cope with the transition to a semi-independent existence.

Doreen's early diary entries reveal a mixed set of feelings. Her comments express pride in her new-found independence, but tempered with a dose of caution as she faithfully records her every move, as if to report her good behaviour to an invisible reader or supervisor. In 1961 sociologist Erving Goffman published a significant critique of psychiatric institutions in which he argued that long-time residents became so accustomed to life within those walls that they became incapable of adjusting to a non-institutional environment. He suggested that the long-term consequences of being under surveillance created psychological and emotional changes that fundamentally and, often, irreversibly altered human habits and activity such that individual personalities were overwhelmed by the institution and people become disaggregated components of the larger institutional system, or the "total institution" as he called it.[27]

Doreen's diary entries match Goffman's description to some extent, particularly as she continued to perform roles that might have been expected of her in an institutional framework. Cooking, cleaning, attending church, visiting friends, and reporting her activities fit into this picture, whereas there was less focus on expressing emotions or building relationships. Although it is possible that Doreen planned to keep her diary for future readers to examine, she does not initially appear to have regarded it as a secret repository for her innermost thoughts or intimate feelings. Rather, she diligently wrote in it each day as if instructed, or as if she imagined that at some point someone might ask her to account for how she had spent her time. Or, taking Goffman's assumptions seriously, perhaps Doreen had grown so accustomed to life under surveillance that she had not developed a habit of expressing such intimate thoughts or feelings. Her every move and utterance had been subject to scrutiny in the institution; now, left to her own devices, Doreen remained constantly prepared for external judgment.

Foucault, a contemporary of Goffman's, went further in his critique of institutionalized surveillance, arguing that institutions such as asylums and penitentiaries shared similar architectural traits that created the illusion that one was being watched at all times. He lamented that this powerful gaze was an insidious feature of such institutions, as the mere idea of its presence created an institutional form of discipline. In other words, residents or inmates of these facilities internalized a code of conduct or behaviour that was premised upon a fear of judgment or, worse, punishment if they failed to conform to the rules of the institution. The entire system, he suggested, was held in place through the power of assumed surveillance.[28] Doreen's early entries might be interpreted in support of this idea, as she appears to have been prepared to report on all of the tasks she accomplished, while leaving no traces of her attitudes towards her supervisors, group home staff, or peers.

Contrary to contemporary scholarly assertions that institutionalized personalities could not overcome a disciplined, institutionalized identity, however, Doreen's entries and writings begin to change over time to challenge that point of view. By early November 1976, just over two months since she arrived at the group home, her entries become more personal and reflective. On 7 November she records: "I have been receiving a lot of help. I had run into a few of my own personal problems which is no ones fault by mine. It is so nice to have some one to talk too that does know about me."[29] On the next page, she engages in more self-criticism: "If I reject the help that is available to me I will lose the respect of those who tried to help me plus my psychiatrist ... and my relatives .... I must try to help myself."[30] This last segment reads like a well-rehearsed testament to her commitment to independent living, one that health care professionals hoped patients would adopt on their way out of the institution. In this case, it is unclear whether Doreen was encouraged to accept this view of herself upon exiting Deerhome or came to this realization on her own. Her candid reflections, however, underscore the dramatic shift from a collective to an individualized identity, even as she acknowledges that part of her identity or feelings of self-worth continued to be monitored and shaped by her psychiatrist and family.

In this manner, Doreen's story encapsulates a broader and often more subtle set of changes associated with deinstitutionalization. Whether consciously or not, her comments tap into deeper, culturally held sentiments about mental illness and disability, and their individualized versus collective nature. Part of the assumption behind the state's provision of institutional care had rested upon the idea that the state or community had a responsibility to take care of vulnerable citizens, including those who had become sick or disabled, often through no fault of their own, or when they became a danger to themselves or others. This perception, however, started to change in the latter half of the twentieth century as responsibility gradually shifted to the individual. The medicalization of mental illness and disability, for example, emphasized the individual's role in acquiring and maintaining a particular disorder. Legal and political precedents further forged this connection between illness and individual responsibility. Doreen was a product of these socio-cultural shifts, and whether or not she accepted this conceptualization of herself, her language reveals an implicit recognition that she should take responsibility for her problems and actions.

These illuminating passages in her diary, in addition to breaking away from her earlier habit of writing short, perfunctory notes, begin to hint at Doreen's conscious acknowledgment that she was now straddling two different worlds. Her past experiences had been framed almost entirely by an institutional existence. Her new lifestyle retained elements of institutionalization, but it also afforded her additional freedoms and flexibility that she had not enjoyed in the hospital or in care facilities. The foreign world of the group home altered familiar routines and introduced new roles and responsibilities, leaving Doreen feeling more alone than she claimed to have been during her stays in the institutions.

Three months after being discharged from Deerhome, Doreen left the group home. With a characteristic flourish of gratitude she carefully typed letters to each of the staff members, thanking them for helping her in her program of rehabilitation. To Pam she writes: "I just wouldn't feel right not expressing to you how much I had enjoyed your talks and whenever I had problems also helping me with my money programs also arithmetic." She then adds, "I am looking forward to having you and Jack help us out on the sex Programs later on."[31] This is the first mention of sex in any of her correspondence, and although the topic does not resurface in her diary again until the 1980s, it suggests that group home staff were exposing residents to discussions about sex. It also indicates that Doreen was curious about the topic, which raises questions about her familiarity with the sterilization operation or the kind of information that had been supplied to sterilization candidates before and after their surgery.

In 1978, to prepare adult residents for discharge from psychiatric facilities, provincial government psychologists began to provide courses on sex education. The Department of Social Services and Community Health, which designed the courses, felt they were equivalent to those on money management and domestic skills. The courses remained voluntary and subject to the discretion of parents, guardians, and family members, and were conducted in groups with weekly sessions over the course of a six-month period. The curriculum, adopted from a California model, was intended for adults of lower intelligence and covered basic anatomy and physiology so that individuals could learn about their bodily functions. It also included information about menstruation, dating, inappropriate sexual conduct, birth control, pregnancy, venereal disease, and proper hygiene.[32] The program came into effect after Doreen had been released from the Michener Centre and during the height of deinstitutionalization in Alberta. The program's directors were keenly aware of the controversial nature of such education, acknowledging the long-held view that it might promote sexual activity. They argued, however, that "sexual inclination is already there. What we are doing is trying to educate the residents to prepare them and make them responsible enough to handle that sexual inclination."[33]

The introduction of the sex education program coincided with a shifting mentality towards institutionalized and disabled individuals, as their rights were brought into alignment with other human rights campaigns. Lorne Daniel, the director of the sex education program at the Michener Centre, stated in a media interview: "I think you have to realize we are dealing with adults and they do have certain human rights as adults, aside from the fact that they are mentally handicapped."[34]

The Personal Is Political

In 1977 Doreen moved to a basement suite where, for the first time in her life, she lived on her own. She commemorates this moment in her diary with a tiny cutting of the classified ad describing her new accommodations: "1 bedroom suite, refrigerator, stove, includes heat, $290/month."[35] Over the course of the next several months, Doreen's diary entries shift slightly again. In addition to recording her daily activities, the entries grow more personal and assume an increasingly conscious political edge. She retains the habit of profusely thanking everyone from social workers to bus drivers, friends, and landlords, by recording her appreciation of them in her diary and sending them heartfelt letters. But she also adopts a more aggressive tone, through letters to the editor and in more candid confessions in her increasingly personal diary, as she defends the rights of her friends and fellow former patients who sought integration into the community.

During this period Doreen also resumes searching for her biological family, from which she had been estranged for nearly fifty years. This quest leads her down a painful path of reunion, rejection, and, ultimately, a degree of reconciliation, or perhaps merely a resigned acceptance of the insurmountable distance that had developed between Doreen and her twin sister, whom she learned about while she was a resident at the Provincial Training School and whom she had first attempted to contact in 1959. Doreen's diary entries and copies of letters suggest that her sister's response was not overwhelmingly positive. "Ellen" (her name at birth had been Edna), who had been adopted into a family as an infant, seemed reluctant to embrace Doreen or to develop a relationship with her, which she felt might cause harm to her adopted family. She confessed to Doreen that she had known about her since she was a little girl, but assumed that Doreen had died from what she believed had been a grave illness. It was not until Doreen contacted her in 1959 that she realized her sister was still alive. Now, as Doreen took the opportunity to reach out to her only known family member, Ellen remained distant.[36]

Doreen's search for her extended family began in the fall of 1978 when a former neighbour responded to a letter she had published in the *Red Deer Advocate*. The woman saw Doreen's photograph in the newspaper and recognized her resemblance to her former neighbour, Doreen's mother. It was through this woman's phone call that Doreen learned her parents' names and that she had more siblings; she quickly learned that an elder sister lived in the nearby town of Innisfail with her husband and children. Doreen immediately started a separate diary for her family records. In it she confides: "when I received this call from the lady at the twilight lodge I had no knowledge that it [would] bring back my family which has been kept in the closet for years in which I did not know existed … it is still a dream [and] it will be a while yet before I can know all the family personally which will take time."[37]

The day after the mysterious phone call, Doreen telephoned her elder sister in Innisfail. "She was quite surprised to hear that she might be my sister. She was never told by her mother that she used to have twin sisters."[38] They agreed to meet in due course, and in the meantime Doreen began conducting research at the Department of Vital Statistics to verify this newly acquired information. Within a few months not only had she gathered more information on the family, but she also got in touch with other members, including her father's brother and a branch of the family on her father's side. She also tracked down her twin sister again, who, it turned out, was now living in Console, Alberta, and was married with children. These connections were meaningful to Doreen, particularly since she had been cut off from all familial interactions since she was a young child, and even though they aroused painful memories and feelings of rejection. In writing to her twin sister, she admits: "Sis, finding you has meant so much to me and still does. The visits we had together are not to be forgotten and I have very fond memories of all our visits ... Sis, writing this letter is quite painful for me as I am not certain when I can come to see you again."[39]

Doreen savoured the new relationships she developed with her siblings, their families, and a host of previously unknown aunts, uncles, and cousins: "The family has given me something very important in life, the uncles are willing to accept me and make up what I didn't have as a child and fill the family tie."[40] But not everyone welcomed Doreen back into the family willingly. Her elder sister resisted the desire to develop a relationship with her, as Doreen's letters indicate: "I told uncle Phil that you did not wish to get involved with another family as you have more than you can handle right now, and I did not want to bring hurt to you and wish to respect your wishes, they won't bother you Sis I promise." The rejection deeply saddened Doreen: "I am crying while I write this letter Sis, longing to see you all again." She concludes with a deeper set of reflections on the importance of family: "I used to feel hungry for that same kind of family love which I never had as a child, and when I first found you I wanted that love from you that I did not get as a child but it was hard to get close to you and finding out that your family was your only ones that needed your love ... I just had learned to accept just whatever you can give me, no doubt that [Uncle Phil's family] will be able to give me the love you are unable to give me." Finally, she comments on the absolute lack of familial love in the institution: "Me being in mental institutions can not fill the love that is needed in a family home, this is something that a parent is needed for."[41]

Doreen kept a special diary of all of her correspondence with members of the family. She regularly wrote letters to each member with whom she had been in contact, including sending Christmas and birthday cards to all the young children, nephews, and nieces, even those she had not met. Eventually the elder sister resumed correspondence with her, but maintained a cautious distance and discouraged visits. Doreen confides her sense of rejection in her diary, but retains a remarkably positive attitude as she accepts with gratitude such relationship as they had, which at any rate was better than she had experienced in the institution, where she had not even realized she had a family at all. As her young nieces and nephews grew old enough to write, they began corresponding with "Aunt Doreen," and she treasured every scrap of their work, from letters to Valentine's cards to photographs. Although Doreen's reunion with family members did not meet all her expectations, and possibly caused more hurt than relief in the short run, she weaves her interactions with her relatives into her reflections on the importance of family and of strong emotional support for everyone, including those whose families no longer filled that role.

Although she had been living in the community for only about a year, Doreen's self-perceptions were changing rapidly, and her experiences as a handicapped individual became a critical element of her identity. She grew more and more reflective on the subjects of ability, the right to education, and the value of different kinds of social contributions; topics that she came to question as they pertained to the limitations that had been placed upon people like herself who had been sent to institutions and restrained from engaging in a variety of mainstream experiences.

The irony of her reproductive fate in the institution grew more pronounced as she routinely sought work as a domestic servant and as a babysitter for local mothers. She cared for children of all ages, including infants, while assisting with the household chores for a variety of local families. Doreen's diaries do not reveal a specific sense of bitterness about these assignments, despite knowing that her own capacity to raise a family had been curtailed when she was a teenager at the Michener Centre without having been given any information, consultation, or opportunity to resist. Her actions, however, reveal her commitment and dedication to improving the rights of individuals considered intellectually impaired, as she strove to prove that she was indeed capable of making her own choices and taking on responsibilities, even when that involved the care of others.

As Doreen set up her new apartment, she meticulously recorded a list of her entire set of belongings, including notes as to where each item came from or from whom she had purchased them and at what cost. She also kept a page of signatures from all the people who visited her home, including social workers, friends, home care nurses, and Canadian Mental Health Association representatives.[42] She maintained this practice for a decade, and the names and comments from visitors reveal her growing connections in the community and her rising popularity as a local disability rights advocate. A note from a Maxine Blowers reads: "It was so nice to meet you. I have been following your story in the newspaper since it first came out. You have done very well for yourself!!"[43]

This progression from a deinstitutionalized patient to a more confident empowered activist unfolded over the twelve years that she resided in the basement suite, and was triggered by both positive and negative interactions with local organizations and families, including her own. A significant set of influences derived from her experiences working with families seeking domestic support, alongside her volunteer work with individuals who had been denied the opportunity to start their own families and who struggled with the transition to a semi-independent life outside the provincial mental health care system. Shortly after she had been transferred out of the group home, she wrote: "I have gotten to know a lot about myself through the way that other people never would have taken the time to help me with my problems years ago. It has been getting to know just how much we can learn more about ourselves."[44]

Working in the community, Doreen encountered a mixed set of reactions, but typically she responded positively to instruction, which she regarded as constructive encouragement. As she reflects on such moments in her diary, her writing becomes more sophisticated as she reasons through people's reactions and tries to draw lessons from her experiences. On 16 September 1979 she writes: "I have found while working on a daily basis it gives me the chance to meet more people. While attending to their needs it is good to feel needed. I am willing to come in any emergency … I do not have any problems getting along with people, it is just how we approach them."[45] She admits that, taken as a whole, most of the people she had worked with were "good," and that interacting with families in this way helped her get to know them, as they too came to understand her and to realize that people like her could assume responsible roles in the community.

Most of the people Doreen first worked with were single mothers. She displays a significant degree of empathy for these women, who, like her, were struggling to make ends meet, pay bills, often work in a variety of jobs, and manage a household. She also identifies to some extent with the children she takes care of, although working with them reminds her of her own upbringing and absence of family interactions: "It is alarming the number of homes in our city who are just single parents ... I never had the chance to live with my parents."[46] Working in these situations strengthens her convictions that everyone deserves access to education programs and supportive services, whether as an extension of social services, family programs, or health care initiatives. She is particularly concerned with the opportunities available to people whose health or abilities have been compromised and who need help negotiating the available kinds of community support. She states in her diary that she enjoys "my experience working with the mentally handicapped in our community and helping others who have medical problems no matter where they live. Also be[ing] supportive of families who may be having problems getting proper help through government or social workers which do value the rights of education and proper programs, jobs, etc. ... [I]t has been very rewarding working with these precious people."[47]

For the first two months of 1979 Doreen worked as a homemaker for a Mrs Foulston. Although the circumstances surrounding this case are unclear, Doreen appears to have provided a valuable service in supporting this single mother and in helping to organize the household after the birth of a daughter. Mrs Foulston might have had a disability, but that point is not made explicitly. Doreen keeps a careful record of the work, and she notes Mrs Foulston's steady improvement in doing household chores and eventually in caring for her child: "[Mrs Foulston] is becoming more independent also very determined to show that she can do her own work. I also had noticed that Mrs Foulston loves things cleaned. There is bathing the baby, also dressing her, she now can do without too much help. Also she is finding it easier in picking up the baby and holding her so on. Mrs Foulston will be able to handle most household chores without too much help. Even if she has a lady come in once a week."[48]

These kinds of experiences not only introduce Doreen to a number of people, some of whom become her friends; they also encourage her to consider her own abilities and strengths. It is through these interactions that she begins to assert more forcefully her identity as a handicapped person, but one, importantly who is a valued member of society. In her diary she notes with some disappointment that there are several people trying to live on their own after being deinstitutionalized who have not sought help and often do not leave their residences due to a sense of shame and embarrassment. "It is very sad to not want help from society figuring they can make it on their own yet unable to cope in the outside world. Not only for the so called normal persons but also for the mentally handicappis [as she calls them]."[49] In her day-to-day interactions with former patients and in conversations with friends from the Michener Centre, she tries to encourage them to embrace their new lives outside the institution and to leave that other world behind. One of her friends, reiterating this attitude, writes: "Tedda said that Carol wants her to forget about Michener Centre, and to think about the future."[50] Crystal, another friend from Michener, writes expressing her excitement about the new opportunities she experiences as a result of being reunited with her family and, importantly, living away from Michener: "Since [I've] been living at my parents' place, [I] have my own freedoms, can cook or bake when I want to. At least here [I] have lots of good encouragement from my mom and dad, [and a] few really good friends[; they] don't put me down. In the afternoon hours [I] help around the house with vacuuming dusting etc., etc. When it is nice [I] like to work outside."[51]

Although Doreen continued to work with single mothers, she also volunteered her time with fellow deinstitutionalized residents to help them make the transition to a more independent life. Those experiences resonate with her more strongly and she develops a regular routine of assisting more and more people with whom she shares similar experiences. For example, she meets Frances Paller, who had been released into the community of Eckville, Alberta, and was living under the guardianship of a legal trustee. After learning about Frances's poor condition from a friend, Doreen concludes that the trustee has not satisfied the requirements of his obligations to Frances, and that further action is required: "So because I am concerned for all persons who have special needs that I feel is not being met, I took it upon myself to get involved."[52] After visiting Frances, Doreen reports in her diary that she was appalled at the conditions the woman had been forced to live in, and had no doubts as to the reasons behind the growing concerns about her mental state. As she describes, the crux of the problem is not a matter of abilities but of support:

Frances owns her own trailer but she wanted it fitted up but Buster would not allow her. Frances had no equipment to work with. Her stove which is 9 amps had been hooked up but could not get help with the pipe work. Sink leaked also and toilet that had rusted out over the years it was just barely holding up by coffee cans. The social workers had gotten her a new toilet seat a few years ago but never was put up. Her furnace filters was never changed on a daily basis. I took over by getting her toilet back in proper order. She got her new toilet up furnace cleaned and stove [fixed]. Frances got rid of a lot of junk she did not want. [I had] to get her a broom, dustpan and vacuum. She had no cleaning supplies. Buster denied her all rights. Frances could not even spend money on some items she wished to have for herself. We worked together and had fun out of it also she just took so much pride in her trailer since I'd been in. Frances can work and she loves it as long as she isn't denied the necessities to work with.[53]

She does not refer to Frances again in her diary or elsewhere, but the case illustrates the way Doreen tackles what she recognizes as inadequacies and gaps in the social services system. More importantly, it demonstrates how she assumes personal responsibility for addressing such shortcomings.

Doreen seems to have moved into this role naturally. In one diary passage, she confesses that "ever since I was a very young girl I had the opportunity of taking care of all types of handicappi people. All had different disabilities. It has been a wonderful experience for me as well as rewarding. There has been a lot of sad cases, some confined to wheel chairs. Others who are bed ridden, some whose bodies are badly deformed while others are just mildly handicappi."[54] In her characteristically self-reflective tone, she generates strength and dignity from these interactions, often taking pride in her own abilities and marvelling at the way that bodies and abilities differ from person to person. The key to individual success, she surmises, rests upon access to a social network of support, which varies from one person to another but always involves a tailored combination of medical, legal, financial, and, importantly, emotional and familial support. The real challenge, she believes, is that, for people whose support systems had been tied to institutions and those whose connections with their families had been damaged or severed, the need for friends and assistance is greater but often more difficult to secure. That role, she feels, is one she can fill: "There are some handicappis who have no family friends no outside contact[s] and are very lonely. Others do have some family friends. My life is dedicated to help those who are less fortun[ate] than myself both physically and mentally. I shall continue to help these people while my health permits."[55]

Over the course of her writings in the late 1970s and through the 1980s, Doreen adopts the habit of referring to deinstitutionalized and disabled individuals as "handicappis." It is unclear if she developed this term herself or borrowed it from elsewhere, but she uses it consistently to refer to individuals who require some support systems and for whom, she feels, empowerment is key to their success. She identifies herself as a "handicappi," and applies the term with pride, recognizing that, although it usually denotes some kind of mental or physical deficit, any such deficit can be and usually is overcome with a wealth of abilities in other areas. For example, she prides herself on her ability to help others, to connect single mothers or deinstitutionalized residents with social workers, to cook meals for her friends, and, increasingly, to write letters that attract media attention and help to raise awareness about the diversity of abilities in the community.

This change in Doreen's language coincides with a growing, self-consciously political, and even radical perspective on the rights of allegedly disabled individuals. For example, in a 1981 letter to the University of Alberta, she forcefully asserts that the "disabled are abled" and that the "disabled are considering themselves consumers and are willing to show [what] they can do for themselves."[56] Building upon this rhetoric, she also joins a trend in disability rights movements that insists upon a "people first" mentality – one that prioritizes the individual over the disability. In a letter to the editor about the poor attendance of interdenominational clergy at a conference for people with handicaps and the church, Doreen laments that "some clergy have an offensive patronizing attitude which discouraged handicappi people from going to church."[57] She explains that the conference had been established, according to Martha Dobbin, who helped to organize the event, to "sensitize clergy and parish workers to the handicapped people as people first." Doreen spoke at this meeting about the time she had spent at the Michener Centre, the lack of spiritual lessons in that environment, and the virtual shunning of "handicappi" people from churches in Red Deer: "God accepts these people as people first and handicapped second, why can't we do the same?"[58] These kinds of public appearances and memorable appeals seem to leave an impression on others, but they also reinforce her own convictions as she continues to write letters to a wider circle of readers and speak to a variety of community groups.

As her confidence in this area grew, she channelled her thoughts into writing and expressed her gratitude as well as her frustrations publicly. Her letters were often published in the *Red Deer Advocate*, but her letter-writing campaigns extended beyond the local press. In 1981 she wrote to the Queen, first expressing her congratulations on the marriage of the Prince and Princess of Wales, then quickly moving on to draw Her Majesty's attention to the plight of individuals with handicaps. Lady-in-waiting Kathryn Dupdale responded, thanking Doreen for her letter and explaining that, "in this country Her Majesty held a Garden Party at Buckingham Palace for several thousand disabled people which was a great success. The different countries of the British Isles are all helping to raise money and trying to integrate the disabled into society." Dupdale closed by adding that "[t]he Queen thought it was very kind of you to write to her and she was most interested to hear how you had overcome your difficulties and managed to make such a useful and worthwhile life."[59] Although the tone is somewhat patronizing, the letter nonetheless pleases Doreen and encouraged her to continue her work in the community.

By the early 1980s Doreen's writings had attracted the attention of other people who found themselves in similar conditions. In 1981 a Newfoundland woman wrote to thank her and to share her own experiences: "I was told that I have a learning disability, but I am not letting that stand in my way of doing the things that make me feel good about myself ... We have to be strong and fight back with courage and perseverance when anyone tries to discourage us from doing something that will help us help ourselves."[60] From as far away as Blackpool, England, a woman wrote to tell Doreen that, although she was severely disabled, she had learned to play the drums and was now in a percussion band.[61] Other letters arrived from Alberta, including from families of children with disabilities who sought Doreen's advice as to how they might best support their children.[62]

In 1981 Doreen's work and activism captured the attention of local filmmakers, who produced a twenty-five-minute documentary on the life and experiences of Doreen Befus. The film, "If I Can Do It, You Can Do It," features a number of former residents of the Michener Centre, but zeroes in on Doreen's life, which had culminated in independence, activism, and community service. The short film even covers the topic of eugenics and the forced sterilization that Doreen and others endured. "They'd just send you up there and you'd have no say in it," Doreen told newspaper interviewers concerning her meeting with the Eugenics Board at age eighteen.[63] The film attracted media attention and triggered a speaking tour for Doreen. She visited Alberta secondary schools and spoke to students about the value of education, the people first movement, and the sting of discrimination.

Conclusion

Reconstructing Doreen Befus's life and situating her in the history of mental health institutionalization and subsequent deinstitutionalization not only personalizes this history; it also helps to explain the growth of patients' rights groups and the proliferation of rights-based activism in the community mental health movement. Doreen's life is remarkable in its own right, but because she kept close records, including a personal diary in which she describes her daily activities and thoughts, her story offers a candid set of insights into a former patient's perspective on this history. Doreen's story is a rare glimpse into the case of a woman who survived the institution and became a strong advocate for patients' rights, particularly for individuals with intellectual disabilities. As a patient under the sexual sterilization legislation, Doreen's records also reveal her thoughts on motherhood, care giving, and human rights. Once released from the institution, Doreen searched for her estranged family, and her records of that quest offer an intimate perspective on her feelings of rejection, her anger towards her family, and her reflections on family values in the context of her own life.

Doreen's contributions to disability rights campaigns raised public awareness about disabilities, mental health, and mental deficiencies. Her public profile began to challenge the conventional view that individuals with disabilities were a drain on the public purse or genetically inferior, attitudes that harkened back to the origins of the eugenics laws. Her capacity to work in the community and to communicate her ideas clearly and convincingly also raises questions about the meaning of a test that originally pegged her IQ at 55, which is at the low end of the scale.

Negative attitudes towards people with intellectual disabilities, however, were not overcome so easily. In 1973, shortly after the Sexual Sterilization Act was repealed, a group of women formed an organization called Unifarm. This allegedly influential prairie-based organization called upon the newly elected Conservative government in Alberta to revisit its position on eugenics and to consider retaining sexual sterilization policies directed at individuals with mental and intellectual disabilities. The government resisted this suggestion, claiming that contemporary research proved that "retarded persons can give birth to normal" children; moreover, resurrecting the eugenics program would be "a contravention of human rights."[64] Members of Unifarm countered by suggesting that, despite genetic data to the contrary, the social tendency of less intelligent people to engage in relationships with other individuals of lower intelligence meant that children raised in these environments suffered.[65]

These attitudes were reminiscent of 1920s perspectives on degeneracy and the value of intelligence, but they failed to confront the reality that many individuals, like Doreen, had learned to thrive in the community, challenging the constructed nature of intelligence as understood by labels of intellectual disability. Moreover, as Doreen Befus flourished in her independent lifestyle, she demonstrated that, even though diagnosed as mentally deficient, she had become a valued member of her community as a domestic caregiver, supportive friend, and loyal relative.

Chapter Six

Appendectomy to Queen's Court Settlement: Leilani Muir

In 1996 Leilani Muir successfully sued the Alberta government for wrongful sexual sterilization. As a teenager in the late 1950s Leilani, then living at the Provincial Training School for Mental Defectives in Red Deer, had been told that she needed to have her appendix removed. When the surgeon took out her appendix, however, he also cut out her Fallopian tubes, rendering her permanently incapable of bearing children. Under Alberta law at that time, the physicians assigned to this task were not obligated to inform Leilani of this second operation, nor did they need to obtain her consent to the procedure. In fact, at the point of committal, Leilani's stepfather had signed a consent form as part of the admission process, permitting surgical sexual sterilization if and when the Eugenics Board deemed such a procedure necessary.

Years later, after Leilani had left the institution, married, and attempted to start her own family, she still did not know that she was physically unable to conceive. The eventual realization of her situation came after years of emotional turmoil and broken relationships, followed by psychological and medical examinations that finally provided conclusive proof that her failed attempts to conceive a child were the fault of the eugenics program. The judge in Leilani's case ruled that, although the program was legal at the time of Leilani's surgery, the sterilization had nonetheless caused catastrophic damages, including personal humiliation and undignified treatment. Ultimately Leilani Muir received a million-dollar settlement, and soon after the trial she emerged as a new face among human rights campaigners in Canada.[1]

Leilani's painful and very public ordeal introduced Canadians to a real person behind Alberta's historic eugenics program. Her trial reminded television audiences and newspaper readers that, as recently as the 1970s, some Canadian authorities remained committed to a sexual sterilization program that denied basic human rights to individuals deemed mentally incompetent, deficient, or disabled. The majority of the men and women who underwent eugenic sterilization had been institutionalized, and therefore lived under the daily scrutiny of medical staff. The implications of Leilani's trial in the 1990s raised the profile of anti-discrimination campaigns, patients' organizations, and family support groups by exposing some of the injustices faced by institutionalized individuals whose rights had been stripped away at the doors of the hospital. At the same time, the publicity cast a dark shadow over the image of mental health care and treatment by connecting it with the draconian measures associated with eugenics, which many people assumed had disappeared after the Second World War. Leilani Muir thus shared many experiences with Doreen Befus, but where Doreen channelled her energy into helping individuals cope with life outside the institution, Leilani set her sights on challenging the province legally to recognize its role in denying fundamental human rights to institutionalized individuals.

Following Leilani's legal success, hundreds of other sterilization victims in Alberta, including Ken Nelson, who appears in Chapter 4, came forward in an attempt to force the province to compensate them for similar damages. Alberta's then-premier Ralph Klein, anticipating a long, expensive, and unflattering public exposé of Alberta's pro-eugenics past, tried to invoke the Constitution's notwithstanding clause to sidestep the legal issue, claiming that the current government and Alberta's taxpayers should not be held responsible for decisions made in the past. Although his legal manoeuvre ultimately failed, the escalating class action suit also lost its momentum and eventually was settled out of court. The result produced a meagre provincial payment to be shared among hundreds of sterilized victims, with a substantial portion devoted to paying the sizeable legal expenses. The relative failure of this collective action further elevated Leilani's status as the sole visible public figure in the contemporary human rights struggles associated with eugenics in Canada. In particular, her role in these debates raised the profile of the issue for individuals in the mental health system and their right to make decisions about their reproductive futures.

In this chapter I draw on the extensive records of Leilani's experiences, including her medical records from her time spent at the Provincial Training School, court documents that involve both the historical papers and more contemporary observations of medical and legal experts, the newspaper accounts of her trial, the National Film Board's documentary on "The Sterilization of Leilani Muir," and Leilani's own reflections on her case. Although Leilani's story shares some of the features of those of other individuals in this book, her struggle to bring that story to the public through legal channels sets her apart from many others who survived the eugenics program. The wealth of documentation, its public access, and Leilani's continued efforts to bring attention to these issues also make Leilani a critical player in the history of eugenics in Alberta.

Leilani's path from an institutionalized girl to a celebrated human rights activist was not easy. Her determination to make her experiences public meant enduring a bout of humiliating testimony, including having to admit openly to spending many years in a mental institution and facing the potential stigmatizing consequences of such a confession. Although, at first, Leilani admitted to feelings of shame and a very low level of self-confidence, over time her feelings changed. The results of the trial brought new degrees of satisfaction and pride, and the responses since then have opened up a world of possibilities for this now motivational speaker, public lecturer, author, and unshakeable human rights activist. Some regard Leilani as a role model, but she might say to them that her reasons for doing what she did had less to do with making a name for herself and much more with ensuring that these kinds of circumstances are never repeated. To that end, Leilani has become an important player in local and international debates about the rights of individuals, which she insists not be compromised or limited due to assumptions about mental, physical, or emotional abilities. In short, choices about reproductive futures should rest with the individuals themselves, not with an impersonal state or a patronizing health care or social service worker, no matter how altruistic their intentions.

Placed in an even broader context, Leilani's powerful sentiments reflect a change in rights-based discourse. When considered in the context of reproductive rights, they also represent a shift away from explicit feminist perspectives to language that self-consciously embraces ideals of inclusivity and ability. This is not to say that the reproductive rights movements of the twenty-first century have shed their feminist veneer, but to suggest that, rather than regard the development of such rights as a linear path from maternal feminism through second-wave campaigns and into the era of decriminalized abortions, the history of choice is much more complicated. Leilani's story helps to reveal one of the ways in which reproductive choice was constrained by some of the same political forces that worked to overturn laws prohibiting contraception.

She exists as a poignant reminder that campaigns for reproductive options continued to deny or ignore implicit assumptions about ability, disability, and any lingering remnants of connections such value judgments might have for reproductive futures. Leilani's story also demonstrates that choice remains highly personal, and that its value rests upon access to information, consent, and social support that allow people to make decisions that best fit their individual needs.

Entering the Institution

Leilani first came to the attention of psychiatric authorities at age seven and a half. At this early age the Guidance Clinic at Red Deer examined her and began piecing together her family history as part of her diagnostic summary. The attending psychiatrist, Dr Leonard J. Le Vann, whom we met in Chapter 4, recorded that she was a "problem child" considering that she "steals 3 or 4 lunches per day from school children [and] eats it all."[2] As an adult Leilani defended herself, stating that, although these accusations were true, she was routinely sent to school without food and her meals at home, if any, were meagre. As Le Vann continued to investigate Leilani's circumstances, he asked her mother, Marie Scorah, about the child's conditions at home. In a series of letters, Leilani's mother provided conflicting information, but began by admitting that she herself had difficulties with alcohol and that her husband, Leilani's stepfather, Harley Scorah, also succumbed at times to heavy drinking. She insisted, however, that she had been sober for the past two years.[3]

Whether or not a direct result of the drinking, the Scorahs' marriage appeared to be a contentious relationship that offered Le Vann clues as to Leilani's behaviour. Since Leilani's birth the family had remained in poor economic circumstances; Marie claimed that she and her husband lived on a combined income of $130 per month and had several children to look after, including Leilani's two elder and one younger brothers. Leilani's natural father had not been seen for several years, and Mr Scorah had taken custody of Leilani and her elder brothers when he married her mother. Scorah's family openly disapproved of his marriage to Marie, which she confessed caused her anxiety. Allegedly, they did not have stable support from a more extensive family network.

Despite Marie's insistence that their relationship had improved since she and her husband had been sober, she admitted to taking measures to avoid having more children, although at first she did not elaborate. By then Marie had given birth to four boys (one boy died at age three from

pneumonia) and Leilani. She had also had a miscarriage, which she recorded as an "accident [when she was] struck by a windshield."[4] As
Marie grew concerned about Leilani's behaviour, which she viewed as
slow or underdeveloped, she further worried about her ability to have
and care for more children. Moreover, Marie told the doctors, Leilani
quarrelled with her brothers, perhaps indicating that the four children
were difficult to manage. These factors, in combination with poverty, encouraged Marie to question her ability to raise future healthy children.

   Marie later told Dr Le Vann that, although she took no direct contraceptive measures, she regularly douched and had not experienced an
orgasm in over a year. It is unclear if Marie felt that this helped to reduce her chances of becoming pregnant, but she further explained that,
in addition to not wanting any more children, she no longer enjoyed
sex with her husband, and might have believed erroneously that the
lack of an orgasm helped to ward off future pregnancies. She admitted
that she and her husband had separated from time to time and that
their sexual relations had suffered; as she stated in her report to the doctor, the "sexual act lasts five minutes [but] feels as if it lasted indefinitely."[5] It is unclear if this admission was related to her fear of having
another child, but there is no doubt that she harboured anxieties about
having more children and about the emotional and financial stability of
her marriage.

   In 1951, when Marie admitted these circumstances to Le Vann, contraception was still illegal. Marie was also a self-identified Catholic,
which might have influenced her decision to seek out contraceptive
methods, although, as discussed in Chapter 3, her Catholicism did not
necessarily mean that she avoided birth control either. Her statements
to Le Vann are nonetheless revealing for what she intimates regarding
her apprehension about conceiving future children.

   The information Le Vann gleaned about Leilani and her mother convinced him that a deeper investigation into Leilani's upbringing was
necessary before he could offer a comprehensive diagnosis, and he suggested that the family return to see him in a week's time; they failed to
reappear. He later admitted that, based on this brief interaction, Leilani
was likely a mental defective, and he began filing an application for her
committal to the Provincial Training School on the assumption that he
would see Leilani the following week.[6] When they did not return to
the clinic, he sent the forms for Leilani's committal directly to Marie for
her to fill out. The application forms failed to appear, so he sent another
set several months later.[7]

According to the Provincial Mental Defectives Act, as amended in 1937, a mentally defective person was anyone living in a "condition of arrested or incomplete development of mind existing before the age of eighteen years, whether arising from inherent causes or induced by disease or injury."[8] The Act thus pertained to Alberta minors who exhibited abnormal, slow, or deficient development in intellectual and/or physical characteristics. Assumptions about the abilities of such individuals were then evaluated more closely through a combination of psychometric and intelligence quotient (IQ) tests and physical examinations, which functioned as part of the preconditions for entering institutional care, but also served as the background for identifying children whom the Eugenics Board later would see and consider for surgery under the Sexual Sterilization Act.

Despite Le Vann's attempts to bring Leilani into institutional care, her parents continually failed to respond. Successive letters returned unopened indicated that the family in fact had moved out of the district. Several months later, however, Leilani once again came in contact with the mental health system, this time following a referral from a guidance clinic in the Foothills region near High River. On this instance she was again reportedly stealing lunches, but her theft had increased now to include "stealing from shops and from home, especially food."[9] The school officials did not corroborate this story, however, claiming that she had not presented herself as a problem at school. Leilani later would testify that this was because her teachers had noticed that she was hungry and brought extra lunches for her, which alleviated her hunger and thus her need to steal food from her classmates.

The renewed Leilani-related activity and her reappearance at the guidance clinic encouraged Le Vann to resume his pressure on the family to commit their daughter to the Provincial Training School. In March 1953 he adopted a more proactive approach and contacted the municipality directly in an effort to address the issue of Leilani's admission to the institution. Leilani's stepfather had worked for a time for the municipality, and initially Le Vann hoped he could contact Scorah through his employer, but by the time Le Vann's letter arrived, the family had moved again, to the village of Black Diamond. This time Le Vann approached the municipality directly in an effort to get the authorities there to sign the committal forms. Black Diamond's secretary-treasurer, however, did not relish the thought of signing the forms out of concern that the municipality might be held financially responsible for Leilani's health care expenses.[10] Although, according to provincial law, families were responsible for any health care costs, including fees associated with institutional confinement, a 1942 amendment to the Mental Defectives Act had stipulated that "the city, town, village, municipal district, improvement district or special area of which the mentally defective person had his abode at the time of his admission may recover from such person as a debt by action or by distraint of any of his goods."[11] If families could not pay the fees, however, the responsibility for paying them fell to the municipality in which the patient resided, using the legal channels just noted to recover the expenses. Thus, in Leilani's case, the municipality could be held legally responsible for her health care costs even up to six months after the family left the district. In such a case the burden of payment would then become a struggle between the municipality and the family, rather than directly between the family and the institution.

Upon receiving Le Vann's request, Black Diamond's secretary-treasurer responded by explaining that, in fact, the village's legal responsibilities in the case were rather complicated. Its officers were reluctant to act as signatories to Leilani's committal given the financial obligations involved for a family that no longer lived in the district. Although Le Vann had already signed a Municipal Approval Certificate and had obtained signatures from the municipality when Scorah was still an employee in the district, the question of payment remained unresolved after Scorah quit his job. Le Vann pressed on, however, suggesting to the municipal authorities that the required $15 per month it would cost to keep Leilani at the Provincial Training School might yet be recovered from the family. Scorah reportedly had had a profitable year of farming, so Black Diamond need not worry about its financial liability over the long term. Le Vann then suggested that the municipality sign the forms without further delay.[12]

Encouraged by the progress he seemed to be making towards Leilani's committal, Le Vann redoubled his efforts to reach the Scorahs and again sent committal forms directly to the family. Finally, he received a response from her stepfather indicating that, although it was true that the harvest had given the family some additional money that year, he did not have sufficient funds to cover hospital expenses. Further, as the financial return on his crops had been rather modest, after a pattern of lean years, he did not intend to return the committal forms or bring Leilani back to the clinic.[13] Le Vann remained fixed in his determination, however, and responded by sending yet another committal request to the Scorahs.[14]

One year after Le Vann first saw her, Leilani returned once more to the guidance clinic in Red Deer, this time with committal forms completed by Harley Scorah. The forms provided a number of personal details and concentrated on the nature of Marie Scorah's pregnancy with Leilani. The application explained, for example, that Leilani was Irish-Polish and Roman Catholic. She had been born early after prolonged labour and the birth had proceeded only with medical intervention and the use of instruments. In response to several stock questions about early childhood development – for example, does the child walk well or clumsily; at what age did the child walk; and is he/she vigorous and active in getting about or indolent? – Scorah had entered nothing unusual, indicating without elaborating that Leilani was a bit slow to develop. Further on, Scorah reported that Leilani suffered from "staring spells," terminology that he borrowed directly from the forms. Another set of questions focused on the family's financial situation, including the patient's estate or property, the capacity of the family to maintain itself financially, and the total estimated value of the family's personal property, in answer to which Scorah reported a total value of $2,600.[15]

It is unclear from this case alone if Leilani's committal was typical. Le Vann made a concerted and even aggressive attempt to bring Leilani into the institution, even at a time when most administrators complained about overcrowded conditions and politicians lamented the heavy expenses associated with large-scale hospitals. Le Vann's persistent and multifaceted approach to securing Leilani's admission seems to have run counter to these broader concerns, although it is difficult to determine how often he persistently pursued potential patients.

Finally obtaining the authority to evaluate Leilani properly and commit her with the submission of these forms and questionnaires, Le Vann set about making his diagnosis. He declared that her mental condition was that of an "intelligent moron."[16] His notes indicate that Leilani was "not insane but mentally deficient and a proper subject for admission to the Provincial Training School for Mental Defectives at Red Deer." He continued that her appearance was "pleasant" and that she "talks easily and volubly."[17]

The family history collected from her parents reveals very few details about them, except that her mother was born in Poland and that her biological father had been in the Army and was overseas during Marie's pregnancy with Leilani and ultimately for her birth in 1944. There is no further mention of him in her file.[18] Further interrogation of the family, however, produced a few more details concerning Leilani's condition. A second set of forms arrived by mail from Marie Scorah, who indicated that Leilani's mental peculiarities first became observable at the age of three. The next set of standard questions – Has [she] ever practised self-abuse? Does [she] hide, break or destroy things?[19] – prompted Marie to make short responses in the affirmative. Then came more questions:

Question: What are [her] amusements, interests and reactions?
Answer: Stealing, then denies same.
Question: Any evidence of abnormal interest or practice in sexual matters?
Answer: Self abuse.

Marie then followed instructions requesting that she underline the terms that applied to Leilani's behaviour at home: "self-centred, quarrelsome, inconsiderate of others, vain, sensitive, easily discouraged, suggestible, stubborn, seclusive, suspicious, indolent, emotionally unstable, ill-tempered, vindictive, sulky, swearing, use of obscene language, cruelty, stealing, lawlessness. [She then added in her own writing] given to lying, cruel to babies and smaller children."[20]

The forms themselves left little room for interpretation or elaboration. Marie faced a list of terms and phrases that, by simply underlining keywords, contributed to the background information that later helped to inform the diagnosis. The questions emphasized distinctions between normal childhood development – for example, "walks well" and "walks clumsily." Other contradistinctions, such as active or indolent in combination with leading questions about a child's intelligence, ability to understand, and peculiar physical features were then followed by questions about blood lines and family history. In each space provided, respondents were given room to include a few words for elaboration, but the majority of the questions sought a yes or no response or the identification of a particular judgment: abnormal or normal; well or clumsy; intelligent or slow. Although these kinds of forms undoubtedly helped to standardize the admissions procedures and perhaps facilitated the initial sorting of patients into rudimentary categories of need, they also encouraged parents to make judgments about their children's abilities and potential need for institutional care. Presumably, as was later determined in Leilani's case, if parents wanted to admit their children to the Provincial Training School, they needed to identify a number of abnormal features on the forms to convince the admissions staff that their child required such expensive care. Leilani's parents were not alone in seeking this kind of care, nor were they alone in requiring care they could not afford. The forms the Scorahs filled out convinced Le Vann that Leilani's case was severe enough to warrant admission, whether or not they contained accurate information.

The day Leilani was formally committed to the Provincial Training School, 12 July 1955, her parents were presented with one final form to complete the application. This form involved a single sentence, a signature line, date, and witness. The sentence read: "I am agreeable that sterilization be performed on my child [space to provide name] if this is deemed advisable by the Provincial Eugenics Board."[21] The form in Leilani's file contains the signature of Harley Scorah. Completing this form at the point of admission gave the Training School blanket authority to recommend children under its supervision to the Eugenics Board, and it further sped up the process of clearing patients for surgery once the Board reached an affirmative decision. Although the revised Sexual Sterilization Act of 1937 did not require the consent of patients who were recommended for sterilization and who fell into diagnosed categories of mental defectives, the pressure placed on families to sign such a form seemingly as a condition of admission gave the institutional authorities a greater capacity to recommend surgical sterilization in cases where patients did not fit in the approved categories. As a result, annual health reports and institutional records indicate that several patients were sterilized even though they were not considered mentally defective but suffered from schizophrenia, epilepsy, or a long list of psychotic and other disorders.

The packet of forms required to institutionalize an individual and the kinds of questions presented to Marie Scorah gave the Provincial Training School sufficient information to begin to make a diagnosis. Even if the child's character traits were described sincerely, they were taken so out of context as to be potentially misleading. For example, while her mother indicated that Leilani had a habit of stealing food, the form contains no further room to consider or interrogate the family about meals provided at home. Questions about family income were limited to determining its ability to pay, rather than considered in relation to the descriptions of abnormal behaviour. Under these circumstances, the addition of a consent form for future sexual sterilization emerged as part of the admission process and, potentially, as a condition of that process. The combined effect of this paperwork served to relinquish parental control over Leilani to the will of the institution, its staff, and its policies. The resultant snapshot of a child's life at the time of committal, while brief and often constrained by the layout of the forms, played a substantial role in the subsequent assessment, classification, and eugenic consideration of each child who entered the institution.

The Institution, the Family, and the Patient

Leilani Muir lived in the Provincial Training School for the next decade. During that time Le Vann, as both superintendent and chief psychiatrist overseeing the children, became an important figure in Leilani's life. Her relationship with her family grew even more strained, and as the letters and visits grew more and more sporadic it became clear that her relationship with her mother and stepfather had been tense from the beginning. Marie Scorah oscillated between expressing remorse and longing for her only daughter to displaying elements of resentment and anger. Since each letter came through Le Vann, he remained keenly aware of the shifts in their relationship and at times shielded Leilani from the letters; at other times he claimed to protect her through the rehabilitative qualities of the institution, which he suggested counterbalanced the instability she experienced in her family. Although it seems clear that staying with her mother had produced a series of hardships, life at the Training School introduced its own set of challenges.

Over the next few years Leilani occasionally visited with her family, sometimes for several days at a time. At other times her mother delayed returning Leilani to the institution or failed to show up in the first place. Le Vann became frustrated by the way these erratic visits disrupted his careful schedule for his patients and seemed to steer Leilani off her rehabilitative course. Leilani often returned upset from these family visits, sometimes ill, and at other times aggressive towards other trainees.[22] Marie reinforced this image of her daughter, complaining in her written reports to Le Vann that Leilani was difficult to handle at home and caused trouble for the family: "Leilani is a problem child and [I have] a baby to look after ... I believe she is more a baby than he is ... Please keep the vacancy for her. I don't know what or where to turn to next."[23] In a postscript she recalled that Leilani had got hold of some rat poison during her last home visit and had poisoned the family's four dogs; she was relieved that Leilani had not also poisoned her infant son. Stressing Leilani's difficult behaviour and the family's reliance on the institution for her care, Marie offered elaborate explanations of her troublesome activities, and expressed her relief and gratitude for Le Vann's willingness to look after her daughter.

On other occasions, however, the Scorahs remained negligent in their responsibilities towards the institution and risked having Leilani return home to them permanently. In autumn 1956 Le Vann wrote to Marie to inquire about her daughter's whereabouts: "Leilani went home for a month's holiday in July and was due back in August. Since she has not returned, I wonder if it is your intention to keep her at home?"[24] He warned that if he did not hear from the family before long, he would have no choice but to discharge Leilani to the care of her family. The nature of this correspondence – both the elaborate accounts from Leilani's mother about her home visits and the rather threatening tone with which Le Vann insisted on compliance from the family – subtly underscores the power Le Vann wielded over the Scorahs. If he refused to take Leilani back under institutional care, the Scorahs risked harm, they claimed, from Leilani's careless and even malicious habits. But if they failed to conform to the institution's schedule, Leilani would be sent home indefinitely. In short, if the Scorahs wanted Leilani to remain in custody, they would have to comply with Le Vann's demands.

The correspondence also reveals, however, that Leilani received little if any support from her family during her first years at the Provincial Training School. In summer 1956 the school's matron, concerned about Leilani and her growing feeling of abandonment during her first months there, wrote to Leilani's parents: "It has been such a long time since Leilani heard from you that she has become most anxious and has not been able to do her best work at the School. She is beginning to feel you have forgotten her and that you won't be coming to see her."[25] The matron also noted that, despite the anxiety caused by being separated from her family, Leilani was doing very well and participated in all of the school's activities.

The school's reports and correspondence often contradicted the letters arriving from Leilani's family. At school she was regularly described as polite, alert, cooperative, and cheerful. Although she reportedly got into quarrels with other girls on the ward, her behaviour was nonetheless considered normal for a girl her age living at the school, and she did not acquire any incidence reports during the first year of her stay.

Throughout the remainder of Leilani's time at the Provincial Training School, Marie Scorah occasionally wrote letters and sent her daughter small gifts, usually clothes, although the parcels were often rather meagre – for the Christmas after Leilani's sterilization operation, her mother sent a gift of two pairs of panties. The family spent the following summer holidays at a cottage in Ontario, but felt that such an excursion might put too much stress on Leilani.[26] Le Vann agreed that Leilani's time could be better spent concentrating on her training at the school, but often reminded Marie that Leilani also required more resources from her family.

In 1960 the Training School staff, sensing that Leilani was not being well served by her family and knowing that she was in desperate need of the new clothes that her mother failed to provide, referred Leilani's case to the child welfare authorities. Her family had since moved to Ontario and its connections with Leilani became even more sporadic and strained. Le Vann also wrote to the family and later to the department requesting an inquiry into the Scorah family and its capacity to provide for Leilani. The department responded, assuring Le Vann that it had confronted the parents and that support was forthcoming: "If in future they do not carry out their obligations toward their child please advise us and we will again contact the Ontario Welfare Department to impress upon the parents the responsibility of providing for their child."[27]

The Provincial Training School followed this set of exchanges with a long list of clothing and financial needs for Leilani, including a request for bi-weekly payments of five dollars. When the family left these requests unfulfilled, the Ontario authorities intervened. Marie Scorah responded by claiming that, during Leilani's previous visit with the family, she had confided to her mother that she had been carrying on an affair with two men at the Training School. Whether Marie fabricated this accusation to alarm the Training School staff about Leilani's alleged sexual activities or mentioned it out of sincere concern for her daughter's well-being, she maintained that this conduct appalled her and had contributed to her subsequent refusal to provide gifts, money, or clothing for Leilani.

Le Vann reacted to this news by referring the case once more to the Alberta welfare authorities. They reminded Marie that Leilani was still a child and, difficult though she might be, she had been staying at the institution with insufficient familial and financial support. The lack of resources available to Leilani, including clothes, made it difficult for her to focus on her training and produced unnecessary anxiety in a girl who was already struggling with the challenges she faced as a trainee.[28] The correspondence suggests that, at this point, Leilani's welfare remained in jeopardy while her mother's credibility came under scrutiny.

The relationship between Leilani and her family continued to deteriorate during her time at the Provincial Training School, which prompted local social workers to register their concern for Leilani's well-being and at times to involve themselves directly in her home visits. Her family moved around the country, spending time in Ontario periodically before returning to Alberta. Over the course of Leilani's institutional stay, her mother frequently sought employment to supplement the family income. Meanwhile her stepfather developed a heart condition that restricted his employment prospects as well as his ability to farm. In 1964 Marie Scorah looked to improve the family's financial situation by seeking training in the United States. Leilani, who had been visiting the family and helping to care for her younger brother, wanted to remain at home with her stepfather while her mother was out of the country. Her social worker reported to Le Vann that the "Father seems to want Leilani," but stated that "he follows his wife's orders." The social worker elaborated by explaining, "Mrs. Scorah was very definite that she didn't want Leilani. She emphasized the financial reasons but I feel she has little affection for Leilani and just can't face a future in which the supervision of Leilani would be permanent."[29]

Leilani's strained relationship with her family was punctuated by her mother's inconsistent communication, which was primarily directed at her daughter and her upkeep. Although Marie occasionally sent encouraging and even affectionate letters urging her daughter to come home or explaining how much everyone missed her, her letters to Training School staff often lamented the family's dire financial situation, Leilani's challenging behaviour at home, or, at times, Marie's concern about Leilani's sexual activities. This kind of correspondence, coupled with long absences or periods of silence from the Scorahs, put both Leilani and her caregivers in a difficult position. Leilani often endured Christmas without gifts from her family and had few resources in the form of clothes or spending money.

Because Leilani later sued the Alberta government and because she has allowed historians and lawyers to review her personal case files, we know intimate details about her past and the conditions that led to her institutionalization and subsequent sterilization. Through these records her story offers us an intimate perspective of a young girl from a somewhat dysfunctional family. Her mother played a critical role in Leilani's fate. At times she relied heavily on the institution to care for her daughter, who she felt was difficult to handle at home amid chronic financial stresses, her husband's poor health, and the raising of three more or less healthy boys. Although Leilani maintained a relationship with her family, unlike the case of Doreen, who was treated as an orphan, the tense familial connection did little to alleviate the pressures of institutional life or the consequences of being labelled mentally defective. Leilani's story thus embodies what in fact might have been a common set of experiences associated with life at the Provincial Training School in mid-century Alberta.

Encountering the Eugenics Board

Twenty-seven months after being admitted to the Training School, Leilani appeared before the Eugenics Board. Her diagnosis, as provided to Board members, indicated that she was a "mental defective moron" with an IQ of 64,[30] sufficient grounds for the Board to authorize her sexual sterilization without seeking further information or consent if it deemed this action necessary.

Her report stated that, at eight years old, Leilani had still been at the grade one level in regular school, although she was excelling at the Training School: she "is good in spelling and arithmetic and is a good reader. Leilani is excellent in dramatization and neat in all her work." Such comments suggest that, regardless of her intellectual abilities, she was demonstrating composure and discipline in the Training School environment, making her a good pupil in the structured setting of the institution. Those qualities and achievements, however, had no bearing on her overall diagnostic assessment or her intelligence rating as far as her eligibility for sterilization was concerned. On Leilani's general behaviour, the report noted that "[s]he is quick tempered and finds it hard to take correction, but is making an effort to become a better loser."[31]

Like the committal forms, these short descriptions, though more elaborate than her mother's responses, failed to place in context the conditions surrounding Leilani's behaviour – most notably, her family's poor economic circumstances and lack of proper meals while she attended normal school. Since arriving at the Training School and receiving regular sustenance, her behaviour and performance in learning and habits had improved. She continued, however, to display bouts of aggression. As the report indicated, "she is hard to manage and is nearly always off privileges because of her bad temper, imprudent and quarrelsome ways. Leilani is lazy and requires constant supervision to see that she looks after her personal appearance and clothing and she has little respect for other children's toys and belongings."[32] Despite these difficulties, Leilani also displayed strong social and some leadership skills, even if at times the leadership came across as headstrong.

As to her continuing at the Training School, the report stated that "Leilani is young and needs considerably more training in self control, good work habits and personal care habits before it is possible to consider discharge for her."[33] The question of her possible discharge readily raised the spectre of the Eugenics Board's involvement. The Sexual Sterilization Act stipulated that any individual considered for discharge from a mental hospital, including the Provincial Training School, would have to be "examined by or in the presence of the [Eugenics] Board."[34] Moreover, in cases where the individual was deemed mentally defective and where the Board unanimously agreed that "the exercise of the power of procreation would result in the transmission to such person's progeny of any mental disability or deficiency," the Board "may direct, in writing, such surgical operation for the sexual sterilization of such mentally defective persons."[35] The 1942 amendment to the Act had expanded the categories of disease and deficiency that fell under this clause, first to include patients diagnosed with psychotic disorders, which included schizophrenia, neurosyphilis, and some dementia-related illnesses, and later categories such as non-psychotic neurosyphilis, epilepsy, with either psychosis or mental deterioration, and Huntington's chorea.[36]

In the mid-1970s, following the repeal of the Sexual Sterilization Act, law professor Bernard Dickens described this legislative progression as the culmination of anti-science, suggesting that the expanded categories of disability targeted for eugenic sterilization increasingly borrowed from cultural understandings of human value. He also argued that, in addition to stepping beyond the boundaries of the acceptable genetic science of the day, the program sought to limit the reproductive capabilities of individuals with conditions, such as Huntington's chorea, that present themselves later in life, often after an individual's reproductive period had ended.[37] Moreover, in cases of mental deficiency, the assessment rested largely upon the results of a dubious intelligence test.

Leilani's experience would later challenge the application of such tests, but even before her case came before the court, Dickens criticized these tests for their significant cultural bias. For example, a woman was sterilized in 1969 based on the results of an IQ test suggesting that her intelligence was low grade and that she would be incapable of intelligent parenting, yet she subsequently completed grade twelve. Other people who were a perceived genetic threat also raised concerns about cultural perceptions and the scientific basis for the program. Children diagnosed with so-called mongoloidism – more commonly referred to as Down's syndrome or trisomy 21 – for instance, were sterilized legally under Alberta law even though they had less than a 60 per cent chance of survival to adulthood.[38] In consequence many of these surgeries were unnecessary; they also incurred costs to the province that the program supposedly was established to avoid. The hypocritical nature of the program thus raised questions about the science underpinning the eugenics program and encouraged medical experimentation on unwitting patients, as described in Chapter 4.

Leilani's case fell into the more traditional category of mental defective, meaning that, by 1957, her potential sterilization would form part of the regular routine associated with a program that had been in existence for almost thirty years. Her diagnosis, however, like that of others, rested on an IQ test. A copy of that test or notes from an oral exam have not survived – or at least have never been located – but the results were a key factor in the Eugenics Board's decision to approve her sterilization. She received a score of 70 on verbal IQ, which was borderline feeble-mindedness, and a score of 64 for performance, which was below acceptable. A final analysis, or full-scale assessment, resulted in a score of 64, placing Leilani well within the bounds of mental deficiency as determined by the Board. The notes accompanying the assessment suggest that the Board was confident in these values: the "level is considered accurate. Her top level of function would be only slightly higher," presumably when she reached adulthood.[39] The analysis also noted that her "thinking is primarily concrete, although there is sporadic use of functional concepts. Her memory is fairly good; her judgment tends to be poor. Social anticipations are weak. Visual motor skills are average for her level of ability."[40]

This assessment of Leilani's abilities and future prospects of ability trumped other cultural considerations that might have confounded the results. Her childhood circumstances – growing up in poverty and in what by all accounts was a broken home and dysfunctional family – did not enter into the discussions. Leilani's successes in the institution also were not taken into account; the Board simply regarded her a "danger of transmission to the progeny of mental deficiency or disability, also incapable of intelligent parenthood."[41]

The IQ test, or psychometric examination, played a key role in eugenics programs throughout North America. Historian Paul Lombardo has determined that, by 1924, public officials in the United States already had become critical of the application of IQ tests, also referred to as Binet tests, after their creator, French psychologist Alfred Binet. The test allegedly provided scientifically verifiable proof of an individual's capacity for intelligence and, conversely, for feeble-mindedness. Lombardo explains that, in the 1920s, a US survey found "98 per cent of unmarried mothers to be mentally deficient."[42] This and other findings drew attention to the environmental factors that confounded intelligence tests and the shortcomings of such examinations for producing useful indicators of parenting abilities or human worth.[43] Moreover, these contemporary analyses drew attention to the ways poverty itself had become woven into the pathology of feeble-mindedness – impoverished conditions appeared synonymous with mental deficiency.

In North Carolina, where nearly 7,000 individuals were sterilized between 1929 and 1975, warnings about the uneven use of psychometrics or IQ tests were ignored. Eugenicists there and elsewhere believed that the externally validated IQ test generated scientific legitimacy for the sorting of individuals into intelligence categories, and they continued to function as a barometer of mental ability and a key factor in determining an individual's suitability for sexual sterilization.[44] In Alberta after 1937, assessments of feeble-mindedness also allowed the Eugenics Board to sidestep the issue of consent, as such individuals were considered incapable of offering or ineligible to offer consent to the operation. Many, like Leilani, were not even informed of the operation.

In January 1959, at age fourteen, Leilani underwent a bilateral salpingectomy and an appendectomy under anaesthetic. She was also administered mecostrin, a muscle relaxant, before the surgeon proceeded to remove her appendix and cut out her Fallopian tubes. A bilaterial salpingectomy can involve simply cutting the Fallopian tubes, which produces the desired effect, but it also creates the potential for reversing the surgery, however rare such a request might be. In Leilani's case, however, the Fallopian tubes were all but entirely removed, which conclusively denied any future possibility of reversal. Surgeon M. Parsons removed seven centimetres and nine centimetres, respectively, of Leilani's left and right Fallopian tubes.[45] The surgery began at 9:45 a.m., and thirty-five minutes later she was wheeled out of the operating room and taken to a recovery wing. A week later her cotton sutures were removed. The post-operative report indicated that hers was a "routine operation."[46]

Leilani remained at the Provincial Training School until she was discharged "against medical advice" in 1965.[47] Similar to Doreen's experience, sterilization as a way to facilitate discharge from the institution did not hold true in Leilani's case. Although there is no systematic study of the rates of sterilization and subsequent discharge, these anecdotal cases suggest that the operation did not necessarily result in a more independent life, as early reformers had promised.[48] At the time of her committal,

Leilani had been described as an "intelligent moron." A physical examination revealed that she was healthy, had good posture, and appeared to
have normal physical development. Mentally her chart described her as
"alert," "pleasant," and "cooperative."[49] Upon her discharge she remained in the category of "moron" and was reportedly healthy, but she
was not told that her Fallopian tubes had been removed.

Family Planning on the Outside

At age twenty-one, a year after leaving the Provincial Training School,
Leilani began living with a man who later became her husband. After a
short courtship they decided to start a family of their own, but repeated
failed attempts at conception encouraged Leilani to seek medical advice.
In April 1966 Leilani's attending nurse at an outpatient clinic wrote to
the Training School's medical officer inquiring into her medical history.
The nurse indicated that Leilani had been complaining of gynecological
problems and was beginning to suspect that she had been sterilized during her time at the school, though she could not confirm any such operation: "I would be interested to know what operation was performed in
order that I may tell Miss Scorah exactly what has happened. At this
time she herself is not certain whether she was sterilized."[50]

The school forwarded a copy of Leilani's medical report to the clinic
confirming that she had undergone a bilateral salpingectomy at age
fourteen.[51] Her new doctor at the clinic discovered, however, that she
had developed a pelvic inflammatory disease, which might have arisen
due to complications caused by the sterilization surgery.[52] In response,
Le Vann assured Leilani's doctor that she had been healthy during her
time at the Training School and that her sterilization had been justified
based on the likelihood of her transmitting mental deficiency to future
children and on her inability to act as a responsible parent.[53]

A few years later Leilani moved to British Columbia and again began
inquiring about her reproductive capacity. Once again a doctor there
wrote to Le Vann to ascertain precisely what kind of operation had been
performed and to determine if it could be reversed: "This girl came to
see me September 28, 1971 complaining of the fact that she had some
pain in her abdomen and also wanted to know whether or not she
could give birth to children."[54] Again Le Vann defended the operation
on the basis that Leilani had been of "moron intelligence" when admitted to the Training School and insisted that, under his care, she had remained in good health. He reminded the inquiring physician that

Leilani had left the institution against his advice and had not been formally discharged, suggesting that he was no longer responsible for her current medical condition.[55]

Although Le Vann remained the primary gatekeeper at the Provincial Training School, others upheld his general views on sterilization in the local media. An article in the *Edmonton Journal* from the 1960s stated: "Two doctors said yesterday that mentally retarded persons should be sterilized particularly if they are contemplating marriage."[56] The argument, by Herbert Pascoe, a psychiatrist at the University of Alberta, rested upon the idea that "mentally deficient men and women become 'very poor' parents and a union of retardates will likely produce retarded children." Trotting out a much older set of arguments, the psychiatrist alleged that individuals with mental deficiencies were more prone to sexual promiscuity, a point that social reformers and early eugenicists had been raising since the 1920s. The "stress" of motherhood, he added, was overbearing for individuals who had difficulty even taking care of themselves. The newspaper article also reported the argument of Dr R.A. Kinch, chief of obstetrics and gynecology at the Montreal General Hospital, that current sterilization legislation did not go far enough. He recommended relaxing the birth-control and abortion laws to provide surgeons a greater range of options when confronting young women deemed mentally deficient and pregnant.[57]

By emphasizing the link between psychiatry and gynecology and adding abortion and birth control to the mix, these medical professionals articulated a set of more widely held values. I explore these connections in more detail in the next chapter, but importantly, in the late 1960s they began to alter the discourse on reproductive rights. The views these physicians expressed represented a minority perspective, since they focused primarily on concerns about mental deficiency, but their attitudes nonetheless gathered momentum in a much wider set of debates on reproductive rights. Women like Leilani, however, did not fit neatly into this emerging discourse, instead offering some physicians a different set of reasons to support the decriminalization of contraceptives and abortion.

Leilani's medical inquiries fell silent for a few years following the disappointing results in British Columbia. Her next recorded interaction with the medical profession came in 1975 when Leilani, now in her second marriage and with a new surname, Draycott, sought psychiatric help. The visit and its case report indicate that Leilani's relationship with her mother had deteriorated even more since she left the Provincial

Training School and that she had grown desperate for some kind of emotional or psychological support in the wake of the realization that she was unable to have children. "The problems Mrs. Draycott complains of and wishes help for are pretty unhelpable. She complains that she has difficulty in accepting the fact that due to sterilization in her early teens she is unable to have children. I pointed to her that this was a fact and had to be accepted. Her unhappiness in regard to it is understandable and in no sense pathological."[58] Although her psychiatrist appeared to sympathize with Leilani's situation, neither the general health nor the mental health services were able to provide any satisfaction to a woman grieving the loss of her ovaries.

Leilani's experience points to the reality faced by hundreds of women who had come through the eugenics program in Alberta, many of whom were not informed about the sterilization procedures performed on them as teenagers. In Leilani's case, her lack of awareness of and information about the operation contributed to marital discord and amplified the resentment that had already come to characterize the relationship between Leilani and her mother.

After 1937 the eugenics program sterilized teenagers with regularity. Under these circumstances it is likely that other men and women faced similar kinds of stresses as Leilani did after they left the institution. Many former patients and trainees had been instructed as to how to behave in mainstream society, including paying bills and doing domestic chores. Having a family arose as another feature of mainstream existence and one that several individuals tried to embrace in their attempt to fit into an allegedly normal society. It became clear, however, that the program's rhetoric and function did not always match. One contradiction was evident in the way in which trainees were kept at the Provincial Training School after they were sterilized, which ran contrary to the original discourse that suggested sexual sterilization offered a cost-saving measure by allowing individuals with mental deficiencies to live in society without incurring the risk of procreation. Yet trainees were not necessarily given guidance or even information that might help them cope with the realities of a sterile existence once they left the institution. As both Doreen's and Leilani's cases illustrate, as formerly institutionalized people established a life in the community, the support they received shrank to minimal levels, both financially and emotionally. Leilani's quest for psychiatric help, although ultimately unfulfilled, suggests that individuals learning to cope with their new procreative futures had to come to terms on their own with their new identity as a sterilized person. A mental health system that once had overseen the plight of individuals deemed at risk now turned its back on those who struggled to come to grips with post-sterilization and post-institutionalization trauma.

Alberta's Eugenics on Trial

In 1987 a forty-two-year-old woman with cerebral palsy sought legal recourse from the Alberta minister of social services for wrongful treatment at the Provincial Training School stemming from the 1960s, when she had been a ward of the provincial government. Her accusation rested upon the claim that she had received a crude diagnosis as a "high grade defective" with "brain damage," and that this label led to her sexual sterilization at age fourteen. Like Leilani, she had not been informed of the procedure; instead, she had been told that she needed her appendix removed, but the surgeon who performed the appendectomy also sterilized her. Although the plaintiff was only a young teenager at the time of the operations, she stated in an affidavit that she had no recollection of ever having been questioned by the Eugenics Board or interviewed as part of the routine assessments that were supposed to occur before a sterilization surgery could be legally authorized. By the time of her claim against the Alberta government, she had graduated with high honours from Mount Royal College in Calgary, and had convinced her lawyers and the staff at Alberta Social Services and Community Health "that she is an extremely articulate and competent individual."[59]

Although this case ultimately was settled out of court, it helped to set a precedent for Leilani and others who, in the 1990s, began challenging the Alberta government's past use of the Sexual Sterilization Act. Leilani became the first and, as it turned out, the only individual successfully to challenge the eugenics law in court. Her case, however, drew upon common themes that had appeared earlier and were later echoed in the mounting class action suits that developed in the wake of her legal victory. As the earlier case demonstrated, contradictions had emerged in several areas. Diagnoses no longer seemed to match intellectual ability when individuals were tested in adulthood. Although social scientists and psychologists had long questioned the validity of the IQ test as a legitimate scientific instrument, even while it was being applied readily to potential sterilization candidates, the legal scrutiny of the 1990s brought sustained attention to its weaknesses. The matter of consent also arose as a key factor in the legal examinations. Despite contemporary laws that allowed for blanket consent at the point of admission or alleviated the need for consent altogether in the cases of people deemed mentally defective, the combination of inconsistent diagnoses and the lack of sophisticated consent procedures proved difficult to defend.

The case that eventually went to trial pieced together expert reports and advice from a host of perspectives, including legal, psychological, medical, genetic, community, and historical. Historians played a key and perhaps unprecedented role in this process, as defendants attempted to dismiss past events as products of a bygone era borne out of misinterpretations and a lack of understanding of modern genetics. The resulting investigation collected a mountain of material, filling rooms in multiple legal offices and occupying several years of time spent by teams of researchers dedicated to interpreting the eugenics law in its appropriate historical context. The trial opened up Alberta's eugenics program to much wider scrutiny and teased apart its origins from its maturation and its policies from its practices, all the while centring on the fate of the plaintiff, Leilani Muir.

Several years after Leilani's unsatisfactory attempts to seek gynecological help and after further escalating tensions with her mother, bouts of severe depression, and feelings of loneliness and dejection, Leilani decided to sue the Alberta government for the treatment she had received at the behest of the Eugenics Board. Her efforts, however, did not immediately gain traction with the legal community. Her first attempt to seek legal support occurred in December 1987, when she contacted a law firm and received a lukewarm response. A letter from an articling student explained that she had no legal recourse in this case because it exceeded a two-year statute of limitations clause. She might, therefore, consider another avenue for advancing this case by seeking political action.[60] Other lawyers seemed equally reluctant to take the case. A letter from another law office told her that, since the Sexual Sterilization Act in effect at the time had included a clause prohibiting legal action against the members of the Eugenics Board or the surgeons involved, "accordingly, we regret to advise that it is our position that no action lies because of your sterilization."[61]

Another lawyer, Lenore Harlton, adopted a different approach, moving beyond the initial set of statements and collecting more evidence before dismissing the case altogether. For example, she contacted Leilani's mother, who outlined the chronology of events as she had remembered them:

Leilani was not a moron or mental case. We put Leilani in their (sic) for being Kleptomaniac. Its why she was in the (institution) And it was temperary. Months later Dr. Le Vann and Mrs. McRae [the nurse] suggested she have her tubes tied. No more was said we believe that's what she had. But I signed no papers. In my opinion Mrs. McRae and Dr. LeVann made the decisions on their own. I'm upset the way the institutions were run. No one to check on the officials that run the place. As we know now the Gov, never looked into such things going on. As mistreating the children. Believe me that's why we took my daughter out of there. Little I relized what really has happened to her. But I did not sign any papers to have her Sterilization. [In fact I never signed] for her tubes to be tied.[62]

Marie's letter seems out of sync with the description of events that unfolded in Leilani's own records and those of the Provincial Training School expressing her concern for her daughter's welfare, but she undeniably and emphatically stressed that she did not sign a consent form nor was she made aware of the sexual sterilization procedure that had been performed on her daughter. Harlton then further ascertained that Mr Scorah also denied signing any such forms, although lawyers later discovered his signature on the consent form that accompanied her admission to the Training School. This point later highlighted the confusion surrounding blanket consent or consent at the point of entry into the Training School, since parents seemed preoccupied with the admission of their child and might not have received a thorough explanation of the consequences of signing the forms.

At this point Harlton began formulating a case. She recognized that, if "the majority of all female persons admitted to the hospital were somewhat routinely sterilized, that would in my respectful opinion call into question the 'good faith' of any persons involved."[63] Setting off to examine the statistical history of the provincial eugenics program, she seized upon the opportunity to launch a suit against the government based on what appeared to be sloppy consent procedures combined with a more pathological approach to sterilizing women who entered the Training School. Her inquiry met with some resistance due to the overwhelming numbers of cases and consequent legwork involved. The director of social services explained that there would be over a thousand cases to review and insufficient staff to carry out such an analysis. After consulting informally with his staff, he estimated that, during the period in question, 1955–65, 95 per cent of the women in residence at the Training School had been sterilized.[64] This crude

estimate convinced Harlton that a case might be made against a program that systematically discriminated against women.

Seeking additional support, she then approached the Women's Legal
Education and Action Fund (LEAF) in search of financial resources to
retain further researchers and to support Leilani's case as a potential
example of gender discrimination. LEAF had been established in 1985
following the introduction of the Charter of Rights and Freedoms,
which guaranteed gender equality in legal matters. Developed through
the foresight of feminist lawyers who recognized the structural limitations placed upon women in the eyes of the law, the founders of LEAF
dedicated the fund to supporting feminist causes. Its founding mother,
Doris Anderson, had also been the president of the Canadian Advisory
Council on the Status of Women, which had led the charge against the
federal government in 1981 to have gender added to the Charter as a
guaranteed right equal to male and female persons.[65] Anderson had
first-hand experience as a single mother of three who also maintained a
high-profile feminist career as editor of *Chatelaine* magazine. Throughout
the 1960s the magazine gave women "an education on all the key issues
of second wave feminism: equal work legislation, birth control, abortion, divorce legislation reform, working wives and mothers," especially in Anderson's editorials.[66] Her legal organization appeared as a likely
candidate for extending support to a woman whose reproductive ca-
pacities had been removed by a patriarchal state.

Harlton astutely identified Leilani's case for its strong potential to support the spirit of LEAF and to expose injustices and discrimination towards women. As Harlton explained in her application, "without her
consent or knowledge [Leilani] was sterilized while so confined. Virtually,
all of the female patients and virtually none of the male patients at mental hospitals were sterilized."[67] She further argued that Leilani's case contained a number of ingredients that lay at the heart of contemporary
feminist concerns, including, and foremost, that "a woman should not be
stripped of her right to reproduce simply to meet the convenience of others." She described eugenics legislation as "perhaps, the blackest mark
upon our history of civil rights and women's rights."[68] Upon closer scrutiny, the estimates provided by the director of social services turned out to
be false, or at least more one-sided than the casual assumptions had first
appeared, but the evolving feminist argument that arose from this line of
reasoning provided an initial entry point into the case.

One historical irony might have been lost on the feminist lawyers
who assembled in support of the case. More than seventy years prior to

the founding of LEAF, leading feminist lawyers and women's rights advocates had successfully lobbied the Alberta government to pass the Sexual Sterilization Act in the first place. Indeed, their focus relied much more heavily on assessments of women and their parenting potential than on men. The original feminist argument rested upon assumptions of class and moral and genetic differences among women that necessitated extreme interventions and policing. By the 1980s, however, feminists viewed all women as part of a patriarchal system in which gender overrode class as a marker of experience. In her application to LEAF, Harlton pleaded for sympathy from her sister lawyers: "All were sterilized and many live today as normal, middle-aged women who lost their right to bear children as a result of arbitrary action. It could have happened to any of us."[69]

The feminists of the 1920s would not have shared this view. As described in Chapter 1, Emily Murphy, the Edmonton judge, feminist, suffragist, and renowned member of the Famous Five, embodied a different blend of feminist values than would her feminist descendants of the 1980s.[70] Where Murphy's feminism emerged from a challenge to the federal government that hinged upon acquiring voting rights for women of status, Anderson's feminism grew out of an insistence that gender be included as a Charter right, a distinction that extended well beyond enfranchisement. Both women operated in legal territory to stake out feminist claims to human rights, but the consequences for everyday women played out differently and relied on competing ideals of feminism. Leilani's gendered experiences sat historically in the period between these two expressions of women's rights in legal discourse. Her case, therefore, not only contained the potential to bolster claims by contemporary feminists about the systemic discrimination women faced; it also underscored how the politics of feminism had changed. LEAF, ultimately, argued that its mandate focused on new legal precedents, and therefore it was not in a position to support injustices from the past, egregious though they might have been.[71]

The case was thus forced to take a different approach, and the opportunity to put Canadian feminism on trial did not unfold as the initial build-up suggested. Upon closer examination, the charges of sexual discrimination coupled with allegations that nearly all women and no men were sterilized did not hold. Men, it turned out, were also recommended for sterilization in proportions almost equal to women over the course of the program's four decades in operation. Faced with this kind of evidence, an argument for systemic discrimination and a rallying cry for collective feminism dissolved.

Leilani nonetheless persisted and found a new team of lawyers who subsequently developed a different approach. Field Law in Edmonton reviewed the case in 1989 and began its own line of research into the eugenics law and how it had been applied to Leilani. The firm began by consulting a psychologist for his professional opinion on her mental and intellectual status. Psychologist Peter Calder, in conducting a comprehensive review of Leilani's medical records from the Provincial Training School, discovered that a calculation error had mistakenly placed her in the category of moron, which had resulted in her sterilization. Her true score, based on the component scores listed in her 1957 file compiled from the tests she took at age fourteen, should have been averaged to produce an overall IQ rating of 71. The cut-off for individuals deemed mentally defective was 70.[72]

Calder also explained that assessments in cases of individuals deemed retarded or intellectually impaired needed to be combined with emotional and educational considerations, and could not be conducted competently in the absence of this contextual information. He reasoned that the learning potential of children from emotionally disturbed homes regularly caused them to perform poorly on these kinds of tests. Leilani's situation fell squarely in this territory and should have received additional adjudication before resulting in a definitive score, particularly one with consequences leading to sexual sterilization. He criticized the institution for failing to meet the needs of its patients, in this case by altering the learning environment or, at the very least, reassessing Leilani after further periods of adjustment to the Training School, and combining IQ tests with evidence gleaned from her training reports, the majority of which showed strong improvement and academic achievement.

Finally, Calder conducted an assessment of his own, involving a number of academic colleagues, in an effort to produce a current intelligence assessment. He stated: "it was our shared belief that Ms. Muir could present her ideas in a clear logical fashion consistent with the level of senior high school students; however she made numerous grammatical and spelling errors that were more typical of an individual with only mid elementary level schooling." After further interviews and assessments, the team of psychologists gave Leilani another IQ test, which revealed that "[h]er overall IQ was 95, placing her in the average range of intelligence. Her verbal score IQ was 85 (low average range), and reflected to some degree her lack of formal education; her performance IQ of 112 placed her in a high average range within the top third of the general adult population."[73] In addressing the discrepancy in scores, Calder suggested that because Leilani originally had been labelled in the moron category, she had not been given suitable educational opportunities, and her performance in the first category had suffered as a result.

This new assessment gave a tremendous boost to the mounting legal case, and Field Law lawyers began seeking additional evidence to support this line of argument. They began by piecing together Leilani's history, her familial relations, her committal to the Provincial Training School, and her behaviour while in Le Vann's custody. They quickly discovered that Leilani's childhood experiences and relationship with her mother qualified as fitting into a disturbed category and should have been handled more delicately by her psychiatric assessors, even according to then-prevailing regulations. They also learned that Le Vann, who had been directly in charge of the Training School and its residents and trainees, had significant gaps in his education and training that raised serious questions about his qualifications and expertise. Indeed, the College of Physicians and Surgeons of Alberta had discovered in the late 1970s that Le Vann "had no formal specialist qualifications, just experience."[74] The lawyers concluded that, although his qualifications as a physician had been acceptable, his psychiatric specialization seems to have been drawn from experience alone, and remained as such until his retirement in 1974, even though he had claimed to have clinical training in psychiatry.

The lawyers began developing a case that initially focused on errors that applied even to the law in force at the time, rather than attempting to find a mechanism with which simply to criticize it. They fixed upon the broader misapplication of the IQ test as a weak indicator of intelligence and as a poorly applied assessment tool in the face of contemporary evidence to support the need for a more comprehensive analysis. Relying heavily on historical evidence to build the context for its use, Leilani's lawyers emphasized that, even according to readily available information and best practices from the late 1950 and 1960s, Leilani's assessment and miscalculated scores revealed a profound injustice. The inappropriate reliance on these scores became more evident when coupled with evidence drawn from correspondence between Leilani and her mother, and between her family and the Provincial Training School, which suggested that she had suffered emotional abuse and a lack of support from her family. Finally, they drew attention to the pain and suffering endured by victims of the sterilization program, for whom there was little follow-up support and for many a complete lack of information about the procedure they had undergone and its consequences for reproduction.

Leilani's case went to trial on 12 June 1995. Six months later the Honourable Madame Joanne B. Viet ruled in Leilani's favour and awarded the plaintiff $740,780 and her lawyers $230,000. Viet judged that Leilani's sterilization had proceeded wrongfully, that the institution had treated her unfairly, and that the accumulated effects had resulted in a loss of dignity and civil rights.[75] In the wake of this precedent-setting legal victory, more than seven hundred individuals came forward with similar grievances against the Alberta government associated with its application of the Sexual Sterilization Act. These cases never went to trial.

Leilani's case catapulted the issue of Canadian eugenics into the public discourse and elevated Leilani's status to that of a human rights heroine. Her story attracted significant media attention, became the feature of a National Film Board documentary, and resulted in casting a dark shadow over the history of early Canadian suffragists, Alberta politics, and mental health institutions. Some of these players had already been implicated in controversial historical decisions, but the connection to feminists raised new questions and criticisms. Leilani's case ultimately encouraged Canadians to develop a deeper understanding of the connections among reproductive rights, women's rights, and human rights.

Chapter Seven

Abortion, Sterilization, and the Eugenics Legacy: Jane Doe

Jane Doe came to the attention of the Therapeutic Abortions and Sterilization Committee at the Foothills Hospital in Calgary on 18 November 1974. Jane was single, pregnant for the first time, and fifteen years old. Her ex-boyfriend, John Smith, was twenty, and had left town shortly after learning about Jane's pregnancy. By the time Jane arrived at the hospital, John had moved to northern Alberta in search of employment in the oil patch. She explained to the obstetrician that they had not used contraception during their relationship, but that she would begin taking the birth-control pill if she were approved for a therapeutic abortion.

Although John had fled, Jane did not face the prospect of teen parenting alone or attempt to conceal her fate by secretly terminating the pregnancy. Her parents, who divorced when she was four years old, came together in their support for her through this challenging time. After her parents' marriage had dissolved, she spent most of her time with her father in Calgary and only occasionally with her mother, who had moved to the United States. She sometimes quarrelled with her parents, and when her fighting with one reached a breaking point, she would pack up and cross the border to live with the other. Faced with this pregnancy, however, she sought support from both parents.

Her frequent trips between the two countries had made it difficult to keep up with her education or to maintain a genuine interest in her studies. Several months before becoming pregnant, Jane had completed grade eight, a year later than her peers. She then stopped going to school altogether. As she approached the therapeutic abortion committee in Calgary, she maintained that her relationships with her mother and father were excellent and overall supportive. Indeed, her mother had returned to

Calgary upon hearing about Jane's pregnancy and had promised to stay with her until things settled down, one way or another. Both parents ultimately agreed that she should get an abortion, and escorted Jane to the Foothills Hospital to meet with the Therapeutic Abortions and Sterilization Committee with that singular objective in mind.

By the time Jane came to the hospital she was in her twelfth week of the pregnancy, and the consulting obstetrician recommended that she proceed with an abortion "on social grounds," which were compounded by looming psychiatric symptoms.[1] In her interview with the doctor Jane appeared depressed about her situation and rather bitter towards John, who had impregnated and then abandoned her. She explained to the charge nurse that she was anxious to return to school and embark on a healthier lifestyle after the abortion. Knowing that her mother was planning to remain in Calgary for a while gave Jane comfort and support. Her parents' presence convinced Jane, or at least helped her to convince the hospital staff, that she could no longer escape from her problems in Alberta and instead would become more responsible, if she could terminate the pregnancy and concentrate on her own process of maturing before becoming a mother.[2]

The gynecologist who examined Jane filled out a perfunctory report, stating Jane's name, address, and other personal details, before running through a checklist of questions designed to elicit her emotional, psychological, social, and physical well-being. The stock questions considered the woman's marital status, religious denomination, her and her husband's – assuming that most cases applied to married women – understanding of the procedure, the involvement of parents, and her mental health. In Jane's case, when asked to consider how she might react if the committee denied the procedure, the gynecologist reported that Jane already exhibited severe anxiety and depression, and would probably seek an abortion elsewhere. It is not clear whether the gynecologist implied that Jane would secure an illegal abortion, visit an unaccredited venue, seek an untrained service provider, or travel outside Alberta – likely to the United States – but any of these suppositions might have influenced the committee's final decision.[3] As for why Jane was a good candidate for the surgery, the gynecologist explained that it was chiefly due to her age and immaturity.[4]

Before the committee could assess Jane adequately, the hospital required her, in addition to undergoing these physical and psycho-social examinations, to fill out numerous forms and questionnaires attesting to her personality and past behaviour. For example, she was asked to complete the Cornell Medical Index health questionnaire, which began with questions directed at her eyesight, hearing, past illnesses, and physical health and fitness. By page two, the questions gradually shifted to information about family illnesses and nervous habits, including the familial instances of epilepsy, the propensity to bite one's nails, stuttering, and stammering.[5] The third page zeroed in on anxious reactions, and Jane answered affirmatively to having difficulty sleeping, to finding it impossible to take regular rest periods or to get regular exercise, and to smoking more than twenty cigarettes per day. On the next page she responding "yes" to questions about anxiety and depression, including trembling during exams, becoming "nervous and shaky" when approached by superiors, experiencing muddled thinking, performing tasks slowly to avoid making mistakes, being afraid of "strange people and places," being nervous while alone, being clumsy, being sad at parties, crying often, and feeling outright depressed. By her own admission, Jane described herself as nervous, shy, and easily irritated.[6]

A second self-administered form asked Jane to comment on her family situation, based on a series of multiple-choice questions. Her responses reveal that she held her parents in high regard, that she felt comfortable and secure in their care, and that she had experienced a middle-class, urban upbringing even though her parents lived in two different countries and she had travelled between the two households frequently. Her own life, however, had suffered from her parents' divorce – for example, because of travelling between one parent and the other, she had attended seven different schools by the time she reached grade eight. As a child she had been exposed to daily disagreements between her parents, which she felt had not conditioned her to forming her own strong, stable relationships.

Perhaps some of that instability had led her to seek romantic relationships from an early age, yearning for some sense of belonging and attraction. She began dating between the ages of eleven and thirteen, and by fifteen she was dating weekly. She felt somewhat guilty about her premarital sexual encounters, but confessed to having had more than five sexual partners by age fifteen. She stated that she had never had any feelings of homosexuality. She had never been in trouble with the law, and although she identified several friends who had been, she provided no details about them. She admitted to having taken illegal drugs once in her life, but denied alcohol use or the persistence of any psychiatric problems – although she confessed she had once tried to commit suicide.[7]

Jane's emotional and psychological profile, based on her responses to the questionnaires, gave the committee an image of a young girl struggling to find her way in the world and battling with issues of self-esteem and stability. The committee believed motherhood would pose a tremendous challenge for Jane and could create future challenges for her child, and it recognized that an abortion might offer a significantly different path for her and any future children.

Before making its decision, however, the committee gave Jane a booklet outlining the procedure and its current legal status. The booklet, prepared by the committee in concert with the Department of Obstetrics and Gynecology at the Foothills Hospital, summarized the physiological developments in pregnancy and identified the risks associated with an abortion, calling it unsafe after twenty weeks' gestation and describing the various methods used at other gestational periods. It defined the legal parameters permitting a therapeutic abortion, emphasizing that abortion was legal only if proceeding with the pregnancy would be dangerous to the woman's life or health; as the booklet stated, "there is a strong natural reluctance of the Therapeutic Abortion Committee to see a therapeutic abortion being viewed by anyone as an alternative to contraception."[8] Although hospitals in Calgary and elsewhere in the country interpreted these stipulations differently in the immediate wake of changes to the federal abortion law, Jane, like other women who sought abortions during the 1970s, had to convince hospital authorities that proceeding with her pregnancy constituted a danger to her health. Defining what constituted a justifiable health risk occupied physicians, parents, patients, lawyers, hospital administrators, and anti-abortion lobbyists in intense debates over health, life, autonomy, and the morality of these decisions.

Jane Doe is, of course, a pseudonym for a real patient whose name was changed by the charge nurse who recorded her case when she arrived at the Foothills Hospital as a minor, approximately two and a half months pregnant. John Smith, the ex-boyfriend, is also a pseudonym. Jane's case was a relatively typical one, as she fit into the growing category of teenaged patients who were the majority of abortion cases reviewed by these Calgary hospitals in the 1970s. Her story also exemplifies the discussions that took place among Albertans about reproduction and the emerging language of choice in the wake of the decriminalization of abortion in 1969 and the end of Alberta's sexual sterilization policy in 1972. As the number of teenage women seeking abortions grew steadily, public and medical discourse grew reminiscent of the debates in the 1920s concerning feminine virtue, promiscuity, and responsible motherhood, and seized upon mental health and psychiatric indications as suitable markers to justify abortions.

Moral judgments about illegitimacy also merged with earlier eugenic ideas, and revisited concepts of biological and environmental ingredients that colluded to produce so-called defective children.[9] Physicians voiced their disgust that a married middle-class woman would seek an abortion, but they accepted a more humanitarian argument when it came to a young unmarried woman or one with mental or physical disabilities. Although the context had changed over the decades, persistent concerns about intelligence, maturity, mental health, and suitable motherhood remained a part of these debates and continued to justify abortion and sterilization policies aimed at women who were marginalized or had mental and intellectual disabilities. In these debates, men once again vanished from view as potential fathers or genetic stock.

The Legal History of Abortion in Canada

The 1892 Criminal Code of Canada prohibited abortion, along with abortificients and any devices or advice leading to abortion. Section 237 of the Code read:

> (1) every one who, with intent to procure the miscarriage of a female person, whether or not she is pregnant, uses any means for the purpose of carrying out his intention is guilty of an indictable offence and is liable to imprisonment for life. (2) every female person who, being pregnant with intent to procure her own miscarriage uses any means or permits any means to be used for the purpose of carrying out her intention is guilty of an indictable offence and is liable to imprisonment for two years.[10]

The law was not significantly revisited until August 1969, when the Trudeau government decriminalized contraception and abortion under certain circumstances. The amended law included exceptions to the original law, namely:

> (a) a qualified medical practitioner, other than a member of a therapeutic abortion committee for any hospital, who in good faith uses in an accredited or approved hospital any means for the purpose of carrying out his intention to procure the miscarriage of a female person, or (b) a female person who, being pregnant, permits a qualified medical practitioner to

use in an accredited or approved hospital any means descried in ... for the purpose of carrying out her intention to procure her own miscarriage.[11]

The change in the law further specified that a woman could obtain an abortion if she had the approval of a therapeutic abortion committee demonstrating in writing that in its "opinion the continuation of the pregnancy of such female person would or would be likely to endanger her life or health."[12] Historian Christabelle Sethna has argued that the change did very little to improve access to abortions, as many physicians felt that the risk of criminal liability remained a serious concern. As Sethna points out, however, before and after this change in the law, Canadian women sought abortions; the amended law, it seems, merely gave more people a rallying point around which they could articulate a series of grievances.[13]

The number of abortions performed in Alberta grew precipitously after the change in the law, and by 1972 the Alberta Hospital Services Commission reported that twenty-three of its hospitals performed abortions. During the first year of the amended law, Alberta ranked third in Canada, after Ontario and British Columbia, in the total number of abortions performed, and maintained that position for the next several years.[14] Those rankings also matched the relative numbers of live births in each province, but the Alberta data indicated that many women from outside of Alberta travelled there to obtain abortions due to the services provided.

Soon after the change to the Criminal Code, Alberta hospitals responded by establishing therapeutic abortion committees, which, like the Eugenics Board, relied on a multi-professional assessment of a case that then determined the validity of an abortion request and ultimately made a referral for the procedure if approved. Most of these committees included a medical-social worker, a psychologist, and three qualified medical practitioners, who then examined the various questionnaires and sometimes interviewed the woman and her husband or parents before making a decision.[15] These relatively advanced and sophisticated services meant that Alberta became an attractive destination for women seeking abortions from other, less well serviced areas. For example, 39 per cent of the abortions in 1972 were performed on women who lived in the Northwest Territories, 33 per cent on women from British Columbia, and 23 per cent on women from Saskatchewan,[16] which might have reflected Alberta's quick response to the change in the abortion law and other provinces' comparatively slow development. By the middle of the decade, however, over 97 per cent of abortions were performed on women residing in Alberta.[17]

Initially, 61 per cent of the women who obtained abortions in Alberta's accredited hospitals were single, 28 per cent were married, and the rest separated or divorced. The vast majority of the pregnancies were of teenagers between the ages of fifteen and nineteen, most of them single.[18] The therapeutic abortion committees justified nearly 60 per cent of the abortions for psychiatric reasons; in only a relatively small number of cases were abortions approved because of health risks or, even more rarely, exclusively on social grounds. These trends continued into the mid-1970s.[19]

Non-Catholic hospitals in Calgary and Edmonton provided the bulk of the services and soon complained about an inequitable workload. The Royal Alexandra Hospital in Edmonton reported that it had performed ten therapeutic abortions in 1969 and already twenty-four in the first six months of 1970.[20] In comparison, however, there had been 4,594 live births at the hospital, 12 per cent of which were reportedly born to mothers out of wedlock. The Department of Social Services indicated that, despite the therapeutic abortion committees' figures, the number of unwanted pregnancies in the province had steadily increased among married women, even more so than among single girls.

The language of "women" and "girls" used explicitly in these reports further separated the categories of people seeking abortions as well as the official judgments applied to their situations. Single "girls" were assumed to be younger, foreshadowing a focus on teenage abortions, while "women" connoted an older, possibly more mature individual whose foray into motherhood might be forestalled with an abortion due to her allegedly irresponsible behaviour or her attempts to control fertility in her marriage. Given the recent decriminalization of abortion and findings elsewhere suggesting that the rate of legal abortions hovered between 20 and 25 per cent of the number of live births, Edmonton officials anticipated that the annual demand for abortions at the Royal Alexandra alone would soon exceed one thousand. Such a need would place significant surgical demands on the obstetrical staff with no sign of abatement. To complicate matters, women in their thirties, particularly those who already had two or more children, began asking for both an abortion and sterilization to secure their reproductive future completely.[21] The increased demand on surgical time would also create the need for new administrative pressures and challenge hospital boards to prioritize and reallocate their resources. Furthermore, staff at the Royal Alexandra Hospital worried that they would inherit a disproportionate surgical burden given the refusal of local Catholic hospitals to perform similar operations.

Of the more than four thousand women who obtained abortions in Alberta hospitals in 1972, 13 per cent were also sterilized at the same time, not including a few for whom hysterectomy was the method of abortion.[22] Six months later the figure had risen to 15.5 per cent.[23] Most of those who sought sterilization in combination with abortion already had children, and most were between the ages of twenty-five and thirty nine, although women as young as fifteen also underwent sterilization.[24] Although only a minority of women demanded both procedures, such cases highlighted the surgical burden on hospital staff. Usually, the decision to combine the two surgeries rested with the women themselves, but in some cases it fell to parents or the medical professionals to determine the likelihood of responsible parenthood.

Throughout the 1970s, as abortion attracted increasing media and public attention, the debate about parenthood refocused on women: their bodies, once again, came under medical and public surveillance as the site of contests over reproductive morality. Some women celebrated the steps taken towards greater autonomy and reproductive choice that the decriminalization of abortion offered. Others – pregnant teenagers and those considered mentally incapable of autonomous living and responsible parenthood – instead encountered greater scrutiny.

One way in which the new abortion laws appeared inadequate centred around issues of access and privacy. As historian Christabelle Sethna demonstrates, intensely private and invasive questioning formed a routine part of the abortion assessment exercise for women like Jane Doe, even after the decriminalization of the procedure; consequently, abortions remained out of reach or unappealing for many women.[25] The Vancouver Women's Caucus, for example, protested Canada's limp new law by staging a trek to Ottawa, intentionally modelling its cross-Canada parade after the on-to-Ottawa-trek of unemployed men during the Depression. Unlike its precursor, however, the Abortion Caravan, as it became known, succeeded in reaching Ottawa and stalling Parliament as these activist women forced the issue of abortion access into the public spotlight.[26]

As Sethna also shows, Canadian women, both before and after the change in the abortion law, travelled extensively – often abroad – in search of medically sanctioned therapeutic abortions, but the expense of doing so meant that safe abortions remained out of reach for those who lacked sufficient means.[27] Beth Palmer finds that western Canadian women tended to travel south to the United States, rather than across the Atlantic, and that they identified the lack of services and access as their key concern.[28] Moreover, in Alberta, the hospitals that offered abortions were clustered in Calgary and Edmonton, leaving meagre resources for women outside those two major cities.

These Canadian studies on abortion emphasize the connections between abortion legislation and a more radicalized response from women. Protests such as the Abortion Caravan showed that Canadian feminists regarded the Trudeau government's omnibus bill as a paltry measure that insufficiently acknowledged women's modern reproductive rights. Their response stemmed particularly from the second-wave feminist movement, which had already begun articulating a more explicit expression of personal autonomy and reproductive health under women's control.

Feminists and family planning advocates, including physician Henry Morgentaler,[29] led the charge for better access to decriminalized abortions based on the language of personal autonomy and reproductive choice. Amid the chorus of support for an issue that increasingly became defined as one of women's rights, however, some women's voices remained quiet. In the period leading up to the change in the federal abortion law, for example, the number of Aboriginal and Métis women being sterilized in Alberta picked up pace. These women became overrepresented in Alberta's eugenics program in the last few years of the program, as discussed in Chapter 2, and did not routinely join the ranks of outspoken feminist women who wanted greater access to abortions or contraception.

For women such as Leilani Muir and Doreen Befus, who remained under the scrutiny of medical authorities for most of their lives, the language of independence in the 1970s meant independence from medical surveillance and the promise of a life outside an institution. Although Leilani and Doreen became human rights advocates in their own ways, they did not fit the typical image of a 1970s feminist engaged in campaigns to improve access to therapeutic abortion or to ensure better advice from their doctors regarding reproductive health. The politicization of these debates suggests that, beyond divisions along class lines, different kinds of feminism and various progressive perspectives on human rights coexisted. Rather than characterizing the movement as strictly middle class or feminist, the politics of choice reengaged individuals and families in discussions of intelligent, responsible parenthood.

The legacy of eugenic sterilization, especially as it affected marginalized women, meant that, in the language of autonomy, third-party advocates made choices for women that were considered "in their best interests." Women deemed incapable of making autonomous choices included those considered mentally incompetent due to mental illness or disability, but increasingly that category included teenage girls. As the number of teenage pregnancies rose in the province, parents, doctors, and legal guardians subsequently came to govern the reproductive futures of these minors. Even though the publicity afforded abortion altered the context of discussions about reproductive rights and focused on women as the guardians of reproduction, for some women, including teenagers, that responsibility allegedly was too much to handle. For them, a more protective mentality re-emerged that viewed them as the new models of immature and inadequate motherhood.

The records of therapeutic abortion committees in Calgary and Edmonton hospitals and letters from obstetricians help to show how the public debates about abortion and a woman's right to choose overshadowed the more pernicious practice of sterilizing women and aborting fetuses carried by women deemed unfit for parenting. Obstetricians and hospital administrators appeared caught in a moral or ethical quandary. On the one hand they were upset by the rising tide of requests for "abortion on demand," which they connected with irresponsible middle-class feminists who were challenging traditional family values and over which they wished to retain medical authority. On the other hand, they appeared less conflicted about proceeding with abortions, in combination with or separate from tubal ligations, on women and teenage girls for whom parenthood, in their view, presented serious challenges. Some members of the medical community took umbrage to the feminist view of reproductive rights while shielding themselves with humanitarian language when it came to denying those same rights to young, marginalized, impoverished, or disabled women. The issue of choice in this sense effectively absorbed an essential grain of eugenics philosophy and continued to rely on the authority of the medical profession to determine who made good parents, either biologically or socially.

Rather than usher in a new discourse on reproductive rights and choices, the medical profession returned to an older set of attitudes that blamed women and combined elements of sexuality with accusations of immorality. Morality, in the 1970s, remained tethered to attitudes about middle-class families: the moral path led to a middle-class, heterosexual marriage with healthy children. To achieve that goal, abortions and sterilizations remained a necessary way to weed the proverbial garden. Such attitudes also blended with newer, more empowering connotations associated with reproductive choice and the appeal of abortions and sterilization surgeries for women seeking to exercise their recently acquired power and rights. Many women recognized that access to such surgeries might help to ensure they, too, took the path of morality and grew up to be suburban wives and mothers.

Jane Doe's experience opened a new chapter in the discussions of reproductive rights, but concerns about eugenic sterilization continued beyond the end of Alberta's formal sexual sterilization program. At the same time, concerns about abortion centred on young, single women who sought to terminate their pregnancies, while for individuals deemed mentally incompetent, the medical profession donned updated language to describe ability and disability and continued to emphasize the supposedly humane and responsible need to sterilize them.

Defining Health

Health risks remained a critical factor in determining a woman's eligibility for an abortion, and psychiatric and medical concerns trumped all others in Alberta's hospitals. In the period immediately following the legal changes to the status of abortion and for the two years before the repeal of the Sexual Sterilization Act, the spectre of eugenics crept into the debate on acceptable abortions. This overlap created a moment in which the two sets of surgeries comingled in the medical-legal discourse on reproductive choices and their relationship to mental and physical health.

The definition of health became crucial in determining the legal status of an abortion. The World Health Organization (WHO) defined it as "a state of complete physical, mental and social well-being and not merely the absence of disease or infirmity."[30] The Alberta Medical Association (AMA) recommended this definition of health, and suggested that it should apply in the determination of acceptable abortions. Dr Robert Clark, executive secretary of the AMA's board of directors, argued that "social well being" was key and, if applied, "would definitely widen the criteria for therapeutic abortions."[31] As Clark admitted, accepting this interpretation of health effectively would create opportunities for therapeutic abortions under almost any circumstances. He estimated that, annually, as many as eight thousand women in Alberta wished to terminate their pregnancies.[32] The major stumbling block, for him and for the province's chief of obstetrics, remained a question of resources and personnel.

In August 1969 the Ontario Hospital Association had issued a memo addressing the recent legal changes regarding abortion.[33] The memo

reminded physicians that the new law indicated that "abortions to preserve the life or health of the mother are permissible in certain circumstances in 'accredited' hospitals."[34] Cleaving to the language of the
federal bill, the memo emphasized the issue of maternal health risks
and the use of accredited facilities. It drew attention to the somewhat
ambiguous terms "life" and "health," which most physicians acknowledged required further interpretation. The medical organizations in
Ontario and Alberta thus agreed to widen the interpretation with additional specificity: "life" expanded to include survival or health, and
"health" involved both physical and mental health.[35]

A few months later Alberta hospitals began responding to this expanded definition but further wrestled with how best to interpret the
murky language surrounding "certain circumstances" and "health
risks." The Foothills Hospital in Calgary took an early position on the
issue, claiming in an internal memo that it would provide abortions only
for therapeutic reasons, which it narrowed to include consideration for
"medical, psychiatric, social, economic, eugenic and humanitarian" purposes.[36] In particular, the memo stipulated that social, economic, or humanitarian grounds alone were insufficient reasons for an abortion
without further close scrutiny of family history. Indeed, medical and
psychiatric reasons were singled out as the only legitimate reasons for
abortion, although the grip on those contributing factors loosened upon
the realization that such issues had a cascading effect on economic and
social well-being.

Hospital administrators were also reluctant to rule out eugenic reasons. The Foothills Hospital claimed that it only "recommended [abor-
tions] on medical or psychiatric grounds. However, it must again be
stressed that the social, economic, eugenic and humanitarian factors are
assessed in each and every case."[37] Teasing apart these various justifica-
tory categories proved increasingly difficult, and women became particularly adept at presenting themselves in a manner that conformed
with these acceptable reasons even if abortion committees attempted to
use them as a filtering mechanism.[38]

Within a year the Foothills Hospital, much like the Royal Alexandra
in Edmonton, was complaining that it had been overwhelmed with requests for abortions and worried that it had developed a reputation for
its liberal response to the change in the law. Dr Harry Brody, Director of
the Department of Obstetrics and Gynecology at the Foothills Hospital,
suggested that his department had taken a "unique stand" with regard
to abortions, even prior to the change in the law. "As it has turned out,"

he explained, "we anticipated this change in social thinking of our society ... [Yet] in the last year this problem has snowballed to such an extent that we have been overwhelmed with the number of requests."[39] Brody sought advice and a clearer definition from the provincial health minister on how best to interpret "health" so that his department could better predict its workload: "Should the Minister of Health leave the definition to the profession, then the recently passed motion of the Alberta Medical Association defining health in the broadest terms will be utilized by physicians in this Province. On that basis I can predict with almost certainty a further increase in demands for therapeutic abortion."[40] He suggested that the abortion committees had the resources to review only five cases per week. He also emphasized the need to focus on prophylactic and preventative public health measures to avoid resorting to abortions in the future. If anything, decriminalizing abortion appeared to have had a concurrent influence on the number of medical professionals demanding better public health education that emphasized the importance of contraception. This was, he added, partly because "nursing personnel have occasionally balked at assisting a therapeutic abortion, especially in pregnancies that are advanced. I might add that I personally find the procedure of therapeutic abortion a repugnant one, especially after 10-12 weeks gestation."[41]

While acknowledging the change in the Criminal Code, the AMA abhorred the loose definitions attached to the amendment. In a statement issued at its annual meeting, the AMA suggested that the decision should be left to the physician's discretion and professional judgment, though it reiterated that the Association would not support abortion on demand.[42] Brody agreed with this sentiment, but he also reiterated that doctors and policy makers should place greater emphasis on prevention and public education regarding contraception.[43] The notion of abortion on demand, associated with irresponsible women who were too lazy or self-righteous to practise birth control, affronted many physicians.[44] Alternatively, abortions for women who were unlikely to want additional children, or be capable of providing for them, was a humane response to the much larger social problem of unwanted pregnancies.

The AMA called an emergency meeting in the fall of 1970 to address the growing demand for abortions and the corresponding lack of resources or clear guidelines on how best to proceed with what appeared to be a ballooning problem. One obstetrician laid out some of the many controversies inherent in interpreting health risks and the liabilities doctors would shoulder if they agreed to be responsible for abortions and sterilizations:

Health is a liberal thing. Do we have to define health? We have to think if we do this liberally, do we change the population of this country which is not over-populated; we have to think of war; we have to think of many things. Secondly, he thinks it is wrong to utilize this procedure unless for a medical pathological reason; it is wrong to use top flight beds – we should have a clinic for this purpose. He agrees that the figures are frightening. Hospitals might be disassociated from the mass sterilization – perhaps the matter of having this done in a clinic might overcome the problem.[45]

Another attendee indicated that most of the hospitals in Calgary had already adopted a rather liberal view of health and permitted abortions and tubal ligations, and even expected the Catholic hospitals to start participating in these operations within a year, given the demand for and public acceptance of such procedures.

The question of abortion on demand attracted more discussion from the AMA members. A liberal interpretation of health, including subscribing to the WHO's definition, in effect allowed abortion on demand. The problem, according to some physicians, was that such an interpretation put the decision for an abortion in the hands of the patient and removed control from the physician. One member suggested that, no matter what the medical community decided, abortions on demand likely would go ahead, and since they would no longer be a medical problem, they should be set up by other agencies, such as social services.[46] The issue of control assumed an interesting dimension in the discussion, with some physicians readily admitting to wanting to retain control over the decisions they made and the surgeries they permitted, while others wished to absolve themselves of any responsibility associated with population control.

Brody vehemently argued against this point, claiming that, by refusing abortions, on demand or otherwise, the medical profession was merely contributing to a growing and complicated social problem. Women with means, he argued, obtained abortions somehow, suggesting that restricting the procedure fundamentally punished poor and young women who had insufficient resources. He had extensive experience studying the mental health concerns both of women who successfully obtained an abortion and of those who were denied the operation. He published his research in the *American Journal of Obstetrics and Gynecology* in 1971 where he emphasized the difference between psychiatric or emotional disturbances among women who had obtained abortions and among those whose request for the procedure had been rejected. His research showed that, although women in various studies and regions reported elements of regret, self-reproach, and guilt after a legal abortion, the number who developed serious psychiatric disorders following their abortions was extremely low – indeed, the majority of women were reportedly "pleased and grateful."[47] The same, however, was not true for women whose requests for abortion had been denied; in 6 to 25 per cent of those cases psychiatric complications had arisen. These surveys suggested that an abortion to end an unwanted pregnancy might help to alleviate stress, and thereby mitigate the development of a psychiatric disorder.[48]

Brody had concluded that abortion created a health problem and a set of social disparities that needed to be addressed, and physicians had a social responsibility to participate in that discussion: "For every unwanted child born it places a burden on our economy with regard to the care of the infant and the problem that arises for that family that cannot cope. It is cheaper to see that there are no unwanted children than to deal with them if they are unwanted and are here."[49] Despite Brody's argument, physicians at the meeting generally displayed deep disgust with the idea of having to perform an operation they felt contraceptive methods could avoid. Nonetheless, discussions circled around the issue of medical responsibility and liability for a mounting set of social problems tied to population control in the wake of the new abortion legislation. For many members of the medical community, the issue came down to the inherent authority vested in their profession to make these decisions.

The other major issue for the AMA centred on the psychiatric justifications that lay behind demands for abortions. Contemporary statistics indicated that "about 90% [of the abortions] are for psychiatric reasons."[50] Some speakers conflated illness with a whole host of challenges, which combined to trigger psychiatric problems. For example, one doctor exclaimed: "It is a big problem. It has to be done. These people are sick. It does not matter how they are sick – socially, economically and morally, or physically – they are sick."[51] To many participants, separating out psychiatric from other health risks seemed futile. Brody reinforced this idea by showing that women who sought an abortion developed significant anxieties and depressive traits when faced with the stress of an unwanted pregnancy. Whether that stress culminated in a full-blown disorder or a physical response, the health risks escalated and became acutely difficult in communities where women had limited resources at their disposal. Faced with social, economic, and potentially physical challenges, psychiatric risks were soon to follow. The meeting ended with an explicit acknowledgment that the demand for abortions was on the rise without an adequate increase in the resources allotted to hospitals, a clear definition of what constituted health, or a legal interpretation of what "certain circumstances" included. The medical community seemed to be reeling from these changes and lacked clear guidelines on how best to proceed.

Brody continued to play a leading role in these debates as they unfolded in the final months of 1970. In December he wrote again to the Foothills Therapeutic Abortions and Sterilization Committee requesting further clarification on the age of consent for the operations. He indicated that women over the age of eighteen and living away from their parents had not so far been required to provide additional consent.[52] Borrowing this precedent from the Canadian Medical Protective Association (CMPA), Brody stressed, however, that the physician retained the ultimate authority over these and other cases: "The question of obtaining consent or informing the parents and actually doing the procedure is a matter up to the responsible physician."[53] For Brody, the issue of medical control loomed large in these debates. He appeared more concerned with the fate of physicians losing their status as moral authorities – with their right to make decisions about who deserved or required reproductive surgeries – than with emerging cultural assumptions about the morality of abortions writ large.

The rising numbers of young women demanding abortions continued to plague the discussions and introduce new challenges. Brody noted that young women over the age of eighteen did not need to inform their parents if they gave up an illegitimate child for adoption. Therefore, he reasoned, the same logic should apply to consent in an abortion case.[54] Throughout these discussions Brody maintained his emphasis on abortion as a social problem: "I feel that if the hospital takes the posture that they must inform the parents of nursing students in matters such as therapeutic abortion that we will simply drive these girls underground to have illegal procedures done or will have it done in some other fashion. This would lead to the detriment of many individuals and I feel is morally not acceptable to me."[55] Ultimately, though, he preferred to maintain the position and authority of the physician in determining the best course of action regarding abortion: "May I also point out that we will see patients at any age, even fourteen without their parents, however, it is up to the physician who does the procedure to see that he is legally protected whenever a procedure is contemplated."[56]

Partly owing to Brody's influence, Calgary hospitals opened the door for justifying medical abortions by concentrating on the psychiatric consequences of denying the procedure. The Foothills Hospital subsequently assumed a leading role in providing abortions. By 1971 it had a separate centre devoted to the practice and had acquired a reputation for providing abortions quickly and efficiently. Martha Weir, president of the new Calgary Abortion Centre, told the *Calgary Herald* that "we've noticed a switch from having a very good reason to grant an abortion to having to have a good reason for not granting one."[57] Dr Robert Lampard, the Foothills Hospital's assistant medical administrator, also told the paper that "the new procedures would allow abortions to be performed in the emergency ward, without anaesthetic. The patient would be released the same day."[58] In a survey conducted by the Centre, 79 per cent of the women interviewed agreed that "it is a basic human right of a woman to control her own reproduction without fear of legal or social recrimination. Therefore, all laws that would force any woman to bear a child against her will must be eliminated."[59]

The public face of the abortion issue, or at least the way in which it was reported in the local press, reinforced its character as part of a women's rights campaign or a natural extension of feminist lobbying in the wake of women's health concerns. Physicians, however, even while participating in the expansion of plausible justifications for performing abortions, continued to register their abhorrence of the operation. One psychiatrist resigned from the Therapeutic Abortion Committee at the Calgary General Hospital after serving on it for nearly five years, citing his disapproval of the philosophy behind abortions. He felt that the complex comingling of psychiatric, social, and economic reasons for abortion made it difficult to satisfy a moral position on the debate.[60]

By 1973 some Calgary doctors had grown concerned by the number of women suffering from serious mental and emotional disorders, and teenage girls like Jane Doe who were seeking abortions, the latter often with the assistance of their parents. These doctors felt that the strain associated with teenaged pregnancy, which was almost invariably illegitimate, and its implications for the girl's future, was sufficient to warrant a psychiatric indication. One doctor stated:

in my experience, too little attention is paid to the feelings of the patient and their immediate family and now that abortion is recognized as a well known alternative to going to term with an illegitimate pregnancy, it is one that particularly teenaged children are turning to increasingly. For example, I have had a well known "pro-lifer" present with her 15 year old daughter seeking a therapeutic abortion and when confronted with her public attitude, remarked that when it happens to your own children it is different.[61]

The admission of a change of heart by a known pro-lifer offers a revealing indication that wielding such views more often pertained to casting judgment on other people's choices, but when it came to pregnancy in one's own family, the issues were perhaps more complicated.

The president of the Therapeutic Abortions and Sterilization Committee at the Foothills Hospital, Ralph Coombs, complained in 1973 that demands for abortions continued to grow, threatening to reach a ratio of ten abortions for every one hundred live births.[62] A Calgary-based pro-life organization published shocking figures suggesting that the rate of abortions was nearing that of live births in the province.[63] In fact, as Lampard corrected in the local news media, the actual ratio was one abortion to every three live births, and all of these abortions "were done for medical reasons and involved cases where either the life or health of the mother was at stake."[64] Even as the definition of health the hospitals adopted included an expansive list of ailments, including social and economic ones, the responses by physicians, pro-life organizations, and anti-abortion advocates stressed the flimsiness of this approach, lambasting women and doctors for their flagrant disrespect for human life.

Sterilization and Mental and Physical Disability

The twinned issues of sterilization and abortion for eugenic purposes had been two sides of the same coin for some time. In 1958 the *Canadian Medical Association Journal* outlined the psychiatric reasons for abortion as approved in Sweden, including the suggestion that "eugenic indications exist where it may, with reason, be presumed that the woman or the father of the expected child will transmit to the offspring, through hereditary channels, insanity, mental deficiency or serious physical disease. These cases must, however, submit themselves to compulsory sterilization."[65] The author of the article, D.E. Zarfas, an Ontario physician, summarized the international situation by claiming that "Denmark, Norway, Sweden, Japan and Russia consider that there are eugenic and humanitarian indications for therapeutic abortion, while in England, United States and Canada these indications are not considered."[66] On the issue of psychiatric indications, however, he noted that Canada followed the same logic as the Scandinavian countries, meaning that, in the majority of cases, therapeutic abortion was approved where women exhibited signs of psychiatric disorders. One Ontario case involved a thirty-four-year-old mother of two children who had given herself an abortion. Her file suggested that "she exhibited masculine protest and an obsessive ruminative personality with an adolescent depression ... Her abortion was carried out, sterilization was done and her mental health was considered greatly improved."[67] In another case, a woman suffering from post-partum depression with psychosis – or what some doctors referred to as the schizophrenic type of depression – had undergone "delivery by Caesarian section and sterilization at the time of operation," as recommended by her physician, in consultation with a psychiatrist.[68]

Other cases, however, escaped sterilization and abortion, despite their falling within the traditional target categories. A twenty-four-year-old pregnant woman, described as a "single, mentally defective girl with an IQ of 69," did not appear to understand the consequences of her actions. She appeared undisturbed by her pregnancy and had not developed psychiatric conditions; as a result, the physicians ruled there were "no legal grounds for termination."[69] She might not have escaped sterilization had she been a resident of Alberta, where this diagnostic picture could have triggered a response from the Eugenics Board. In Ontario, however, where the woman lived, the relationship between IQ and sterilization did not produce an automatic response, even though women with psychiatric disorders became candidates for sterilization surgery. Zarfas suggested that post-partum psychosis warranted "sufficient grounds for therapeutic abortion," whereas if the mental illness had reached full-stage schizophrenia, both an abortion and sterilization should occur.[70] Zarfas concluded that Canadians required clearer guidelines on the psychiatric and medical indications that might trigger the need for an abortion and sterilization. Although Zarfas might have based his conclusions on presumptions about intelligent parenthood, his focus on major psychiatric disorders, rather than mental development or intelligence, implicated a different pool of sterilization candidates. Consequently, his interpretations relied on a fundamentally different understanding of the risks involved in pregnancy and parenthood.

Daniel Cappon, a psychiatrist at the University of Toronto, shared some of Brody's concerns that the greatest health risk to pregnant women was posed by criminal abortions, or underground, non-medical, non-approved methods: "Likely the woman who presents herself for abortion and demands it vigorously is one of the most adequate, ego-strong, aggressive types among those with psychopathology connected with pregnancy, therefore one of the least likely to break down if the abortion is refused. The greatest danger in her case [is] her seeking criminal abortion or interfering dangerously with herself."[71] Tapping into some of the social arguments surrounding abortion, Cappon seized upon the psychological and emotional consequences of desperation and anxiety over carrying a child to term. In an attempt to explain the chain of events in pathological terms, Cappon indicated that pregnant women were already bordering on psychopathological behaviour, and carrying an unwanted fetus could present an unmanageable psychological burden, which arguably necessitated medical intervention.

The point at which the medical profession became obligated to intervene, however, raised significant questions about liability. Law professor Bernard Dickens argued that "it is not necessarily illegal for a therapeutic abortion committee to decide that a given pregnancy should be terminated only on condition that the woman agrees to be sterilized at the same time. If the medical indications are that a woman will be able to have only one more child, and if it will be considerably more hazardous for her to have it later, an abortion committee may in these special circumstances inform her of her option to have another child 'now, or never.'"[72] Dickens's interpretation of the legal context placed the authority for this decision squarely with the medical profession, which, he believed, then could respond proactively by determining the likely risks associated with future pregnancies and act accordingly by recommending sterilization for some women who sought an abortion. His views fell in line with those of physicians who continued to show concern for their professional authority in the unfolding debate.

The crux of this issue, for Dickens, was the interpretation of the health of the mother. Concerns for the child's potential health or disability were secondary in these discussions. As Dickens explained,

regarding the child's likely inheritance of physical or mental abnormality, therefore, the key to legal termination of pregnancy will be the fear of those attending the mother that her awareness of this likelihood would or would be likely to cause her distress endangering health. Since the law focuses on the condition of the mother and not that of the prospective child, there need not be 'substantial risk' of the prospective child being 'seriously handicapped,' [as it is in British law].[73]

The emphasis on maternal health helped to draw a line in the debate by narrowing the focus on the mother. The minutes of the Therapeutic Abortion Committee at the Calgary General Hospital for 1974 indicate that its members wished to retain this focus in addressing the cases that came before it. In the past, the committee claimed, the probability of a fetal abnormality was a credible reason to approve an abortion, but the committee moved that such an indication be struck from the allowable list, leaving medical conditions and significant depression concerning the mother the two remaining justifications.[74]

These kinds of discussions firmly reinforced the emphasis on women as sites of pathological behaviour. Although women had campaigned for better access to abortion services, the trade-off came with a greater effort on the part of obstetricians and gynecologists to ensure that they could cite psychiatric reasons or risks that necessitated an abortion. Although this approach partly represented a humanitarian and progressive interpretation of women's health autonomy, it eroded the privacy of the doctor-patient relationship by introducing abortion committees, legal advisors, and psychiatric consultants into the decision-making process of approving or denying abortions.

Sterilization and Disability: The Legal Issue

The congruent issues of autonomy, privacy, and consent coursed through the abortion and sterilization debates, but applied unevenly to different groups of women. By the late 1970s the language of human rights and civil liberties helped to galvanize support for several marginalized groups in society, not the least of which were women seeking autonomy over reproductive health. The sentiment did not necessarily extend, however, to embrace women with disabilities. In 1978 Dr Norman Brown of the CMPA wrote to Dr Ian Burgess, Vice-President of the Salvation Army Grace Hospital in Calgary, in response to an inquiry about sterilization surgeries for "mentally retarded juveniles." Brown explained, "as you may know, there are those who believe sterilization of a mentally retarded person is an infringement on civil liberties of the person and that consent for it cannot be properly given by anyone." He continued by offering legal advice to Burgess and suggested, "although we do not wholly agree with this point of view it must be acknowledged nevertheless that there may be groups or individuals who object strenuously to the principle of sterilization because of mental incapacity."[75] The biggest concern, he cautioned, emerged in the potential for legal complications in the future stemming from the sterilized woman, her family, or companions. He went on to explain that, despite these challenging legal concerns, the CMPA recognized the "pressing social reasons as well as medical and psychiatric indications for sterilization of mentally retarded persons."[76] Moreover, "the Association has concurred with decisions for sterilization of mentally retarded minors," in cases where both parents were in agreement with the decision – in fact, only when parents recommended the operation.

The CMPA stated emphatically that doctors should not initiate such a discussion. In a sustained effort to avoid future legal challenges, the association recommended a thorough set of assessments by a variety of medical professionals, including family physicians, psychologists, psychiatrists, and possibly social workers to ensure that there was sufficient documented professional support for a decision.[77] Building upon past legal precedents, he added that the procedure should be explained to the child before proceeding, if all other parties are in agreement. Women such as Leilani Muir and Doreen Befus had been victims of an older practice that ignored this feature of the sterilization process, and they later took the province to task for this gross oversight. A new generation of women in the mental health system, however, faced a different regime.

The directions and guidelines stipulated by the CMPA reflected its familiarity with the challenges posed by the eugenics program and its legacy, particularly for its lack of consent considerations, which ran roughshod over patients who had been deemed mentally incapable of providing consent: "We are particularly concerned about anything which might appear as an established program for 'wholesale' sterilizations of these patients ... We would be particularly concerned about the sterilization of a child unless the operation were requested by interested, concerned and attentive parents."[78] Whether responding to local sterilization policy or international programs that had garnered significant attention, the legal advice doled out to physicians by this time clearly stressed the need for consent as a sacrosanct feature of modern medical interventions.

By the end of the 1970s, the issue of sterilization surgery for adolescent children with severe mental and physical disabilities was attracting more publicity and becoming the focus of a review by the Law Commission of Canada aimed at providing legal guidance on the ethics of sterilization. Among the variety of proposals it received from across Canada was one from Ontario health minister Dennis Timbrell, who suggested abolishing all sterilizations of minors and individuals with mental disabilities. Timbrell's proposal followed the release of a report from Dr Zarfas, by then a special consultant on mental retardation with the Ontario Ministry of Community and Social Services, indicating that, in the absence of a clear policy on the matter, 608 individuals deemed mentally incompetent had been sterilized in 1976 without their consent, although the hospitals concerned had obtained consent from next of kin. Only fifty of the cases were men and boys.[79]

After thoroughly reviewing the proposals and existing and previous laws on sterilization, including those of Alberta and British Columbia, the commission concluded that individuals with mental illnesses "should not be sterilized against their will." Indeed, mentally handicapped persons "should have the same rights as other persons to consent to or refuse sterilization as long as they can understand the nature and consequences of the operation." The commission even went so far as to state that "sterilized mentally retarded persons tend to perceive sterilization as a symbol of reduced or degraded status."[80]

Building upon the themes of protection and autonomy, the commission noted that, "[i]n the zeal of the law to protect, what has occurred is protection 'against' rather than protection 'for' such categories of persons."[81] The language of protection assumed different meanings in the context of autonomy, and the commission further reminded Canadians of the need to "both protect such persons and still give adequate scope for individual choice to be expressed and to prevail. People who are mentally handicapped simply constitute a group with special needs. Self-respect, dignity, and self-determination must be guaranteed for each individual, including those with limitations. The law should not only uphold but also enhance these essential human qualities."[82]

None of the agencies in Alberta participated directly in the Law Commission, although many hospitals continued to seek clarification of their legal capacity to proceed with these operations. The legal team retained by Grace Hospital in Calgary, for example, reiterated the commission's advice, reminding Calgary-based physicians that Alberta had once maintained sterilization laws that had come under intense scrutiny: "with the repeal of that Act, there is no statutory provision expressly governing the sterilization of any persons, whether competent or incompetent."[83] Indeed, the commission had drawn attention to Alberta's sterilization laws, meaning that the province might face more sustained national scrutiny as a result, and any future policies in this area would require a careful balance of civil liberties.

With the repeal of the Sexual Sterilization Act, Alberta needed new legislation, and in 1976 it introduced the Dependent Adults Act, which laid out provisions for the guardians of dependent individuals over the age of eighteen. Guardians assumed the power and authority "to consent to any health care *that is in the best interests of the dependent adult* [emphasis in original]."[84] Health care had been defined in the earlier act to include "any procedure undertaken for the purpose of preventing pregnancy." The new legislation introduced different features of consent by elevating the status of third-party decision makers and fundamentally triangulating the politics of choice as it concerned reproductive autonomy. Indeed, in many cases, the issue was not whether a woman ultimately might bear children, but whether she passed through puberty with all of her sexual hormones and organs intact.

In the early 1980s Grace Hospital administrator David Luginbuhl, in concert with the Women's Social Services Secretary, and in an effort to embrace the case-by-case analysis recommended by the Law Commission, brought up three cases that he hoped would clarify the issue of sterilizing incompetent minors. The cases were those of girls who had been considered incompetent, incapable of controlling their bodily functions, and "unable to look after their personal hygiene." The parents in each case had requested hysterectomies for their daughters when they reached puberty, due to the challenges in dealing with their menses. The sterilization committee approved these operations, but Grace Hospital's administrators overruled the decisions, claiming a court order was needed before they could proceed. Luginbuhl expressed his exasperation that much paperwork had been filled out and time wasted, only to have the requests refused, to the frustration of the parents and doctors who had initiated the process. He maintained that such cases should be judged individually and that consideration be granted particularly in cases where a hysterectomy would alleviate the challenges posed to caregivers in dealing with the patient's inability to conduct personal hygiene.[85]

In such cases sterilization arose as an ethical and procedural issue. Although consent from parents and guardians appeared less difficult to obtain, the legal position remained murky. In the 1980s Grace Hospital struck a Medical Executive Sterilization Committee to review such files and adjudicate them on a case-by-case basis, as Luginbuhl had recommended. One woman in her twenties, whose case notes suggested she was plagued with a number of health concerns, among them glaucoma and hearing problems, appeared before the committee at the behest of her parents. Her mother had put her on the birth-control pill, but, believing it had contributed to her having a mild stroke, decided she should be sterilized instead. Under further examination during a CT scan, the patient appeared to exhibit an abnormality in her right brain hemisphere. No specific details explained the implications of this potential abnormality, but her mother felt that her general functioning had deteriorated since the stroke. The assessment concluded: "Mother doesn't feel that she can look after herself with her heavy menses, and in view of the multitude of problems I would be glad to agree that she should be considered as a candidate for hysterectomy."[86] A committee of four ultimately reviewed her medical and social situation and approved her for a total abdominal hysterectomy. In that case, her file also contained a consent form, signed by the patient herself, indicating that she understood the nature of the procedure and that she authorized a named surgeon to perform the operation "and any alternative procedures as he in his judgment deems advisable."[87]

Another case involved a young woman who had recently entered puberty and had considerable difficulty managing her personal hygiene. In correspondence between doctors, she was described as "markedly retarded, and slowly degenerating in this field. She is a semi cripple, deaf, has bi-lateral congenital glaucoma and many other small problems. I concur that a panhysterectomy and appendectomy ... is the recommended procedure of choice."[88]

Other such cases arose at the request of public guardians or foster parents. The foster mother of an eighteen-year-old girl described as "retarded" sought a total hysterectomy to stop her from menstruating. The girl had been in the custody of the Child Welfare Department for some time, and other caregivers had made several attempts to have her sterilized, but both Grace Hospital and the Calgary General Hospital had refused those requests. Her case notes reveal that her IQ had been assessed as 45 – ten points lower than Doreen Befus's – and she was therefore considered "severely mentally handicapped." Given the girl's status as a foster daughter and her seeming inability to comprehend the importance of hygiene during menstruation, her doctor sought advice as to the legality of performing a hysterectomy.[89] The Department of Social Services and Community Health responded two and a half months later, explaining that, under the Dependent Adults Act, the girl's legal guardian had sufficient authority to consent to such an operation. Department officials recommended, however, that her foster parents obtain a court order first, to ensure that all legal angles had been covered before proceeding. The department also encouraged her physician to consider several other factors before confirming that a hysterectomy was the most suitable solution, including whether the girl was even capable of reproduction, the extent of her exposure to sexual contact that might result in pregnancy, the feasibility of alternative forms of contraception, the availability of less-intrusive sterilization options, and the potential for future scientific advances that might address the girl's mental disability.

The department also spelled out a number of concerns that resembled those raised in connection with the now-defunct eugenic law: Could the dependent adult care for a child? Is the handicap hereditary or congenital? Are there confounding medical factors that might create a high risk pregnancy? If the hospital refused to perform the operation, would the family look elsewhere for the surgery?[90] Her doctor had already written to the sterilization committee at Grace Hospital stating that "I feel it is a very reasonable request that a hysterectomy be performed on [her] as the possibility of her ever being able to look after children is unthinkable and unrealistic."[91] Although the girl's legal guardians and her doctors recommended her for sterilization, the hospital administrators upheld the decision to refrain because they could not determine if the surgery would be in the patient's best interest. Thus, in this case, legal protection was extended to a "severely mentally handicapped" minor, but such protection dissolved once an individual no longer was covered under the dependent minors clause. The girl's doctor thus had the option of waiting until she turned eighteen and could be considered under the Dependent Adults Act, when her guardian could provide consent and the operation performed.[92]

These kinds of cases posed challenging medical, humanitarian, and legal questions, and although successive hospital policies attempted to erect strict guidelines to direct physicians and families, the case-by-case analysis meant that additional loopholes continued to arise. Grace Hospital changed its policy on sterilization throughout the 1980s in an attempt to distinguish between voluntary sterilizations sought by married or divorced women and those thought necessary for incompetent adults and minors. The Dependent Adults Act further separated these groups by age, with eighteen functioning as the dividing line. The sterilization committee reviewed the cases of incompetent minors, but insisted that parents or guardians obtain a court order before presenting such cases.

With these precautions the issue of autonomy slipped away from individuals and into the hands of guardians and medical and legal authorities, whose actions were guided more by concerns of liability. Subsequent changes to the policy retained this component, and thus helped to shield the hospital, physicians, and families from any legal retribution arising from a sterilization case. Competent minors and "incompetent adults," conversely, required no such court order before their parents or guardians could present the case to the sterilization committee.[93] These changes in policy in the 1980s regarding minors reflected a subtle shift in the power and authority, away from the state and the medical community exclusively, and ultimately back to families and guardians.

Despite successive revisions to the policy, involuntary sterilization remained difficult to standardize. In 1987 the issue emerged once more at Grace Hospital, this time involving a sixteen-year-old girl described as "profoundly retarded." Although she was capable of taking care of herself, of managing her menses, and even of some basic learning, her mental state was somewhat static, and her doctor stated explicitly that "she just really could not bring up or look after a baby."[94] Thus, despite being otherwise capable and healthy, the girl's apparent inability to parent meant her potential sterilization. Her case helps to illustrate one of the ways in which eugenics language remained part of the conversation about sterilization as it pertained to assumptions about responsible motherhood.

Conclusion

At the end of the 1980s the Supreme Court of Canada amended the Criminal Code to remove the health risk clause from the abortion section. Chief Justice Brian Dickson declared that "[s]ection 251 clearly interferes with a woman's bodily integrity in both a physical and an emotional sense. Forcing a woman, by threat of criminal sanction, to carry a foetus to term unless she meets certain criteria unrelated to her own priorities and aspirations, is a profound interference with a woman's body and thus a violation of security of person."[95] Thus, as the twentieth century neared its end, the politics of reproductive choice became infused with the language of liberalism and autonomy. For some women, exercising reproductive choice meant retaining access to medical services without judgment. For others, however, it meant freedom *from* medical intervention. For women caught in the web of social services and welfare, the repeal of sexual sterilization laws and the decriminalization of abortion did not usher in an uncomplicated era of reproductive choice or introduce new degrees of autonomy. Instead, women such as Jane Doe, who at fifteen entered the Foothills Hospital in search of a sympathetic obstetrician to relieve her of the burden of teenage motherhood, increasingly came under the purview of the medical services.

In the 1970s the relaxation of the legal use of contraceptive devices, abortion, and even sterilization altered the meanings of reproductive language and created new opportunities for women. In the initial steps down that path, a degree of medical-legal authority over women was retained, as abortions became permissible only when a team of medical experts could identify health risks to the mother. Women who sought an abortion or sterilization still had to surrender themselves to the judgment of medical and legal authorities about their choices, their futures, and, ultimately, their likelihood of becoming responsible mothers. Medical and legal dominance of the language of morality combined with the view that teenage girls and women with disabilities would make poor mothers and that married women denigrated the role of motherhood if they sought to restrict their natural fertility. These debates contributed to the further medicalization and pathologization of women's bodies and behaviour even as women attempted to secure a measure of autonomy over their reproductive choices.

Chapter Eight

Conclusion

In 1972 the newly elected Conservative government of Peter Lougheed struck down Alberta's Sexual Sterilization Act, claiming it no longer served its purpose. During his time as leader of the opposition, Lougheed had received letters encouraging him to make this move once elected. The head of genetics at the University of Alberta, Dr Jan Weijer, for instance, complained that the Eugenics Board no longer had the expertise to make a genetic judgment on cases, and its actions "no longer reflect[ed] our modern genetical [*sic*] knowledge on these matters."[1] Weijer's letter had been prompted by an article in the *Globe and Mail* about a woman who had been sterilized in Alberta as a teenager, then went on to complete her grade twelve education. The article explained that, although some groups agreed with the idea of voluntary sterilization, compulsory sterilization for people considered unfit defied modern concepts of human rights and medical science.[2] Law professor Bernard Dickens also castigated the outdated law, explaining that "it was permeated with biological and social fallacies, and was more a product of anti-science than of science."[3]

Even as the new government struck down the legislation, some newspaper readers were shocked to learn that it had even still existed. Albertans congratulated themselves on closing the book on a dark chapter of their provincial history and moving towards a more enlightened future, one that cherished human rights and modern medical ethics. Yet, despite these legislative changes, heated debates over reproductive rights continued to attract public attention and remained an issue at the ballot box. As recently as 2012 Prime Minister Stephen Harper came under attack from opposition members as well as from within the ranks of his own Conservative Party for not effectively managing abortion legislation. Fellow Conservatives, including a handful of prairie-based Members of Parliament, publicly demanded that Harper reopen the debate on abortion. Stephen Woodworth, MP for Kitchener Centre, introduced a private member's bill asking that a special committee of the House of Commons be struck to revisit the Criminal Code on the issue of when a "child becomes a human being,"[4] implying that abortion could be considered murder.

In April 2012, following the first reading of the bill, the CBC reported that, "despite Stephen Harper's determination not to reopen the abortion debate, the issue is back in the parliamentary spotlight as MPs consider whether to create a committee to look at the legal definition of when human life begins."[5] The frustration with the prime minister from within his party ranks stemmed from his resistance to reopening the debate and for his failure to register his own views on the controversial topic. Opposition members, and perhaps Harper himself, remained critical of the concept of abortion as murder. Some parties, including the official opposition New Democratic Party, defined their position as pro-choice; their stance did not negate the timing of life after conception, but emphasized a woman's right to choose whether or not to terminate a pregnancy before twenty weeks' gestation in a free, informed, and non-coercive environment. Liberals and New Democrats alike thus officially supported the legislation that has been in place since Trudeau's amendments to the Criminal Code.

Although Prime Minister Harper has attempted to maintain the status quo, factions on the political and religious right continue to pressure his government to reconsider the law in light of new evidence. In the *National Post*, for example, Michael Schouten, director of an organization that promotes a change in the abortion law, offered his political analysis of the situation as it affected election returns, suggesting that "the Prime Minister believes that an abortion debate would hurt his party in the polls. I [an avowed pro-life advocate] submit the opposite." Schouten connected Harper's liberal stance on abortion directly with a dip in his approval rating and the corresponding shift in popularity towards the New Democrats. Schouten concluded his article with a blunt recommendation: "there is still time to heal the damage and to woo back those millions of votes. Let's have the [abortion] debate."[6] Implying that voters had turned their backs on the Conservatives because they failed to take a public and united stand against abortion might be to misread the electorate, but Schouten's article stands as a fierce reminder that the issue of reproductive rights continues to fuel ideological battles.

In the event, the bill was defeated in the House of Commons on 26 September 2012 by a vote of 203 to 91. Among those who supported the bill was Rona Ambrose, then Minister for the Status of Women and MP for Edmonton-Spruce Grove, who subsequently faced public pressure from pro-choice and other organizations in favour of the advancement of women to resign her post since she could not fairly represent and promote the status of women while holding decidedly anti-women and anti-choice views.[7] In her defence Ambrose claimed she had voted for the bill on account of discrimination against girls in sex-selection abortions.

To reopen the abortion debate in the twenty-first century requires examining where to draw the moral line between pro-life and pro-choice perspectives. Pro-life advocates suggest it should be at the point of conception, and any deviation from that stance implies murder, or at least an anti-life response. For pro-choice supporters, the line is a matter of autonomy and individual responsibility; they argue that third-party decision making or top-down authority denies basic human rights and is a breach of modern ethics. Interestingly, both perspectives separate themselves from the dark, even heinous history of eugenics, which has had much less regard for either the definition of life or the concept of free choice or individual autonomy. In this, both sides mount their arguments as enlightened, reasonable steps away from misguided and malicious historical approaches to population control.

These perspectives, however, have become locked in an intractable debate that relies on fundamental differences in how we define reproductive rights and for whom. Both sides select historical precedents to support their arguments, but in so doing they often oversimplify the past to clarify their viewpoints. The respective advocates attempt to assume the moral high ground by distancing themselves from the history of eugenics. Pro-life supporters do so by maintaining a zero tolerance of abortion, and some include sterilization and contraception in their condemnation. Pro-choice advocates seize upon the language of force and coercion that was intimately woven into eugenics programs, whether it existed as a criterion of consent or contributed to broader coercive measures associated with institutionalization. This conceptual framing of eugenics for the purposes of current debates provides a convenient approach for bolstering support for pro-life and pro-choice campaigns, but it fails to appreciate the more complicated historical terrain.

The history of reproductive politics is complicated. Through the swirl of debates surrounding sterilization, contraception, and abortion, loud voices have often been raised to condemn seekers of such choices for their carelessness and irresponsibility. Carelessness has been framed in terms of personal hygiene, proximity to mainstream values – whether Anglo-Saxon, middle-class, or heterosexual – and intelligence or ability. Irresponsibility has been used to justify intervening in people's lives, sometimes coercively, and, in the case of eugenics, to curb their fertility. It has also been applied to people who independently sought ways to control their reproduction and, in doing so, allegedly flaunted their personal autonomy, which to some observers undermined the sanctity of so-called natural or traditional family values. Historically many people and groups have crossed this culturally defined line that distinguishes good behaviour from bad, a humanitarian from an inhumane approach to reproduction. Indeed, the line itself has shifted over time, its position determined by social, political, religious, and medical attitudes that are continually refreshed and revisited, whether by new evidence or by more traditional ideas about the proper conduct of men, women, and families.

Current debates largely ignore this more nuanced past, however, in an attempt to relocate the dividing line and provide a different legislative benchmark. As I have attempted to illustrate by the cases in this book, the politics of reproduction often spill outside the confines of legislation, which suggests that even subsequent legal changes might not diminish fundamentally divisive cultural dispositions towards this contentious topic. Although past laws provided focal points for establishing eugenics programs and defining legal contraception, sterilization and the right to autonomous decisions about reproduction remain contested subjects. Eugenic ideas were not simply contained within the policies of the Sexual Sterilization Act, and debates about human value and reproduction continue in the post-eugenics era. Overturning that specific law was more than just a salutary gesture, but the resurgence of the abortion issue in Canadian politics shows that these issues remain part of an evolving and historically sensitive discourse about reproductive rights.

The current context also reminds us of the fluid nature of political positions in these debates. In 2012, as historically, the ideological terrain was not clear-cut. Pro-life advocates attempt to discredit pro-choice supporters by drawing attention to the ways in which their reform-minded antecedents supported eugenics. Feminists, for example, have been implicated throughout eugenics history as promoters of punitive sterilization laws, but also as supporters of a more autonomous decision-making apparatus for reproductive and human rights. During the lead-up to

Alberta's sexual sterilization laws in the 1920s, reproductive rights were entangled in debates about autonomy for women, which at that time also involved lobbying for political enfranchisement and the right to hold positions of authority as qualified persons. Contemporary feminists, including politically powerful women on the front lines such as Violet McNaughton and Irene Parlby, underwent sexual sterilization operations. Although their operations treated cancerous tumours, and they concealed their experiences from the public, they nonetheless emerged as childless players on the feminist stage during a time when feminism and motherhood went hand in hand. Sexual sterilization then, as later, did not simply represent an application of a eugenics philosophy. McNaughton's and Parlby's decisions, forty years later, might have been celebrated as a strident expression of autonomy and deviation from patriarchal values that confined women to motherhood and domesticity.

Second-wave feminists flung open the metaphorical door to contraception, and their activism put critical pressure on governments in North America to decriminalize acts related to reproductive control. These campaigns did not encompass the views of all women, but they effectively exposed how patriarchal levers of control over reproduction had been distorted under the cloak of medical science. Although Catholic doctrine held firm in its defence of the traditional family and the natural laws of fertility, the medical community at times provided secular evidence to reaffirm the correctness of this position. These odd bedfellows came to represent a patriarchal grip on authority, which helped to galvanize support for collective action framed along the lines of a newly defined feminism and autonomy.

Socialists emerged as another set of progressive players caught red-handed in eugenics history. Co-operative Commonwealth Federation leaders T.C. Douglas and J.S. Woodsworth supported both sterilization and contraception and, in a debate that draws the line at life, these figures fall easily into the anti-life category. Placed in their historical context, however, these reformers viewed eugenics as part and parcel of building a healthy community. For both Douglas and Woodsworth religion had a fundamental role to play in embracing people, while medicine had a social and political responsibility to provide meaningful options for struggling families. Much like debates about the regulation of vice, liberal approaches routinely argue that legalizing or regulating activities such as drug use give society the means to police and discipline such behaviour. Conversely, criminalizing vice forces participants to conceal their activities from the authorities and public health officials.

Clandestine vice, whether sexual or addictive in nature, introduces higher elements of risk and invariably results in greater social and financial costs to society. Douglas and Woodsworth, among others, adopted a similar philosophy when it came to sterilization and contraception. They accepted that families, especially newly arrived immigrants to Woodsworth's Winnipeg or desperate Depression-era farmers in Douglas's Saskatchewan, were taking greater risks to control fertility in pursuit of survival on the prairies. Legalizing and regulating medical services aimed at fertility arose as a responsible way to manage the health risks that imperilled such families.

Players from the other side have been equally implicated in the messy eugenics past. Social Credit governments praised for their conservative stance on resource development and embrace of capitalism borrowed eugenic precepts from the ideological left and transformed them into a politically palatable approach to population control. For families like the Mannings, the issue was intensely personal: Ernest Manning's eldest son lived most of his life in an institution for mentally deficient children. Yet Manning embodied the populist, fiscally conservative, Depression-era politician whose views on cumbersome state institutions complemented those of his peers: such facilities were expensive. Manning articulated a logical justification of sterilization that matched his dual roles as premier and father. Sterilization offered a defensible humanitarian response to the expensive prospect of institutionalizing generations of individuals with mental disabilities or of providing services for orphaned children whose biological parents could not take care of them.

Catholic views likewise have been held up as self-righteously anti-eugenic, particularly given the Church's firm stance on family values and intolerance of all matters of contraception, including sterilization and especially abortion. Papal doctrine in the 1930s, however, bowed to the suggestion that sterilization was justified for social purposes for those considered mentally defective or feeble minded. Although that acceptance was short lived, it nonetheless indicates that, even among some of the staunchest of today's pro-life supporters, a different set of ingredients complicated the issue in the past, particularly with respect to concerns about disability. Indeed, as the debate wore on, rank-and-file Catholics across the prairies, as elsewhere, appeared to ignore papal doctrine when it suited their personal needs. These decisions at the personal level suggest that high-level doctrine, individual practice, and social experiences require different sets of analyses, and warn against assumptions about a unified Catholic response to the issue of reproductive rights.

Historical consideration and context therefore encourage deeper reflections on the enduring meanings of the controversies surrounding the politics of reproductive choice. If one recasts the issue, not as jockeying for the upper hand on the morality of life or maternal autonomy, but as exposing the history of authority over human value, a different picture emerges. Intelligence arises as the dividing line between good and bad, responsible and irresponsible. Good, responsible behaviour in the first half of the twentieth century included conforming to Anglo-Saxon Protestant values, even if that meant assimilating into a new culture or relinquishing traditional practices in a clear expression of subservience to a different set of social and political authorities. Bad, irresponsible behaviour at times also included challenging authorities. It included married women who challenged physicians in their role as health advisors. It also included Aboriginal people who sought the advice of their own healers instead of embracing Western medical solutions even to common health problems. Cultural authorities – whether elite feminists, elected officials, protected surgeons, or seemingly celibate Catholic priests – controlled the discourse on intelligence and responsible behaviour, which reinforced the parameters governing the ability of certain segments of the population to make their own choices.

Although it is tempting to paint a picture of authority with a patriarchal brush, equating authority with males and victims with females would be an oversimplification. Men and women have been on both sides of the equation. Casting them in black and white roles in the context of debates on reproductive rights would perpetuate misleading characterizations that women were the overwhelming victims of the sterilization program or that male physicians were rigid obstacles to women's gaining access to regulated operations. Much like the ideological and religious arguments for and against sterilization, activists on both sides have adjusted their positions in these debates over time.

Concepts of intelligence played an important role in the eugenic classification of institutionalized individuals, particularly those considered feeble minded or mentally deficient. Intelligence quotients indeed functioned as the dividing line in cases where both consent and disclosure hinged upon a subject's presumed ability to comprehend the consequences of the surgery. In that context a different set of victims clearly emerged alongside a more heterogeneous assembly of authoritative voices justifying that categorization. Individuals such as Leilani Muir, Ken Nelson, Doreen Befus, Nora Powers, and George Pierre were among the most marginalized and least powerful in society. Heaping labels of mental deficiency on orphaned, abandoned, racialized, or incarcerated individuals ensured that their perspectives continued to be discounted. On that matter, the rising tide of support for their sterilization or confinement included a motley crew of strange bedfellows that changed over time but included first-wave feminists, Catholics, socialists, conservatives, physicians, psychiatrists, social workers, and voters. People from families in marginal circumstances were subjected disproportionately to sterilization. They faced a strong and, at times, relatively united front consisting of a varied group of cultural authorities who continue to influence definitions of family values and intelligence.

The justifications for sterilizations performed on such people were packaged in various ways, from hereditary arguments to concerns about responsible parenthood, the financial burden on taxpayers and the state, and the need to help parents and guardians coping with disabled children. Cloaked in the language of humanitarian intervention, the subjects of these operations were considered irresponsible or incapable of authorizing decisions affecting their own bodies. They were also considered unqualified to act as full citizens, whether due to their apparent lack of intelligence or maturity or simply their age.

Given the use of intelligence and ability as an enduring barometer of human value, it is all the more remarkable that people such as Doreen Befus and Leilani Muir gained the confidence to speak publicly about reproductive rights and sterilization from their personal perspectives. What is perhaps equally remarkable is that these women refused to subscribe to polarized debates about reproductive rights – of life versus choice – but offered much more nuanced and reflective insights. Doreen's work in the community, often as a surrogate aunt, housekeeper, babysitter, and caregiver, prompted her to confront these issues directly, and fuelled her outrage at a system that had robbed her of her ovaries with no regard for her personal views or capabilities. Both her subsequent work and her thoughtful reflection challenged assumptions that she was unfit to be a responsible mother or insufficiently intelligent to live independently. Leilani's experiences underscore the misapplication of intelligence testing in a manner that went well beyond the inherent cultural biases embedded in such evaluations and redirected her life. Leilani, in fact, proved quite capable of challenging provincial laws at the highest level, and did so on the basis of abuse of authority over institutionalized bodies. That her intelligence quotient had been added incorrectly emerged as a cruel irony.

A social history of the eugenics program in Alberta helps to avoid the temptation to judge debates on reproductive or fetal rights using the language of pro- or anti-choice and pro- or anti-life. Historical distance shows us that the moral terrain has changed over time with the introduction of new information, amended laws, and shifting cultural authority. External influences have been significant in how we understand this moral ground. By considering sterilization, contraception, and abortion against the historical backdrop of eugenics and over the course of the twentieth century, it becomes clear that there is no uncomplicated moral high ground in these discussions; instead, what is revealed is a complex history layered with generations of assumptions about population control, degeneracy, responsibility, intelligence, mental health, and progress. A closer look at these different historical layers reinforces the importance of acknowledging the distinctions between institutionalized and non-institutionalized experiences, the way we comprehend intelligence and its bearing on citizenship, and the gendered assumptions that have influenced our understanding of control and autonomy. Finally, it shows how sexual sterilization, which has been an important feature of modern society, has contributed to shaping attitudes about collective rights, feminism, masculinity, and, ultimately, the politics of reproductive choice.

Notes

Introduction

1 Law Reform Commission of Canada, "Sterilization: Implications for Mentally Retarded and Mentally Ill Persons," Working Paper 24 (Ottawa: Law Reform Commission of Canada, 1979), 29.
2 Ibid., 27.
3 Paul Lombardo, ed., *A Century of Eugenics in America: From the Indiana Experiment to the Human Genome Era* (Bloomington: Indiana University Press, 2011), ix.
4 Daniel Kevles, *In the Name of Eugenics: Genetics and the Uses of Human Heredity*, 2nd ed. (Cambridge, MA: Harvard University Press, 1995), xiii.
5 For examples, see Leonard Darwin, *What Is Eugenics?* (London: Watts and Company, 1928); Frances Galton, *Inquiries into Human Faculty and Its Development* (London: J.M. Dent and Sons, 1907); Julian Huxley, *Essays of a Biologist* (London: Chatto and Windus, 1923); Bertrand Russell, *Marriage and Morals* (New York: Liveright, 1929); and T.W. Shannon, Samuel Fallows, and W.J. Truitt, eds., *Eugenics* or *Nature's Secrets Revealed: Scientific Knowledge of the Laws of Sex Life and Heredity* (Marietta, OH: S.A. Mullikin Company, 1917). See also Pauline Mazumdar's historical study of the British Eugenics Society, *Eugenics, Human Genetics and Human Failings: The Eugenics Society, Its Sources and Its Critics in Britain* (London: Routledge, 1992).
6 Marius Turda, *Modernism and Eugenics* (Basingstoke, UK: Palgrave Macmillan, 2010), 6.
7 See Angélique Richardson, *Love and Eugenics in the Late Nineteenth Century: Rational Reproduction and the New Woman* (Oxford: Oxford University Press, 2003).

8 See, for example, Paul Lombardo, "Anthropometry, Race, and Eugenic Research: 'Measurements of Growing Negro Children' at the Tuskegee Institute, 1932–1944," in *The Uses of Humans in Experimentation*, ed. Erika Dyck and Larry Stewart (forthcoming).

9 For more in-depth examples of US eugenics programs by region, see, in particular, Lombardo, *Century of Eugenics in America*.

10 Scholarship on eugenics has thus tended to focus on the association between eugenics and Holocaust or genocide studies. Within this tradition historians have emphasized how medical and scientific studies were used to authorize the state's involvement in crude human experimentation and annihilation. See, for example, Lombardo, *Century of Eugenics in America*, 1; André Pichot, *The Pure Society: From Darwin to Hitler*, trans. David Fernbach (London: Verso, 2009); Robert Proctor, *Racial Hygiene: Medicine under the Nazis* (Cambridge, MA: Harvard University Press, 1988); and Vivien Spitz, *Doctors from Hell: The Horrific Account of Nazi Experiments on Humans* (Boulder, CO: Sentient Publications, 2005).

11 See Michael H. Kater, *Doctors under Hitler* (Chapel Hill: University of North Carolina Press, 1989); Proctor, *Racial Hygiene*; and Paul Weindling, *Health, Race, and German Politics between National Unification and Nazism, 1870–1945* (Cambridge: Cambridge University Press, 1989).

12 Ian Dowbiggin, *The Sterilization Movement and Global Fertility in the Twentieth Century* (Oxford: Oxford University Press, 2008).

13 For an example of this characterization, see Janice Fiamengo, *The Women's Page: Journalism and Rhetoric in Early Canada* (Toronto: University of Toronto Press, 2008), especially chap. 6 on Nellie McClung.

14 See J.S. Woodsworth, *Strangers within Our Gates* (1909; repr. Toronto: University of Toronto Press, 1972). See also Howard Palmer, *Patterns of Prejudice: A History of Nativism in Alberta* (Toronto: McClelland & Stewart, 1985).

15 See Bill Waiser, *Saskatchewan: A New History* (Calgary: Fifth House, 2005), 249–51.

16 See Ramsay Cook, *The Regenerators: Social Criticism in Late Victorian English Canada* (Toronto: University of Toronto Press, 1985).

17 For more on the rise of the United Farmers of Alberta, see Bradford Rennie, *The Rise of Agrarian Democracy: The United Farmers and Farm Women of Alberta, 1909–1921* (Toronto: University of Toronto Press, 2000).

18 See Sheila Gibbons, "The True [Political] Mothers of Tomorrow: Eugenics and Feminism in Alberta" (MA thesis, University of Saskatchewan, 2012).

19 Amy Samson, "Coercion, Surveillance and Eugenics" (PhD diss., University of Saskatchewan, in progress).

20 Alexandra Minna Stern, *Eugenic Nation: Faults and Frontiers of Better Breed-ing in Modern America* (Berkeley: University of California Press, 2005), 100. Stern also notes that over 80 per cent of the sterilizations took place in two California hospitals in Stockton and Sonoma.

21 Eugenics Board Meeting Minutes, Binder 1, letter to Grand Knight C.C. Connolly, Knights of Columbus, 28 November 1946, 4.

22 Howard Palmer and Tamara Palmer, *Alberta: A New History* (Edmonton: Hurtig, 1990), 198–9.

23 See Amy Samson, "Eugenics in the Community: Alberta's Sexual Steriliza-tion Act, 1928–1972," *Canadian Bulletin of Medical History* (under review).

24 See Terry L. Chapman, "Early Eugenics Movements in Western Canada," *Alberta History* 25, no. 4 (1977): 9–17; Cecily Devereux, *Growing a Race: Nellie L. McClung and the Fiction of Eugenic Feminism* (Montreal; Kingston, ON: McGill-Queen's University Press, 2006); and Angus McLaren, *Our Own Master Race: Eugenics in Canada, 1885–1945* (Toronto: McClelland & Stewart, 1990).

25 Jana Grekul, "Social Construction of the Feeble-Minded Threat" (PhD diss., University of Alberta, 2002). See also Jana Grekul, Harvey Krahn, and David Odynak, "Sterilizing the 'Feeble-minded': Eugenics in Alberta, Canada, 1929–1972," *Journal of Historical Sociology* 17, no. 4 (2004): 358–84.

26 Exceptions include Chapman, "Early Eugenics Movements in Western Canada"; and Robert Lampard, "The Sexual Sterilization Act of Alberta: An Introduction, 1928–1972," in *Alberta's Medical History: Young and Lusty, and Full of Life* (Red Deer, AB: Robert Lampard, 2008).

27 Jana Grekul, "Sterilization in Alberta, 1928–1972: Gender Matters," *Canadian Review of Sociology* 45, no. 3 (2008): 247–66.

28 Timothy Christian, "The Mentally Ill and Human Rights in Alberta: A Study of the Alberta Sexual Sterilization Act" (honours thesis, University of Alberta, 1974).

29 Timothy Caulfield and Gerald Robertson, "Eugenic Policies in Alberta: From the Systematic to the Systemic?" *Alberta Law Review* 35, no. 1 (1996): 59–79.

30 Douglas Wahlsten, "Leilani Muir versus the Philosopher King: Eugenics on Trial in Alberta," *Genetica* 99, no. 2–3 (1997): 185–98.

31 Jane Harris-Zsovan, *Eugenics and the Firewall: Canada's Nasty Little Secret* (Winnipeg: J. Gordon Shillingford, 2008).

32 See, for example, Ruth Schwartz Cowan, *Heredity and Hope: The Case for Genetic Screening* (Cambridge, MA: Harvard University Press, 2008); Dowbiggin, *Sterilization Movement*; Susanne Klausen, *Race, Maternity, and the Politics of Birth Control in South Africa, 1910–1939* (New York: Palgrave

Macmillan, 2004); Wendy Kline, *Building a Better Race: Gender, Sexuality, and Eugenics from the Turn of the Century to the Baby Boom* (Berkeley: University of California Press, 2001); Rebecca Kluchin, *Fit to Be Tied: Sterilization and Reproductive Rights in America, 1950–1980* (New Brunswick, NJ: Rutgers University Press, 2009); Molly Ladd-Taylor, "Sterilizing the 'Retarded': Contraceptive Surgery and Eugenics in the 1970s and 1980s," *Canadian Bulletin of Medical History* (under review); Susan Lindee, *Moments of Truth in Genetic Medicine* (Baltimore: Johns Hopkins University Press, 2005); Paul Lombardo, *Three Generations, No Imbeciles: Eugenics, the Supreme Court, and Buck v. Bell* (Baltimore: Johns Hopkins University Press, 2008); Johanna Schoen, *Choice and Coercion: Birth Control, Sterilization, and Abortion in Public Health and Welfare* (Chapel Hill: University of North Carolina Press, 2005); and Stern, *Eugenic Nation.*

33 Lombardo, *Three Generations, No Imbeciles.*

34 Gunnar Broberg and Nils Roll-Hansen, eds., *Eugenics and the Welfare State: Norway, Sweden, Denmark, and Finland* (Ann Arbor: Michigan State University Press, 2005); Daniel Kevles, *In the Name of Eugenics: Genetics and the Uses of Human Heredity*, new ed. (Cambridge MA: Harvard University Press, 2004); Mazumdar, *Eugenics, Human Genetics and Human Failings*; and Weindling, *Health, Race and German Politics.*

35 Cowan, *Heredity and Hope.*

36 Dowbiggin, *Sterilization Movement.*

1. Vagrancy, Violence, and Virtue

1 Provincial Archives of Alberta (hereafter cited as PAA), Attorney General Files, 75.126, 1309, Box 87, "Crime Report," 12 May 1924.

2 PAA, Attorney General Files, 75.126, 1309, Box 87, memo from Deputy Attorney General to Provincial Jail Warden, re: Mrs Powers, 2 June 1924.

3 PAA, Attorney General Files, 75.126, 1309, Box 87, letter from William Power to Claresholm, to wife Nora Powers; a copy was sent from the jail to the Attorney General, 20 June 1924.

4 PAA, Attorney General Files, 75.126, 1309, Box 87, memo from Deputy Attorney General to Provincial Jail Warden, re: Mrs Powers, 9 June 1924.

5 PAA, Attorney General Files, 75.126, 1309, Box 87, letter from Dr Henry to Provincial Jail Warden, Re: Mrs Powers, 10 June 1924.

6 PAA, Attorney General Files, 75.126, 1309, Box 87, quoted in letter from Deputy Attorney General to Mrs Louise C. McKinney, 23 June 1924.

7 PAA, Attorney General Files, 75.126, 1309, Box 87, letter from Dr T.W.E. Henry, 19 June 1924.

8 Rennie, *Rise of Agrarian Democracy*, 7.
9 This sentiment is expressed in the UFA's records: "Women's most important place is in the home as Mother of the Race" (United Farmers of Alberta, *Annual Report 1916*, 126). Bradford Rennie also explains that the president of the United Farm Women of Alberta, Irene Parlby, stressed that women's roles were best suited not for formal politics but rather for the "politics" of the home "as a mother of the race"; Rennie, *Rise of Agrarian Democracy*, 117.
10 Gibbons, "True [Political] Mothers of Tomorrow."
11 UFA, *Annual Report 1918*, 147.
12 Rennie, *Rise of Agrarian Democracy*, 118.
13 Ibid., 119.
14 PAA, GR 1975.0126/1309, Attorney General Files, 4-M-4, Mental Defectives Act, 31 December 1925.
15 For more on this connection, see Devereux, *Growing a Race*; and Grekul, "Sterilization in Alberta."
16 UFWA, "Minutes of Board Meeting, January 15, 1923," 84.
17 See examples in UFWA, "Reports and Addresses to the 11th Annual Convention, 1925," 22, 23, 27; and idem, "Annual Address of the President of the UFWA, 1925," 21, 22, 38, 39.
18 UFWA, "Reports and Addresses to the 11th Annual Convention, 1925," 21.
19 UFWA, "Board Meeting, 1926," 144.
20 UFWA, "13th Annual Convention, 1927," 127.
21 For a more in-depth explanation of some of the religious and social reformist attitudes behind this development, see, especially, Cook, *Regenerators*.
22 For more on the British side, see, especially, Mazumdar, *Eugenics, Human Genetics and Human Failings*.
23 For a historical review of these studies, see Paul Lombardo, "Return of the Jukes: Eugenic Mythologies and Internet Evangelism," *Journal of Legal Medicine* 33 (2012): 207–33.
24 Paul A. Lombardo, "Davenport's Dream: 21st Century Reflections on Heredity and Eugenics," *Quarterly Review of Biology* 84, no. 2 (2009): 178. Davenport was also the founder of the Eugenics Record Office and thus an influential figure in the US eugenics movement.
25 Charles Davenport, "The Nams: The Feeble-minded as Country Dwellers," *American Philosophical Society*, 2 March 1912, 1844.
26 Ibid., 1845.
27 Richard Dugdale, *The Jukes: A Record and Study of the Relations of Crime, Pauperism, Disease and Heredity* (New York: G.P. Putnam Sons, 1874), 11, 12, where he explains his method in this regard.

28 For more on the photographs, see R.E. Fancher, "Henry Goddard and the Kallikak Family Photographs," *American Psychologist* 42, no. 6 (1987): 585–90. See also National Film Board of Canada, *The Sterilization of Leilani Muir* (Ottawa, 1996).

29 Henry Goddard, *The Kallikak Family: A Study in the Heredity of Feeble-Mindedness* (New York: Macmillan, 1912), 12.

30 Tommy C. Douglas, "The Problems of the Subnormal Family" (MA thesis, McMaster University, 1933), 1.

31 Ibid.

32 Ibid., 2.

33 Ibid., 5, 6.

34 Ibid., 9. He later elaborated on this point, stating: "they tend to set up the mores for their own group rather than to live by the moral standards of society" (16).

35 For more on these elements, see ibid., 20–7.

36 Ibid., 28.

37 Ibid., 26.

38 Ibid., 27.

39 Ibid., 32.

40 Ibid., 32–3.

41 Ibid., 33.

42 This explanation appears, for example, in Angus McLaren, *Our Own Master Race: Eugenics in Canada, 1885–1945* (Toronto: McClelland & Stewart, 1990), 9.

43 See, for example, Tom Blackwell, "Canadians airbrush the truth about Tommy Douglas's enthusiasm for eugenics: MD," *National Post*, 14 March 2012, available online at http://news.nationalpost.com/2012/03/14/tommy-douglas/, accessed 19 March 2012; and Michael Shevell, "A Canadian Paradox: Tommy Douglas and Eugenics," *Canadian Journal of Neurological Sciences* 39, no. 1 (2012): 35–9.

44 PAA, 83.391, File GSE 116, "Mental Health Surveys in Alberta," 1 [n.d., estimated, 1968].

45 For more sustained studies of the social reform movement and its relationship with eugenics, see, especially, Mariana Valverde, *The Age of Light, Soap and Water: Moral Reform in English Canada, 1885–1925* (Toronto: Oxford University Press, 1991); McLaren, *Our Own Master Race*; and Cook, *Regenerators*.

46 McLaren, *Our Own Master Race*, 59.

47 See, especially, ibid., chap. 3.

48 Centre for Addiction and Mental Health Archives (hereafter cited as CAMH Archives), "Mental Hygiene of the Province of Alberta, Canadian

National Committee for Mental Hygiene," October–November 1921, 2. Additional surveys were conducted in 1928 and 1947.

49 Ibid., 6.

50 For more on the notion of Canada as a "dumping ground," see Myra Rutherdale, "'Canada is no dumping ground': Public Discourse and Salvation Army Women and Children, 1900–1930," *Social History* 40, no. 79 (2007): 115–42.

51 Ibid., 142.

52 J.S. Woodsworth, *Strangers within Our Gates* (Toronto: Doreen Stephen Books, 1909), preface.

53 J.S. Woodsworth, *Strangers within Our Gates* (1909; repr. Toronto: University of Toronto Press, 1972), 133.

54 Ibid., 167.

55 PAA, 73A. Premier's Papers, memo to Premier from Alberta Government Liquor Control Board, Enforcement Branch, 26 June 1924.

56 PAA, Attorney General Files, 75.126, 1309, Box 87, letter from [illegible], RR1 Pickardville, to Alberta Provincial Police, 14 April 1924.

57 PAA, Attorney General Files, 75.126, 1309, Box 87, report from Constable, Alberta Provincial Police, File 23 #32, "A" Division, 27 April 1924.

58 PAA, Attorney General Files, 75.126, 1309, Box 87, Police Report: re: William Wallace, Alberta Provincial Police, Lethbridge, 14 March 1923.

59 PAA, 73A, memo from Attorney General's Office to Premier Brownlee, 19 October 1926.

60 Suspicions had been founded in the United States, where a vocal and aggressive Italian anarchist movement flared up in the 1920s. See Paul Avrich, *Sacco and Vanzetti: The Anarchist Background* (Princeton, NJ: Princeton University Press, 1996).

61 PAA, Premier's Office Fonds, 69.289, roll 433, "Report on Conditions in the Foreign Districts," from the Minister of Health to Hon. Mr Greenfield, 13 October 1921, 2.

62 Ibid.

63 Ibid., 4–5.

64 Ibid., 6.

65 PAA, Premier's Office Fonds, 69.289, roll 433, "Report on Conditions in the Foreign Districts," from the Minister of Health to Hon. Mr Greenfield, 13 October 1921, 1.

66 Ibid., 3.

67 Ibid., 5.

68 Ibid., 8.

69 See Samson, "Coercion, Surveillance and Eugenics."

70 PAA, Premier's Office Fonds, 69.289, roll 433, memo from Dr Laidlaw, Department of Health, to Premier Brownlee, 6 November 1924.

71 Ibid.

72 Ibid., 2. There is no further elaboration on race at this instance.

73 PAA, Premier's Office Fonds, 69.289, roll 433, memo from Miss E. Clark (Nursing Branch) to Dr W.C. Laidlaw, Deputy Minister of Health, 10 September 1924, 1.

74 Another case involved a family that had recently given birth to a baby who was a "suspect mental defective," which put the family on the potential for deportation list; see ibid.

75 Ibid., 4.

76 PAA, 73B, report from Commanding Sergeant Albert Chapman to the Alberta Provincial Police (Grand Prairie Division), 31 August 1925.

77 PAA, Attorney General Files, 75.126, 1309, Box 87, letter from Relief Officer, Miss M.A. Carson, to Attorney General's Office, 12 September 1922.

78 PAA, Attorney General Files, 75.126, 1309, Box 87, letter from C.H. Lawford, MD, to C.B. Hill (inspector), Smoky Lake, 2 September 1921.

79 PAA, 73B, memo from the Attorney General to Premier Brownlee, 30 May 1929, 1–2.

80 PAA, 73B, letter from Henry E. Spencer to Premier Brownlee, 9 May 1929, and telegram from Spencer to Brownlee, 10 May 1929.

81 PAA, 74A, memo from the Deputy Attorney General to Premier Brownlee, 14 March 1932.

82 For more on family strategies see: André Cellard and Marie-Claude Thifault, "The Uses of Asylums: Resistance, Asylum Propaganda and Institutionalization Strategies in Turn of the Century Quebec," in *Mental Health and Canadian Society: Historical Perspectives*, ed. David Wright and James Moran (Montreal; Kingston, ON: McGill-Queen's University Press, 2006); and Marie-Claude Thifault and Isabelle Perreault, "Premières initiatives d'intégration sociale des malades mentaux dans une phase de pré-désinstitutionnalisation: l'exemple de Saint-Jean-de-Dieu, 1910–1950," *Social History* 46, no. 2 (2011): 197–222.

83 PAA, Attorney General Files, 75.126, 1309, Box 87, memorandum from Mr English to the Department of Municipal Affairs and the Deputy Attorney General, buildings, 15 April 1924.

84 PAA, Attorney General Files, 75.126, 1309, Box 87, memorandum from Mr English to the Department of Municipal Affairs and the Deputy Attorney General, buildings, 15 April 1924.

85 PAA, Attorney General Files, 75.126, 1309, Box 87, police report, Mrs William Albert Jarvis, Mentally Deficient (Wainwright), 25 August 1923.

86 PAA, Attorney General Files, 75.126, 1309, Box 87, letter from Police Magistrate (on letterhead from Jones, Scott and Carswell, Barristers, Solicitors and Notaries) to R.A. Smith, Deputy Attorney General, 28 April 1924.

87 PAA, Attorney General Files, 75.126, 1309, Box 87, letter from Dr J.B. Mackay to the Deputy Attorney General, 2 October 1923.

88 PAA, Attorney General Files, 75.126, 1309, Box 87, letter from Commanding D Division, Lethbridge, to the Commissioner of the Alberta Provincial Police, 25 May 1923.

89 PAA, 74B, pamphlet, Ralph Spooner, "Mental Hygiene in Ontario," Canadian Workers Association, August 1932.

90 PAA, 74A, "Unemployed taken from list supplied by communist committee," 30 June 1930, 1–3.

91 See Devereux, *Growing a Race*.

92 City of Edmonton Archives, Emily Murphy Scrapbooks.

93 Ibid.

94 PAA, GR1971, 0420/19, Irene Parlby, "Mental Deficiency," address delivered before the UFWA, January 1924, 4.

95 Ibid., 7–8.

96 Ibid., 11.

97 Emily Murphy, *Lethbridge Herald*, June 1926 (Legislative scrapbooks, microfilm, no page number).

98 *Calgary Herald*, January 1928 (Legislative scrapbooks, microfilm, no page number).

99 *Edmonton Journal*, 24 February 1928 (Legislative scrapbooks, microfilm, no page number).

100 For a full breakdown of these debates, see Christian, "Mentally Ill and Human Rights in Alberta."

101 Rennie, *Rise of Agrarian Democracy*, 117.

2. Race, Intelligence, and Consent

1 See Christian, "Mentally Ill and Human Rights in Alberta," 85.

2 For more on this idea, see, in particular, Mary Ellen Kelm, "Diagnosing the Discursive Indian: Medicine, Gender, and the 'Dying Race,'" *Ethnohistory* 52, no. 2 (2005): 371–406; and Maureen Lux, *Medicine that Walks: Disease, Medicine, and Canadian Plains Native People, 1880–1940* (Toronto: University of Toronto Press, 2001), especially 9, 19, 226. For more on how other scholars have examined these questions with particular reference to mental health, see James B. Waldram, *Revenge of the Windigo: The*

Construction of the Mind and Mental Health of North American Aboriginal Peoples (Toronto: University of Toronto Press, 2004).

3 Yvonne Boyer, "First Nations, Métis and Inuit Health and the Law: A Framework for the Future" (thesis, University of Ottawa, 2011), 184.

4 Ibid., 181–6. The remainder of the evidence provided for this claim relied on generalizations regarding the activities and members of the Eugenics Board, as reported in newspapers and magazines nearly forty years later, but contains no direct evidence from contemporary records or oral sources.

5 Paul Primeau, "A Social History of the Eugenic Movement: The Enactment of the Sexual Sterilization Act S.A. 1928 and Its Effect on Indian and Metis People" (thesis, Lakehead University, 1998), 41, where he cites the Blair Report (see note 87 below), although he credits the trial transcript of *Muir v. Alberta*, Alberta Court of Queen's Bench Judicial District of Edmonton (1996) A.J. 37, 18.

6 Ibid., 43, where he cites Christian, "Mentally Ill and Human Rights in Alberta," 22. I could not find this information on p. 22 of Christian's thesis, but a slightly different version appears on pp. 85 and 90.

7 Karen Stote, "An Act of Genocide: Eugenics, Indian Policy, and the Sterilization of Aboriginal Women in Canada" (PhD diss., University of New Brunswick, 2012), 2.

8 Ibid., 116.

9 John D. O'Neil, "Self-determination, Medical Ideology and Health Services in Inuit Communities," in *Northern Communities: The Prospects for Empowerment*, ed. Gurston Dacks and Ken Coates (Edmonton: Boreal Institute for Northern Studies, 1988), 36.

10 Christian, "Mentally Ill and Human Rights in Alberta," 21.

11 Ibid., 85.

12 Ibid., 90.

13 Grekul, Krahn, and Odynak, "Sterilizing the 'Feeble-minded,'" 375.

14 Ibid.

15 For a much more thorough study of this situation, see Lux, *Medicine that Walks*.

16 Maureen Lux, "Care for the 'Racially Careless': Indian Hospitals in the Canadian West, 1920–1950s," *Canadian Historical Review* 91, no. 3 (2010): 409.

17 For more studies on this, see Patricia Jasen, "Race, Culture, and the Colonization of Childbirth in Northern Canada," *Social History of Medicine* 10, no. 3 (1997): 383–400; Mary Ellen Kelm, *Colonizing Bodies: Aboriginal Health and Healing in British Columbia, 1900–1950* (Vancouver: UBC Press, 1999); and Lux, *Medicine that Walks*. For an alternative view, one that examines a more

cooperative exchange among healing women across the colonial contact zones, see Kristin Burnett, *Taking Medicine: Women's Healing Work and Colonial Contact in Southern Alberta, 1880–1930* (Vancouver: UBC Press, 2011).

18 Molly Ladd-Taylor makes a similar point in her study of US eugenics programs, where she argues that mental capacity, intelligence, and "retardation" overruled racial categories in the medical records. Although these criteria comingled and overlapped one another, the social construction of intelligence provides a fruitful avenue of inquiry for teasing apart the racial and clinical elements of this program. See Molly Ladd-Taylor, "Sterilizing the 'Retarded': Contraceptive Surgery and Eugenics in the 1970s and 1980s," *Canadian Bulletin of Medical History* (under review).

19 See Lux, "Care for the 'Racially Careless'"; and idem, *Medicine that Walks*.

20 Lux, *Medicine that Walks*, 8.

21 Ibid., 92.

22 See also Kelm, "Diagnosing the Discursive Indian," 397–8.

23 PAA, Premier's Office Fonds, 69.289, roll 433, "Report of Medical Survey in the Wabasca District" (n.d., but filed with other reports from the late 1920s), 1.

24 Ibid., 3.

25 See Jasen, "Race, Culture."

26 PAA, Premier's Office Fonds, 69.289, roll 433, "Report of Medical Survey in the Wabasca District," 4.

27 Ibid.

28 Ibid.

29 Ibid.

30 Ibid., 8.

31 Ibid., 6.

32 Ibid., 6.

33 Ibid., 7.

34 Mary Percy Jackson, "Midwifery among the Metis," *Alberta Medical Review* 14, no. 3 (1949): 11.

35 Ibid.

36 Ibid., 14.

37 Legislative scrapbooks; and Christian, "Mentally Ill and Human Rights in Alberta."

38 Rennie, *Rise of Agrarian Democracy*, 117.

39 *Edmonton Journal*, 24 February 1928 (Legislative scrapbooks, microfilm, no page number).

40 *Edmonton Journal*, 28 February 1928 (Legislative scrapbooks, microfilm, no page number).

41 The party, under various names, such as the People's League, the People's Party, was likely a fringe communist group. There are no records of the organization in the Provincial Archives of Alberta, or any of its constitutional challenge.

42 Statutes of Alberta, 1928, Chapter 37, The Sexual Sterilization Act. For more information on J.M. MacEachern, see Wahlsten, "Leilani Muir versus the Philosopher King."

43 Eugenics Board Meetings, 1929–1942 (Binder 1), 29 January 1929, 1–2.

44 Eugenics Board Meetings, 1929–1942 (Binder 1), 1 March 1929, 2.

45 Ibid., 3.

46 Eugenics Board Meetings, 1929–1942 (Binder 1), 12 April 1929, 1.

47 Eugenics Board Meetings, 1929–1942 (Binder 1), 17 May 1929, order-in-council.

48 Grekul, "Social Construction of the Feeble-Minded Threat," 102; that figure includes one-year members who covered in cases of illness.

49 Eugenics Board Meetings, 1929–1942 (Binder 1), 25 October 1929, 2.

50 Eugenics Board Meetings, 1929–1942 (Binder 1), 24 June 1930, meeting with the Deputy Minister of Health, 1–2.

51 Eugenics Board Meetings, 1929–1942 (Binder 1), 26 October 1929, 5.

52 Ibid., 6.

53 C.A. Baragar et al., "Sexual Sterilization: Four Years Experience in Alberta," *American Journal of Psychology* 19, no. 2 (1935): 897–923.

54 Ibid., 908–9.

55 Ibid., 900.

56 Ibid., 902; the proportion in this category was 54.2 per cent.

57 Ibid.

58 Ibid., 905.

59 R.C. Wallace, "The Quality of the Human Stock," *Canadian Medical Association Journal* 31, no. 4 (1934): 2.

60 Ibid., 3–4.

61 Ibid., 6.

62 Baragar et al., "Sexual Sterilization," 898.

63 In particular, this arose as a result of the Nuremberg Trials in 1947, which established the Nuremberg Code for Medical Ethics through an international tribunal charged with examining German science under the Nazis. Despite this international agreement, several countries continued to follow their own approaches to ethics, but the Nuremberg Trials nonetheless raised the issue in a visible manner. See, for example, Jenny Hazelgrove, "The Old Faith and New Science: The Nuremberg Code and Human Experimentation in Britain, 1946–73," *Social History of Medicine* 15, no. 1

(2002): 109–35. For a discussion of pre-Second World War approaches and discussions in the American Medical Association, see Susan E. Lederer, *Subjected to Science: Human Experimentation in America before the Second World War* (Baltimore: Johns Hopkins University Press, 1995).

64 Nancy Campbell, *Discovering Addiction: The Science and Politics of Substance Abuse Research* (Ann Arbor: University of Michigan Press, 2007).

65 For further discussion of these kinds of coercive connections between consent and treatment, see, for example, Jordan Goodman, Anthony McElligott, and Lara Marks, eds., *Useful Bodies: Humans in the Service of Medical Science in the Twentieth Century* (Baltimore: Johns Hopkins University Press, 2003). For studies that link these measures specifically to race, see Allan M. Brandt "Racism and Research: The Case of the Tuskegee Syphilis Study," in *Sickness and Health in America*, 3rd ed., ed. Judith Walzer Leavitt and Ronald L. Numbers (Madison: University of Wisconsin Press, 1997); and Keith Wailoo, *Dying in the City of the Blues: Sickle Cell Anemia and the Politics of Race and Health* (Chapel Hill: University of North Carolina Press, 2001).

66 Eugenics Board, Meetings, 1929–1942 (Binder 1), 16 April 1930, 2.

67 Eugenics Board, Meetings, 1929–1942 (Binder 1), 5 June 1931, 1.

68 Eugenics Board, Meetings, 1929–1942 (Binder 1), 3–6 June 1931, 3.

69 Eugenics Board, Meetings, 1929–1942 (Binder 1), 16 March 1932, 1.

70 Eugenics Board, Meetings, 1929–1942 (Binder 1), 16 June 1933, 5.

71 R.R. MacLean and E.J. Kibblewhite, "Sexual Sterilization in Alberta: Eight Years' Experience, 1929 to May 31, 1937," *Canadian Public Health Journal* (1937): 589. Of the cases passed, 501 were of males and 507 were of females.

72 Ibid., note.

73 Ibid., 590.

74 Statutes of Alberta, 1937, "An Act to amend the Sexual Sterilization Act," assented to 14 April 1937, clause 6, 182.

75 Ibid., clause 5(2).

76 Ibid., clause 7.

77 E. Mary Frost, "Sterilization in Alberta: A Summary of the Cases presented to the Eugenics Board for the Province of Alberta from 1929 to 1941" (MA thesis, University of Alberta, 1942), 86, 90. The savings were based on estimated costs of $295 per year per patient for expenses related to institutionalization.

78 Eugenics Board, Meetings, 1929–1942 (Binder 1), 18 March 1932, 2.

79 Eugenics Board, Minutes (Binder 1), 31 May 1937, letter from the Medical Superintendent to the Indian Agent, Edmonton, 29 April 1937.

80 Eugenics Board, Minutes (Binder 1), 31 May 1937, letter from T.R.L. MacInnes to the Director of Indian Affairs Branch, Department of Mines and Resources, 11 May 1937; and letter from G.C. Laight, Indian Agent, Edmonton, to the Director of Indian Affairs Branch, Department of Mines and Resources, 11 May 1937, re: Sterilization of Indian Cases.
81 Eugenics Board, Minutes (Binder 1), 31 May 1937, letter from the Medical Superintendent to the Indian Agent, Department of Indian Affairs, Edmonton, 22 May 1937; the letter includes the request that "*I would ask that you not operate until I further advise you*" [emphasis in original].
82 Eugenics Board, Minutes (Binder 1), 31 May 1937, letter from the Medical Superintendent to the Indian Agent, Department of Indian Affairs, Edmonton, 26 May 1937.
83 Eugenics Board, Minutes, letter from T.R.L. McInnes, Indian Affairs Branch, Department of Mines and Resources, to the Medical Superintendent, Provincial Mental Hospital, Ponoka, 10 September 1942 (responding to the letter from Ponoka sent 25 August 1942 and quoted in this response).
84 Ibid.
85 Eugenics Board, Minutes, Meeting 113, 28 January 1943, 2.
86 Grekul, "Social Construction of the Feeble-Minded Threat," 375.
87 W.R.N. Blair, *Mental Health in Alberta: A Report on the Alberta Mental Health Study, 1968* [Blair Report] (Edmonton: Ministry of Human Resources and Development, 1969), 267.
88 Ibid., 267–8.
89 Ibid., 268.
90 See, for example, Robert Lechat, "Intensive Sterilization for the Inuit," *Oblate Fathers of the Churchill-Hudson Bay Diocese* (fall/winter 1976–77), 5–7.

3. Sterilization Redefined

1 Poem included in R.M. Ellison, "Psychiatric Complications following Sterilization of Women," *Medical Journal of Australia* 2 (1964): 628. Bessie Moses was a well-beloved Baltimore physician who specialized in the contraptions of contraception.
2 For more on McNaughton and a fuller analysis of her feminism, see Georgina Taylor, "Ground for Common Action: Violet McNaughton's Agrarian Feminism and the Origins of the Farm Women's Movement in Canada" (PhD diss., Carleton University, 1997), especially chap. 1.
3 Saskatchewan Archives Board (hereafter cited as SAB), Violet McNaughton Papers, A1. E3, Correspondence: Birth Control, letter from Mrs T.B. Wilson to Violet McNaughton, 6 May 1922, 1.

4 SAB, Violet McNaughton Papers, A1, E3, Correspondence: Birth Control, letter, "Dear Mamma," n.d., 2. Angus McLaren and Arlene Tigar McLaren speculate that the letter indicates inter-war knowledge of birth-control practices, which would date it in the 1930s; see *The Bedroom and the State: The Changing Practices and Politics of Contraception and Abortion in Canada, 1880–1980* (Toronto: McClelland & Stewart, 1986), 28.

5 SAB, Violet McNaughton Papers, A1, E3, Correspondence: Birth Control, letter, "Dear Mamma," n.d., 2.

6 Ibid., 2–4.

7 Angus McLaren, "'Keep Your Seats and Face Facts': Western Canadian Women's Discussion of Birth Control in the 1920s," *Canadian Bulletin of Medical History* 8, no. 2 (1991): 191.

8 Ibid., 193.

9 Ibid., 195.

10 Taylor, "Ground for Common Action," 386; and Library and Archives of Canada, "Violet McNaughton," available online at http://www.collections-canada.gc.ca/women/030001-1117-e.html, accessed 23 February 2012.

11 Taylor, "Ground for Common Action," 165.

12 SAB, A1, D. 54, McNaughton Correspondence with Irene Parlby, Parlby to McNaughton, 12 April 1918, 1.

13 SAB, A1, D. 54, McNaughton Correspondence with Irene Parlby, Parlby to McNaughton, 2 May 1918, from General Hospital in Calgary.

14 SAB, A1, D. 54, McNaughton Correspondence with Irene Parlby, Parlby to McNaughton, 1918 [no specific date], 1.

15 Irene Parlby, "Mental Deficiency" (address to the United Farm Women of Alberta, 1924), 8.

16 Ibid., 11.

17 This phrase was coined by Carol Hanisch, a radical reformer and writer for the New York Radical Women and Redstockings; see, for example, Carol Hanisch, "Struggles for Leadership in the Women's Liberation Movement," in *Leadership and Social Movements*, ed. Colin Barker, Alan Johnson, and Michael Lavalette (Manchester, UK: Manchester University Press, 2001), 77.

18 Another example of these nuances comes in the person of Charlotte Whitton, a leading feminist from Ontario and two-time mayor of Ottawa, who was chiefly concerned with child welfare and women's equality. Her views were considered more socially conservative in some respects, but she too concentrated her reform efforts on issues pertinent to families, particularly in the realm of social services. In 1999 her previously restricted diaries were opened to the public, revealing her close companionship with Margaret

Grier, a relationship that historian Steven Maynard speculates may have been lesbian; see Steven Maynard, "Maple Leaf (Gardens) Forever: Sex, Canadian Historians, and National History," *Journal of Canadian History* 36, no. 2 (2001): 70–105.

19 Linda Revie, "More than Just Boots! The Eugenic and Commercial Concerns behind A.R. Kaufman's Birth Controlling Activities," *Canadian Bulletin of Medical History* 23, no. 1 (2006): 120.

20 See McLaren and McLaren, *Bedroom and the State.*

21 Criminal Code of Canada, 1892, S.C. 1892, c. 29. See also Constance Backhouse, *Petticoats and Prejudice: Women and Law in Nineteenth-Century Canada* (Toronto: Women's Press/Osgoode Society, 1991).

22 McLaren and McLaren, *Bedroom and the State*, 135.

23 Johanna Schoen, for instance, offers a remarkably nuanced account of women's agency in tension with government control over women's reproductive choices in the United States. Teasing apart the class and race elements in these negotiations, Schoen shows how welfare reformers felt caught in a moral quandary regarding the rights of unmarried women, particularly those in the African American, Hispanic, and Native American communities; see Schoen, *Choice & Coercion*. For another study in this vein, see Stern, *Eugenic Nation*; Stern focuses on the state of California and its aggressive eugenics program, which boasted that it out-sterilized other states. Within her analysis is also the subtle reminder that women sought sterilization voluntarily and for health reasons, which she argues was tied to the broader discourse of eugenics and family fitness.

24 Kluchin, *Fit to Be Tied*, 1.

25 Gunnar Broberg and Mattias Tydén, "Eugenics in Sweden: Efficient Care," in *Eugenics and the Welfare State: Norway, Sweden, Denmark and Finland*, ed. Gunnar Broberg and Nils Roll-Hansen (East Lansing: Michigan State University Press, 2005), 111.

26 Substantial work by Angus McLaren moves in this direction, but does not confront the post–Second World War circumstances, nor does he consider the topics of birth control and eugenics against the backdrop of mental health reforms. See McLaren and McLaren, *Bedroom and the State*; and McLaren, *Our Own Master Race*. Ian Dowbiggin examines the relationship between psychiatry and eugenics in his comparative study of Canada and the United States, but does not extend that analysis after the Second World War; see Ian Dowbiggin, *Keeping America Sane: Psychiatry and Eugenics in the United States and Canada, 1880–1940* (Ithaca, NY: Cornell University Press, 1997). By contrast, in a more recent study, he connects the rise of birth control with fertility, particularly in middle- and

professional-class families, thereby extending the Roman Catholic perspective on this topic through the twentieth century; see Ian Dowbiggin, *Sterilization Movement*. McLaren and McLaren began that process in their thorough account of the history of birth control and contraceptives across Canada, and although they find evidence that working-class women in Ontario were sterilized, they emphasize the way in which sterilization as birth control divided Canadian reformers; see McLaren and McLaren, *Bedroom and the State*, 105.

27 Eugenics Board, Meetings, 1929–1942 (Binder 1), 3–6 June 1931, 1.

28 McLaren, *Our Own Master Race*, 94. Helen Gregory MacGill was a judge and mother of two.

29 McLaren, "'Keep Your Seats and Face Facts,'" 190.

30 Angus McLaren writes about McNaughton's women's column in *The Western Producer* in "'Keep Your Seats and Face Facts.'"

31 For more on this history, and for the controversial entry of women into professional medicine and obstetrics, see Jacalyn Duffin, *History of Medicine: A Scandalously Short Introduction* (Toronto: University of Toronto Press, 1999), especially 267–9; and Georgina Feldberg, "On the Cutting Edge: Science and Obstetrical Practice in a Women's Hospital, 1945–1960," in *Women, Health, and Nation: Canada and the United States since 1945*, ed. Georgina Feldberg, Molly Ladd-Taylor, Alison Li, and Kathryn MacPherson (Montreal; Kingston, ON: McGill-Queen's University Press, 2003).

32 For a more in-depth examination of this cultural shift, see, for example, Nancy Christie, *Engendering the State: Family, Work, and Welfare in Canada* (Toronto: University of Toronto Press, 2000); and for a specific analysis of the changing relationship between women and their doctors, see Wendy Mitchinson, *Giving Birth in Canada, 1900–1950* (Toronto: University of Toronto Press, 2002).

33 Ellison, "Psychiatric Complications," 653.

34 See, for example, Allan C. Barnes and Frederick P. Zuspan, "Patient Reaction to Puerperal Surgical Sterilization," *American Journal of Obstetrics & Gynecology* 75, no. 1 (1958): 65–71; Ellison, "Psychiatric Complications"; M. David Enoch and Keith Jones, "Sterilization: A Review of 98 Sterilized Women," *British Journal of Psychiatry* 127, no. 6 (1975): 583–7; Therese Lu and Daphne Chun, "A Long Term Follow-up Study of 1,055 Cases of Postpartum Tubal Ligation," *Journal of Obstetrics and Gynaecology in the British Commonwealth* 74, no. 6 (1967): 875–80; and David R. McCoy, "The Emotional Reaction of Women to Therapeutic Abortion and Sterilization," *Journal of Obstetrics and Gynaecology in the British Commonwealth* 75, no. 10 (1968): 1054–7.

35 J.M.A. Ansari and H.H. Francis, "A Study of 49 Sterilized Females," *Acta Psychiatrica Scandinavica* 54, no. 5 (1976): 321.

36 W.P. Black and A.B. Sclare, "Sterilization by Tubal Ligation – A Follow-up Study," *Journal of Obstetrics and Gynaecology in the British Commonwealth* 75, no. 2 (1968): 219.

37 SAB, A1, McNaughton Collection, "Birth control," letter to the editor, *Women's Forum* (n.d.), 1–2.

38 B.X. O'Reilly, "The doctor has a chance to do much good," *Prairie Messenger*, 19 June 1929, 7.

39 SAB, A1, McNaughton Collection, "Synopsis of the Report of the Provincial Committee on Birth Control, December 1937" (presentation to the United Farm Women of Alberta Meeting, 1938 [no specific date]), 1.

40 SAB, A1, McNaughton Collection, Myrtle H. Roper, "The United Farm Women of Alberta: Amendments to the Criminal Code re: Control of Contraception" (address, 19 January [1938?]), 1.

41 Ibid., 2.

42 Ibid., 3.

43 Ibid., 9.

44 Ibid., 10.

45 SAB, A1, McNaughton Collection, Emilie O. Briggs, "Birth Control: Negative Argument," 8.

46 Cook, *Regenerators*, especially chap. 6.

47 For the most comprehensive studies on this topic, see Richard Allen, *The Social Passion: Religion and Social Reform in Canada, 1914–28* (Toronto: University of Toronto Press, 1971); and idem, *The View from Murney Tower: Salem Bland, the Late Victorian Controversies, and the Search for a New Christianity* (Toronto: University of Toronto Press, 2008).

48 See Valverde, *Age of Light, Soap and Water*.

49 Richard Allen, "The Social Gospel and the Reform Tradition in Canada, 1890–1928," *Canadian Historical Review* 49, no. 4 (1968): 381–99.

50 David Marshall, *Secularizing the Faith: Canadian Protestant Clergy and the Crisis of Belief, 1850–1940* (Toronto: University of Toronto Press, 1992).

51 See Michael Gavreau and Nancy Christie, *A Full-Orbed Christianity: The Protestant Churches and Social Welfare in Canada, 1900–1940* (Montreal; Kingston, ON: McGill-Queen's University Press, 2001).

52 See *Canada Year Book 1939: The Official Statistical Annual of the Resources, History, Institutions, and Social and Economic Conditions of the Dominion* (Ottawa: King's Printer, 1939), 95; and M.C. Urquhart and K.A.H. Buckley, eds., *Historical Statistics of Canada* (Cambridge: Cambridge University Press, 1965), series A114-132, 18.

53 Census data indicate that, in 1921, Roman Catholics (including Ukrainian and Greek) numbered 105,518 people in Manitoba, 147,517 in Saskatchewan, and 97,628 in Alberta; in 1931 there were 189,836 in Manitoba, 234,242 in Saskatchewan, and 168,643 in Alberta; in 1941 there were 150,083 in Manitoba, 182,920 in Saskatchewan, and 134,229 in Alberta; and in 1951 there were 219,900 in Manitoba, 236,629 in Saskatchewan, and 223,826 in Alberta.

54 J. Van der Heyden, "Dangers of birth control told at Dutch congress," *Prairie Messenger*, 25 August 1929, 1.

55 "Eugenics again," *Prairie Messenger*, 25 June 1930, 6 (reprinted from the *Vancouver Bulletin*).

56 "Woman attorney, Catholic, flays birth control," *Prairie Messenger*, 8 October 1930, 8.

57 "Doctors condemn birth control at medical gathering: noted Cincinnati surgeons attack practice as unjustifiable socially, economically, physiologically," *Prairie Messenger*, 17 December 1930, 1, 5.

58 "Refined smut lectures scored in pastoral: warns Catholics against immoral speakers – no scientific basis," *Prairie Messenger*, 11 December 1930, 6.

59 "Vigorous encyclical of Pope Pius on Christian marriage: modern evils of divorce, birth control, sterilization are again condemned," *Prairie Messenger*, 21 January 1931, 1.

60 Ibid.

61 Ibid., 4.

62 Ibid.

63 Ibid.

64 "California birth control bill would legalise hospital treatments," *Prairie Messenger*, 4 February 1931, 8.

65 "The Catholic Church vs. the Federal Council of the Churches of Christ in America," *Prairie Messenger*, 27 May 1931, 2.

66 John F. Noll, "The Catholic Church vs. the Federal Council of Churches of Christ in America III," *Prairie Messenger*, 27 May 1931, 2.

67 Ibid.

68 "Sterilization bill opposed by Catholics, Manitoba Legislature," *Prairie Messenger*, 8 March 1933, 8; "Will Saskatchewan go pagan?" *Prairie Messenger*, 24 January 1934, 11, 37.

69 An Authority on the Subject, "How to meet sterilization," *Prairie Messenger*, 7 February 1934, 11.

70 For a careful and full account of German and Nazi race hygiene, see Weindling, *Health, Race and German Politics*. See also Pichot, *Pure Society*; and Richard Weikart, *From Darwin to Hitler: Evolutionary Ethics, Eugenics, and Racism in Germany* (New York: Palgrave Macmillan, 2004).

71 Matthew A. Michel, "The new marriage act," *Prairie Messenger*, 19 July 1933, 11.

72 For more on this angle, see Gisela Bock, "Racism and Sexism in Nazi Germany: Motherhood, Compulsory Sterilization, and the State," *Signs* 8, no. 3 (1983): 400–21.

73 Michel, "New marriage act."

74 "Sterilization and Hitler," *Prairie Messenger*, 9 August 1933, 11.

75 See, for example, "Signs of the times," *Prairie Messenger*, 7 February 1934, 39, which suggested that the Hitler government "will compel 400,000 so-called 'defectives' between the ages of 10 and 50 years to submit to an operation known as vasectomy."

76 "An expert speaks on sterilization," *Prairie Messenger*, 28 February 1934, 11.

77 "Some thoughts for sterilizers," *Prairie Messenger*, 28 February 1934, 39.

78 Associate Editor, "'Unwanted humanity,'" *Prairie Messenger*, 3 March 1937, 14.

79 "Unwanted humanity," *Prairie Messenger*, 3 March 1937, 43.

80 Quoted in "Mental hygiene," *Prairie Messenger*, 30 March 1938, 15.

81 A.S. Norris, "An Examination of the Effects of Tubal Ligation: Their Implications for Prediction," *American Journal of Obstetrics and Gynaecology* 90, no. 4 (1964): 431.

82 Ibid. The author explains that voluntary sterilizations are only part of the sterilization law in Virginia, whereas another twenty-three had sterilization laws for mental defectives, but no provisions for voluntary use, suggesting that the operation on a voluntary basis was neither legal nor illegal.

83 Johanna Schoen finds similar results in her study of North Carolina; see Schoen, *Choice and Coercion*.

84 "The Legal Aspects of Sterilization, reprint from the Ontario Medical Review," *Alberta Medical Review* 14, no. 3 (1949): 50–3; also printed as "Medico-Legal: The Legal Aspects of Sterilization," *Canadian Medical Association Journal* 58, no. 5 (1948): 512–13.

85 "Medico-Legal: The Legal Aspects of Sterilization," *Canadian Medical Association Journal* 58, no. 5 (1948): 512.

86 "The Legal Aspects of Sterilization, reprint from the Ontario Medical Review," *Alberta Medical Review* 14, no. 3 (1949): 51.

87 Ibid., 53.

88 T.E. Brown, "Cesarean Section in Lethbridge," *Alberta Medical Review* 16, no. 2 (1951): 18–20.

89 Ibid.

90 David Gagan and Rosemary Gagan, *For Patients of Moderate Means: A Social History of the Voluntary Public General Hospital in Canada, 1890–1950*

(Montreal; Kingston, ON: McGill-Queen's University Press, 2002), 87, where they state that, "prior to the depression, only a third of all births in Ontario took place in a hospital. By 1941 the proportion of hospital births had risen to two-thirds, and by 1946 to 80 per cent."

91 Mitchinson, *Giving Birth in Canada*, 255.

92 Ibid., 256. Mitchinson does not suggest that these surgeries were always the woman's decision, and in fact demonstrates that, in circumstances where the woman faced health risks, the decision often rested with the surgeon. It is also clear, however, that women who chose the operation had more control of the situation than had previously been understood.

93 Ibid., 252.

94 In a contemporary US medical study, the authors reached a similar conclusion, arguing that, as surgical sterilizations in females increased, the numbers of Caesarean sections also increased; see Barnes and Zuspan, "Patient Reaction to Puerperal Surgical Sterilization," 65.

95 D. Shute, "Subtotal Hysterectomy in Southern Alberta," *Alberta Medical Review* 17, no. 2 (1952): 23–4.

96 "Birth Control: editorial," *Canadian Medical Association Journal* 57 (1947): 489.

97 Ibid., 490.

98 Thomas Fisher, "Medico-Legal: Sexual Sterilization," *Canadian Medical Association Journal* 76 (1957): 785.

99 Ibid., 786.

100 "The facts about voluntary sterilization," *Calgary Herald*, 10 April 1970.

101 See, for example, Andrea Tone, *Devices and Desires: A History of Contraceptives in America* (New York: Hill and Wang, 2001), chap. 10.

102 "Free male sterilization in British health plan," *Albertan*, 24 April 1970.

103 Calgary Health Services Archives (hereafter cited as CHSA), Calgary General Hospital, 100, letter from J.C. Johnston, Calgary General Hospital Administrator, to L.S. Portigal, City Solicitor, re: Male Sterilization, 10 April 1970, 1.

104 CHSA, Foothills Hospital (FHH)-037, Brief relating to: "Sexual Sterilization and Therapeutic Abortions in the Royal Alexandra Hospital [Edmonton]," presented to the Executive Director, Mr Nye, and the Board of Governors of the Royal Alexandra Hospital, [n.d., but likely 1970], 1.

105 Ibid.

106 Walter Nagel, "Sterilization conditions spelled out for trustees," *Calgary Herald*, 18 April 1970.

107 CHSA, FHH-037, Brief relating to: "Sexual Sterilization and Therapeutic Abortions in the Royal Alexandra Hospital," 2.

108 CHSA, Calgary General Hospital (CGH)-100, Edythe Humphrey, "Steril-
     ization standards set at Rockyview Hospital," *Albertan*, 17 April 1970. See
     also Nagel, "Sterilization conditions spelled out for trustees."

4. Vasectomy, Masculinity, and Hyperactivity

1 Larry Johnsrude, "Province revokes rights; government opts out of Charter, limits sterilization victims' right to sue for compensation; Alberta's
   sterilization solution," *Edmonton Journal*, 11 March 1998, A1.
2 T. Arnold, "Wave of anger, outrage greets proposed law: A time line,"
   Edmonton Journal, 11 March 1998, A1.
3 Ibid.
4 National Film Board of Canada, "Sterilization of Leilani Muir," statements from Ken Nelson.
5 See Grekul, "Social Construction of the Feeble-Minded Threat," 108. Note
   that, between 1929 and 1933, only 23 per cent of males were sterilized
   and in 1972 only 10 per cent were, but these dates correspond with partial
   years of the program.
6 The numbers were compiled by the author using the Annual Reports of
   the Alberta Department of Public Health, Vital Statistics Branch, from
   1927 to 1966, at which point the statistical figures in these reports end.
7 In 1940 and 1942 male sterilizations were only 47 and 48 per cent, respectively, of the recommended total.
8 In 1958 116 males and only 71 females were recommended for sterilization. In all other years between 1944 and 1966, women outnumbered men.
9 Further work needs to be done on this point – in particular, on the ways
   in which mental hospitals were effectively used as proto-welfare institutions during times of acute (and, in the case of the Depression, prolonged) economic stress.
10 Thomas Poffenberger, "Two Thousand Voluntary Vasectomies in California:
   Background Factors and Comments," *Marriage and Family Living* 25,
   no. 4 (1963): 469. India is a notable exception: between 1956, when India
   introduced its sterilization policy as part of a massive national exercise
   in family planning, and 1963, the Indian government authorized 97,583
   vasectomies compared with 81,417 salpingectomies. See, for example,
   R.P. Mohan, "Factors to Motivation towards Sterilization in 2 Indian
   Villages," *Family Life Coordinator* 16 (1967): 35–8, who shows that the
   Indian program contained elements of coercion and financial reward for
   "voluntary" sterilization. For a more comprehensive study of this issue,
   see David G. Mandelbaum, *Human Fertility in India: Social Components and
   Policy Perspectives* (Berkeley: University of California Press, 1974).

11 See, for example, McLaren, *Our Own Master Race*.

12 See Dowbiggin, *Sterilization Movement*.

13 Grekul, "Social Construction of the Feeble-Minded Threat"; and Grekul, Krahn, and Odynak, "Sterilizing the 'Feeble-minded.'"

14 As quoted in Jana Grekul, "Sterilization in Alberta, 1928–1972: Gender Matters," *Canadian Review of Sociology* 45, no. 3 (2008): 249. See also MacLean and Kibblewhite, "Sexual Sterilization in Alberta," 588.

15 Grekul, "Sterilization in Alberta," 252.

16 Grekul found this, too, even within the eugenics program; see ibid., 253.

17 Ibid., 255 and elsewhere.

18 For more on this legal position, see *Bravery v. Bravery* (1954) 3 All ER 59, judgment by Sir Raymond Evershed Denning. The case involved allegations of cruelty in the divorce proceedings of Mr and Mrs Bravery, because Mr Bravery had been sterilized and Mrs Bravery felt the marriage disintegrated thereafter.

19 University of Alberta Archives (hereafter cited as UAA), Leilani Muir Papers, Box 1, Binder: "Files – from PTS – lawyers and doctors from 1979 to 2000," Feminist Theory Underlying the Case.

20 Ibid. This statement included a letter from the Alberta Director of Social Services, 4 November 1988, making this claim.

21 Brian Brennan, *The Good Steward: The Ernest C. Manning Story* (Calgary: Fifth House, 2008), 38.

22 Ibid.

23 As quoted in ibid., 39.

24 Ibid., 38; and Alberta, Department of Public Health, *Annual Report* (Edmonton, 1962).

25 As noted by an anonymous person in an interview by the author, 15 May 2012.

26 Donald J. Dodds, *Voluntary Male Sterilization* (Toronto: Damian Press, 1970), 15, 16, 20–1.

27 Robert L. Dickinson, "Sterilization without Unsexing: 1. Surgical Review with Especial Reference to 5,820 Operations on Insane and Feeble-minded in California," *Journal of the American Medical Association* 92, no. 5 (1929): 373.

28 For more on the California program and an explanation of how it used sexual sterilization in an effort to relieve mental disorders, see Joel Braslow, *Mental Ills and Bodily Cures: Psychiatric Treatment in the First Half of the Twentieth Century* (Berkeley: University of California Press, 1997), chap. 3.

29 Dickinson, "Sterilization without Unsexing," 373.

30 Ibid., 374.

31 Ibid., 379.

32 UAA, Leilani Muir files, Box 2, Binder: Trial Transcripts, 12 June to 20 June 1995 – Robertson examined by Jon Faulds, re: index cards, recorded at 1392.
33 Ibid., recorded at 1401.
34 Ibid., recorded at 1402.
35 Ibid.
36 Ibid, cross-examination by Mr Taylor, at 1539. The item also appears in Eugenics Board, Minutes, Meeting 85, 13–14 October 1937, 2–3.
37 Eugenics Board, Minutes, Meeting 84, 15 July 1937, 2.
38 Eugenics Board, Minutes, Meeting 91, 14 July 1938, 2; idem, Minutes, Meeting 95, 26–28 April 1939.
39 Eugenics Board, Minutes, Meeting 121, 15 June 1944.
40 James Russell Grant, "Results of Institutional Treatment of Juvenile Mental Defectives over a 30-Year Period," *Canadian Medical Association Journal* 75 (1956): 919–20.
41 Edgar Jones and Shahina Rahman, "Framing Mental Illness, 1923–1939: The Maudsley Hospital and Its Patients," *Social History of Medicine* 21, no. 1 (2008): 107–25.
42 Grekul, "Sterilization in Alberta," 254. This shift towards adolescents was also reflected in a growing emphasis on the use of guidance clinics and school programs to detect mental deficiencies or mental health problems. For more on this topic, see Samson, "Coercion, Surveillance and Eugenics."
43 Grant, "Results of Institutional Treatment of Juvenile Mental Defectives," 919.
44 Ibid.
45 Ibid., 220.
46 Ibid.
47 Alexandra Minna Stern makes a similar observation in her study of sterilization in California, finding that eugenicists appeared uneasy assigning gender roles in cases of sexual behaviour that "transgressed heterosexual norms." She explains that "'sodomites' appear in unnamed patient records from the 1920s," which might point to an overlap between homophobia and sterilization. See Alexandra Minna Stern, "From Legislation to Lived Experience: Eugenic Sterilization in California and Indiana, 1907–79," in *A Century of Eugenics in America: From the Indiana Experiment to the Human Genome Era*, ed. Paul Lombardo (Bloomington: Indiana University Press, 2011), 113.
48 The trends in this literature changed over time and place, however. Minna Stern also finds that, in California and Indiana, the initial interest in curbing male sexual behaviour subsided and a growing interest in heredity took its place; see ibid., 97–9.

49 Paul L. Garrison and Clarence J. Gamble, "Sexual Effects of Vasectomy," *Journal of the American Medical Association* 144, no. 4 (1950): 293.

50 Rebecca Kluchin also finds that this association between discharge and sterilization gave men a legal foothold in challenging the state on this practice, which had the effect of dampening the sterilization pressure on men; see Kluchin, *Fit to Be Tied*, 17.

51 This idea played out in California, too; see Braslow, *Mental Ills and Bodily Cures*, chap. 3.

52 Randall MacLean, "Procedures to Be Followed in Obtaining the Admission of a Patient to a Provincial Mental Hospital," *Alberta Medical Review* 7, no. 4 (1942): 23.

53 Braslow, *Mental Ills and Bodily Cures*; Jack D. Pressman, *Last Resort: Psychosurgery and the Limits of Medicine* (Cambridge: Cambridge University Press, 1998); and Edward Shorter, *A History of Psychiatry: From the Era of the Asylum to the Age of Prozac* (New York: John Wiley & Sons, 1997).

54 Shorter, *History of Psychiatry*, 190.

55 For example, Julius Wagner-Jauregg, who introduced the therapeutic application of malaria among patients with dementia paralytica and for which he received the Nobel Prize in Physiology or Medicine in 1927; and Egaz Moniz, who developed the "burr-hole" technique for lobotomies and who received the Nobel Prize in Physiology and Medicine in 1949.

56 Shorter, *History of Psychiatry*, 145.

57 Robert Lampard papers, personal donation, "Medical History of Dr. L.J. Le Vann," curriculum vitae. I am grateful to Bob for allowing me to review his personal collection of Le Vann's papers.

58 UAA, Leilani Muir files, Undertaking #11.

59 Ibid., 8.

60 For more on this trend in psychiatry, see Jonathan Andrews and Anne Digby, eds., *Sex and Seclusion, Class and Custody: Perspectives on Gender and Class in the History of British and Irish Psychiatry* (Amsterdam: Rodopi Press, 2004); Joan Busfield, "The Female Malady? Men, Women and Madness in Nineteenth Century Britain," *Sociology* 28, no. 1 (1994): 259–77; Elizabeth Lunbeck, *The Psychiatric Persuasion: Knowledge, Gender, and Power in Modern America* (Princeton, NJ: Princeton University Press, 1994); Elaine Showalter, *The Female Malady: Women, Madness, and English Culture, 1830–1980* (New York: Virago Press, 1987); and Nancy Tomes, "Feminist Histories of Psychiatry," in *Discovering the History of Psychiatry*, ed. Mark S. Micale and Roy Porter (Oxford: Oxford University Press, 1994).

61 Ilina Singh, "Not Just Naughty: 50 Years of Stimulant Drug Advertising," in *Medicating Modern America: Prescription Drugs in History*, ed. Andrea

Tone and Elizabeth Siegel Watkins (New York: New York University Press, 2007), 137, 138.
62 For more on the way gendered behaviours in children were understood during this period, see Matthew Smith, "Putting Hyperactivity in Its Place: Cold War Politics, the Brain Race and the Origins of Hyperactivity in the United States, 1957–1968," in *Locating Health: Historical and Anthropological Investigations of Health and Place*, ed. Erika Dyck and Christopher Fletcher (London: Pickering & Chatto, 2011).
63 Eugenics Board, Minutes, Meeting 157, 17 November 1949, 2.
64 Eugenics Board, Minutes, Meeting 168, 9 February 1951.
65 L.J. Le Vann, "The Evaluation of Auditory Hallucinations," *Alberta Medical Review* 15, no. 1 (1950): 25–6.
66 Ibid., 25.
67 Ibid., 25–6.
68 For more on the history of electro-convulsive therapies, see Edward Shorter and David Healy, *Shock Therapy: A History of Electroconvulsive Treatment in Mental Illness* (New Brunswick, NJ: Rutgers University Press, 2007).
69 Some of Le Vann's early work focused on alcoholics, but he later developed a greater focus on childhood mental illnesses. See L.J. Le Vann, "A Clinical Survey of Alcoholics," *Canadian Medical Association Journal* 69, no. 6 (1953): 584–8.
70 L.J. Le Vann, "A Concept of Schizophrenia in the Lower Grade Mental Defective," *American Medical Association Journal* 54 (1950): 469–72.
71 As cited in W. Bromberg, "Schizophrenic-like Psychosis in Defective Children," *Proceedings and Addresses of the Annual Session*, American Association for Mental Deficiency, 39 (1934): 226–57; James Russell Grant, "Propfschizophrenia: A Clinical and Physiological Essay," *Alberta Medical Review* 21, no. 3 (1956): 6; and P. Schilder, "Reaction Types Resembling Functional Psychoses in Childhood on the Basis of an Organic Inferiority of the Brain," *Mental Hygiene* 19 (1935): 439–46.
72 The blood test checked for levels of atropine in the blood, as hypothesized by Abram Hoffer, "Effect of Atropine on Blood Pressure of Patients with Mental and Emotional Disease," *Archives of Neurology and Psychiatry* 71 (1954): 80–6; and idem, "Objective Criteria for the Diagnosis of Schizophrenia Exemplified by the Atropine Test," *Confinia Neurologica* 14, no. 6 (1954): 385–90. Hoffer's articles discuss the existence of psychosis but do not make any links to mental deficiency or degeneration, as is suggested by the Alberta study.
73 Grant, "Propfschizophrenia," 8.

74 L.J. Le Vann, "Trifluoperazine Dihydrochloride: An Effective Tranquilizing Agent for Behavioural Abnormalities in Defective Children," *Canadian Medical Association Journal* 80 (1959): 123.

75 Ibid., 123–4.

76 Ibid., 124.

77 Shorter, *Short History of Psychiatry*, 104.

78 L.J. Le Vann, "A Pilot Project for Emotionally Disturbed Children in Alberta," *Canadian Medical Association Journal* 83, no. 10 (1960): 525.

79 Ibid.

80 L.J. Le Vann, "Thioridazine (Mellaril) a Psycho-sedative Virtually Free of Side-effects," *Alberta Medical Review* 26, no. 4 (1961): 144. His thesis was later criticized by US researchers who found that these drugs had serious side effects, especially for children with mental retardation. See Alan A. Baumeister, Jay A. Sevin, and Bryan H. King, "Neuroleptics," in *Psychotropic Medication and Developmental Disabilities: The International Consensus Handbook*, ed. S. Reiss and M.G. Aman (Columbus: Ohio State University, 1998).

81 Marjorie Montgomery Bowker, "Brief on Mental Retardation for a Special Legislative and Lay Committee appointed by the Legislative Assembly of Alberta for the Study of Preventative Health Services in Alberta," December 1965, 3.

82 David Gibson, "Involuntary Sterilization of the Mentally Retarded: A Western Canadian Phenomenon," *Canadian Psychiatric Association Journal* 19, no. 1 (1974): 61.

83 L.J. Le Vann, "A New Butyrophenone: Trifluperidol. A Psychiatric Evaluation in a Pediatric Setting," *Canadian Psychiatric Association Journal* 13, no. 3 (1968): 271.

84 L.J. Le Vann, "Haloperidol in the Treatment of Behavioural Disorders in Children and Adolescents," *Canadian Psychiatric Association Journal* 14, no. 2 (1969): 217.

85 Ibid., 219.

86 L.J. Le Vann, "Clinical Comparison of Haloperidol with Chlorpromazine in Mentally Retarded Children," *American Journal of Mental Deficiency* 75, no. 6 (1971): 719.

87 L.J. Le Vann and R.E. Cohn, "Clinical Evaluation of Norbolethone Therapy in Stunted Growth and Poorly Thriving Children," *International Journal of Clinical Pharmacology, Therapy and Toxicology* 6, no. 1 (1972): 55.

88 L.J. Le Vann, "Neuleptil – A New Phenothiazine," *Modern Medicine of Canada* 27, no. 9 (1972): 1.

89 Eugenics Board, Minutes, letter from the Secretary to the Board, Mrs E.S. James, to Dr A.D. MacPherson, Medical Superintendent, Provincial Mental Institute, Edmonton, 24 June 1963.

90 For more on women activists, see McLaren, *Our Own Master Race*. For more on scientific motherhood, see Denyse Baillargeon, *Babies for the Nation: The Medicalization of Motherhood in Quebec, 1910–1970*, trans. W. Donald Wilson (Waterloo, ON: Wilfrid Laurier University Press, 2009); and Mitchinson, *Giving Birth in Canada*.

91 See also Valverde, *Age of Light, Soap and Water*.

92 Notable exceptions to this trend are Christopher Dummitt, *The Manly Modern: Masculinity in Postwar Canada* (Vancouver: UBC Press, 2007), who considers the challenges men faced under the burden of modernity that at once threatened to reinforce and destabilize gender relations in the post-war period; and Robert Rutherdale, "Fatherhood, Masculinity, and the Good Years during Canada's Baby Boom, 1945–1965," *Journal of Family History* 24, no. 3 (1999): 351–73, who concentrates more on the concept of "domestic masculinity" or fatherhood in middle-class families and focuses on fathers in Abbotsford and Prince George, British Columbia. Judith Walzer Leavitt, *Make Room for Daddy: The Journey from Waiting Room to Birthing Room* (Chapel Hill: University of North Carolina Press, 2009), offers a rich and fascinating account of middle-class fathers and their gradual move into the medicalized birthing process, or from the home through the waiting room to the bedside and the effect this transition has had on ideals of partnership, modern birthing practices, fatherhood, and, to some extent, masculinity. In Canadian studies of masculinity more broadly, see Steven Penfold, "'Have You No Manhood in You?' Gender and Class in the Cape Breton Coal Towns, 1920–1926," *Acadiensis* 23, no. 2 (1994): 21–44; and Jarrett Rudy, *The Freedom to Smoke: Tobacco Consumption and Identity* (Montreal; Kingston, ON: McGill-Queen's University Press, 2005).

93 Leavitt, *Make Room for Daddy*, 18.

94 Ibid., 79, 174–5.

95 David Herzberg, *Happy Pills in America: From Miltown to Prozac* (Baltimore: Johns Hopkins University Press, 2008), 62.

96 Ibid., 63–72. For more on the post-war shift in masculinity and its medicalization, see Lori Rotskoff, *Love on the Rocks: Men, Women, and Alcohol in Post-World War II America* (Chapel Hill: University of North Carolina Press, 2002).

97 Dummitt, *Manly Modern*, 6.

98 Garrison and Gamble, "Sexual Effects of Vasectomy," 293.

99 Ibid., 294.

100 Kluchin, *Fit to Be Tied*, 51.
101 "Birth Control: Editorial," *Canadian Medical Association Journal* 57 (1947): 489–90.
102 G.P.R. Tallin, "The Legal Implications of the Non-Therapeutic Practices of Doctors," *Canadian Medical Association Journal* 87, no. 5 (1962): 210.
103 Thomas Fisher, "Legal Implications of Sterilization," *Canadian Medical Association Journal* 91, no. 26 (1964): 1365.
104 Ibid., 1364.
105 Ibid.
106 Meredith Fleming and Terrence C.R. Joyce, "Elective Sterilization of the Human Male (Vasectomy)," *Canadian Hospital* 45, no. 6 (1968): 2.
107 David A. Rodgers et al., "Sociopsychological Characteristics of Patients Obtaining Vasectomies from Urologists," *Marriage and Family Living* 25, no. 3 (1963): 332.
108 Thomas Poffenberger and Shirley Poffenberger, "Vasectomy as a Preferred Method of Birth Control: A Preliminary Investigation," *Marriage and Family Living* 25, no. 3 (1963): 326.
109 Ibid., 327–8.
110 L.N. Jackson, "Vasectomy in the United Kingdom," *Practitioner* 203, no. 215 (1969): 320.
111 Ibid., 321.
112 Ibid., 323.
113 "Vasectomy in Britain," *IPPF Medical Bulletin* 4, no. 2 (1970): 4.
114 "Voluntary Sterilization for Family Welfare," *Canadian Medical Association Journal* 95, no. 2 (1966): 81.
115 Elizabeth Watkins, *On the Pill: A Social History of Contraceptives, 1950–1970* (Baltimore: Johns Hopkins University Press, 1998), 76–7.
116 As indicated in ibid., 103–4. See also Barbara Seaman, *The Doctor's Case Against the Pill*, 25th anniversary ed. (Alameda, CA: Hunter House, 1995).
117 Watkins, *On the Pill*, 104–5.
118 For a thorough investigation of the Association for Voluntary Sterilization and, in particular, the response to the pill, see Kluchin, *Fit to Be Tied*, especially chap. 2.
119 Heather Molyneaux, "Controlling Conception: Images of Women, Sexuality and the Pill in the Sixties," in *Gender, Health and Popular Culture: Historical Perspectives*, ed. Cheryl Krasnick Warsh (Waterloo, ON: Wilfrid Laurier University Press, 2011), 70.
120 Ibid., 83; she is citing Jack Batten, "Is There a Male Conspiracy against the Pill?" *Chatelaine* (July 1969), 17, 40.
121 On the pill advertisements, see Molyneaux, "Controlling Conception," 74–7.

122 "Vasectomy: 'simplest way' to birth control," *Calgary Herald*, 8 April 1970, 24.

123 As quoted in Kluchin, *Fit to Be Tied*, 57.

124 Calgary Health Services Archives, CGH 100, letter from J.C. Johnston to Mr L.S. Portigal (City Solicitor's Department), 10 April 1970, 1.

125 Dodds, *Voluntary Male Sterilization*, 4.

126 Ibid., 7.

127 Ibid., 8.

128 Ibid., 11.

129 Ibid., 25.

130 Walter Nagel, "Male birth control: vasectomies on increase in city, doctor says," *Calgary Herald*, 7 April 1970, 24.

131 "The Continuing Search for a Male Contraceptive," *Life*, 6 May 1970, 43.

132 Ibid., 42.

5. From Sterilization to Patient Activism

1 Doreen Befus, "Who Says 'Impossible'?" *Decision* (March 1990), 16–17.

2 Red Deer & District Archives (hereafter cited as RDDA), Doreen "Ellen" Befus Files, MG368, Box 4, letter from Doreen Befus to Judge J.K. Holmes, 22 November 1978, 1; and Befus, "Who Says 'Impossible'?" 16.

3 RDDA, Doreen "Ellen" Befus Files, MG368, Box 4, letter from Befus to Holmes, 22 November 1978, 3.

4 Befus, "Who Says 'Impossible'?" 16.

5 Penelope Jahn, "Legal Crusade of the Eternal Children," *McLean's*, 30 November 1981, 20.

6 Grant, "Results of Institutional Treatment," 918.

7 Ibid.

8 RDDA, Doreen "Ellen" Befus Files, MG368, Box 6, news clippings, Jim Lozeron, "Michener Centre laundry problems 'minor,'" *Red Deer Advocate* (1977).

9 See, for example, Jim Struthers, *The Limits of Affluence: Welfare in Ontario, 1920–1970* (Toronto: University of Toronto Press, 1994).

10 See, for example, Raymond Blake, *From Rights to Needs: A History of Family Allowances in Canada, 1929–1992* (Vancouver: UBC Press, 2009).

11 See, especially, Gerald Grob, *The Mad among Us: A History of the Care of America's Mentally Ill* (New York: Free Press, 1994).

12 Geoffrey Reaume, "Patients at Work: Insane Asylum Inmates' Labour in Ontario, 1841–1900," in *Mental Health and Canadian Society: Historical Perspectives*, ed. James E. Moran and David Wright (Montreal; Kingston, ON: McGill-Queen's University Press, 2006).

13 For a comprehensive historical overview of this literature, see Henri Stiker, *A History of Disability*, trans. William Sayers (Ann Arbor: University of Michigan Press, 1999). For a further example in this genre that provides a closer study of specific programs designed to challenge public perceptions of disability and that have confronted legal challenges, see Sharon L. Snyder and David T. Mitchell, *Cultural Locations of Disability* (Chicago: University of Chicago Press, 2006).

14 Geoffrey Hudson, "Regions and Disability Politics in Ontario, 1975–1985" (paper presented at the conference "Putting Region in Its Place," University of Alberta, Edmonton, 26–28 October 2007).

15 Thomas Szasz, *The Myth of Mental Illness: Foundations of a Theory of Personal Conduct* (1960; New York: Harper Collins, 1974).

16 Michel Foucault, *Madness and Civilization: A History of Insanity in the Age of Reason* (New York: Vintage Books, 1965).

17 Befus, "Who Says 'Impossible'?" 17.

18 RDDA, Doreen "Ellen" Befus Files, MG368, diary, 1 September 1976.

19 RDDA, Doreen "Ellen" Befus Files, MG368, Box 4, included in diary collection, letter to the editor, 29 September 1976, 1.

20 Ibid.

21 Ibid., 2.

22 Ibid. The quotation is taken from a handwritten document that is difficult in places to decipher, and represents the author's best attempt at interpretation after reading through the full set of documents and analysing the tone expressed in several boxes of letters.

23 Ibid., 3.

24 RDDA, Doreen "Ellen" Befus Files, MG368, Box 6, diary, October 1976, 1–2.

25 RDDA, Doreen "Ellen" Befus Files, MG368, Box 6, diary, 1 November 1976, 1.

26 Ibid., 3.

27 Erving Goffman, *Asylums: Essays on the Social Situation of Mental Patients and Other Inmates* (Garden City, NY: Anchor Books, 1961).

28 See Michel Foucault, *Birth of the Clinic: An Archaeology of Medical Perception*, trans. A.M. Sheridan (1973; New York: Vintage Books, 1994); and idem, *Madness and Civilization*.

29 RDDA, Doreen "Ellen" Befus Files, MG368, Box 6, diary, 7 November 1976, 1.

30 Ibid., 2.

31 RDDA, Doreen "Ellen" Befus Files, MG368, Box 6, letter to Pam Symons, 2 December 1976, 1.

32 RDDA, Doreen "Ellen" Befus Files, MG368, Box 6, Carolyn Martindale, "Mentally handicapped taught about sex at Michener Centre," *Red Deer Advocate*, June 1981.

33 Ibid.

34 Ibid.
35 RDDA, Doreen "Ellen" Befus Files, MG368, Box 6, diary, "My Experience Living in a Suite at 5622–42 St, Since 1977–78," [n.d.], 1.
36 RDDA, Doreen "Ellen" Befus Files, MG368, Box 3, memo, re: Ellen, note: copied 1975.
37 RDDA, Doreen "Ellen" Befus Files, MG368, Box 4, family records, received 15 October 1978, in response to her letter published in the *Red Deer Advocate*, 16 October 1978, 1.
38 Ibid., 2.
39 RDDA, Doreen "Ellen" Befus Files, MG368, Box 4, letter to "Sis" [believed to be twin sister], no date, 1–2.
40 Ibid., 2.
41 Ibid., 2, 3.
42 RDDA, Doreen "Ellen" Befus Files, MG368, Box 6, diary, "Guest friends who had come to my home, suite B, before Leaving Apartment since 1978."
43 Ibid., 3.
44 RDDA, Doreen "Ellen" Befus Files, MG368, Box 6, diary, no page number.
45 RDDA, Doreen "Ellen" Befus Files, MG368, Box 6, diary, "My experience working in the community on a daily basis," 16 September 1979, 1.
46 Ibid.
47 RDDA, Doreen "Ellen" Befus Files, MG368, Box 6, diary, [n.d.], "My experience working with the mentally handicapped," 1.
48 RDDA, Doreen "Ellen" Befus Files, MG368, Box 2, report on the Foulston family, part 3, 28 February 1979.
49 RDDA, Doreen "Ellen" Befus Files, MG368, Box 6, diary, [n.d.], "My experience working with the mentally handicapped," 1.
50 RDDA, Doreen "Ellen" Befus Files, MG368, Box 3, File A, letter from Tedda, 23 February 1986.
51 RDDA, Doreen "Ellen" Befus Files, MG368, Box 3, File A, letter from Christel, 25 September 1987.
52 RDDA, Doreen "Ellen" Befus Files, MG368, Box 2, report on Francis Paller.
53 Ibid.
54 RDDA, Doreen "Ellen" Befus Files, MG368, Box 6, memo, "My experience working with handicappi people both mentally and physically," 1. See also RDDA, Doreen "Ellen" Befus Files, MG368, Box 6, memo, "My experience working with handicappis, part two."
55 RDDA, Doreen "Ellen" Befus Files, MG368, Box 6, memo, "My experience working with handicappi people both mentally and physically," 1.
56 RDDA, Doreen "Ellen" Befus Files, MG368, Box 6, memo to the University of Alberta, 28 October 1981, "The disabled are abled" (handwritten).

57 RDDA, Doreen "Ellen" Befus Files, MG368, Box 6, letter, "Handicapped seek improved ministry," [n.d.], 1.

58 Ibid., 2.

59 RDDA, Doreen "Ellen" Befus Files, MG368, Box 3, letter from Lady-in-Waiting Kathryn Dupdale to Doreen Befus, 31 August 1981.

60 RDDA, Doreen "Ellen" Befus Files, MG368, Box 3, letter from Karen M. Vardy to Doreen Befus, 4 September 1981, 2.

61 RDDA, Doreen "Ellen" Befus Files, MG368, Box 3, letter from Sylvia Hulme to Doreen Befus, 24 April 1980, 1–2.

62 RDDA, Doreen "Ellen" Befus Files, MG368, Box 3, letter to Mr & Mrs Raymond L'Heureux, Alberta Association for the Mentally Handicapped, 11 October 1983.

63 RDDA, Doreen "Ellen" Befus Files, MG368, Kathleen Engman, "Doreen Befus' story of determination unfolds on the screen," *Red Deer Advocate*, 4 August 1983.

64 John Schmidt, "Unifarm," *Calgary Herald*, 27 March 1973.

65 Gibson, "Involuntary sterilization," 62.

6. Appendectomy to Queen's Court Settlement

1 Wahlsten, "Leilani Muir versus the Philosopher King," abstract.

2 UAA, Field Law Papers Re: Leilani Muir, Files from Provincial Training School, 1940–1978, 1951, Diagnostic Summary by Le Vann.

3 Ibid.

4 UAA, Provincial Training School Clinical Record: Personal and Development History, [completed by Marie Scorah], 12 July 1955.

5 Ibid.

6 UAA, Field Law Papers Re: Leilani Muir, Files from Provincial Training School, 1940–1978, letter from Assistant Superintendent A.W. Fraser to Dr F.W. Hanley (Calgary).

7 UAA, Field Law Papers Re: Leilani Muir, Files from Provincial Training School, 1940–1978, letter from Le Vann to Scorah, 23 April 1953.

8 Statutes of Alberta, 1937, Chapter 46, An Act to amend the Mental Defectives Act, assented to 14 April 1937, 179.

9 UAA, Field Law Papers Re: Leilani Muir, Files from Provincial Training School, 1940–1978, letter from Kibblewhite (Chief Clinical Psychologist) to Le Vann, 14 November 1952.

10 UAA, letter from G.W. Baird to Provincial Training School, 12 March 1953.

11 Statutes of Alberta, 1942, Chapter 47, An Act to amend the Mental Defectives Act, assented to 19 March 1942, 177.

12 UAA, letter from Le Vann to G.W. Baird (Secretary-Treasurer of the Village of Black Diamond), 18 March 1953.
13 UAA, Field Law Papers Re: Leilani Muir, Files from Provincial Training School, 1940–1978, handwritten letter from Harley Scorah to Le Vann, [n.d, likely April 1953].
14 UAA, Field Law Papers Re: Leilani Muir, Files from Provincial Training School, 1940–1978, letter from Le Vann to Scorah, 18 March 1953 and 23 April 1953.
15 UAA, Application form for the Provincial Training School, completed and signed by Harley Scorah, [n.d.].
16 UAA, Field Law Papers Re: Leilani Muir, Files from Provincial Training School, 1940–1978, Ward Admission Record, 12 July 1952.
17 UAA, Physician's Certificate, signed by Le Vann.
18 Ibid.
19 UAA, Provincial Training School Clinical Record: Personal and Development History, 12 July 1955.
20 Ibid.
21 UAA, Provincial Training School, Red Deer, Alberta, 12 July 1955.
22 See correspondence between Mrs Scorah and Le Vann in the UAA files.
23 UAA, letter from Scorah to Le Vann, 3 November 1956.
24 UAA, letter from Le Vann to the Scorahs, 26 October 1956.
25 UAA, letter from matron (unsigned and unnamed) to the Scorahs, 27 June 1956.
26 For example, UAA, letter from Le Vann to Mrs Scorah, 12 May 1958.
27 UAA, letter from A.G. Frauenfeld, Deputy Superintendent, Child Welfare Branch, Department of Public Welfare, to Le Vann, 1 November 1960.
28 UAA, letter from W.D. McFarland, Superintendent of Child Welfare, Department of Public Welfare, to W.H. Bury, Director of Child Welfare (Ontario) and to Le Vann, [n.d.] 1960.
29 UAA, memo from Miss Alford, social worker, to Le Vann, 31 July 1964, 1–2.
30 UAA, Provincial Training School Report presented to Eugenics Board, 22 November 1957.
31 Ibid.
32 Ibid.
33 Ibid.
34 Statues of Alberta, 1937, Chapter 47, An Act to amend the Sexual Sterilization Act, assented to 14 April 1937, clause 4(1), 181.
35 Ibid., 182.
36 Statutes of Alberta, 1942, Chapter 48, An Act to amend the Sexual Sterilization Act, assented to 19 March 1942, 179–80. See also a brief description

of this change in policy in Bernard M. Dickens, "Eugenic Recognition in Canadian Law," *Osgoode Hall Law Journal* 13 (1975): 561.

37 Ibid.

38 For more on the history of "mongoloidism," see Mark Jackson, "Changing Depictions of Disease: Race, Representation and the History of 'Mongolism,'" in *Race, Science and Medicine, 1700–1960*, ed. Waltraud Ernst and Bernard Harris (London: Routledge, 1999).

39 UAA, Psychological Examination, 11 May 1957.

40 Ibid.

41 UAA, Provincial Training School Report presented to Eugenics Board, 22 November 1957.

42 Lombardo, *Three Generations*, 144.

43 For more on the debates surrounding the application of the IQ test, see Richard J. Hernstein and Charles Murray, *The Bell Curve: Intelligence and Class Structure in American Life* (New York: Free Press, 1994).

44 Johanna Schoen, "Reassessing Eugenic Sterilization: The Case of North Carolina," in *A Century of Eugenics in America: From the Indiana Experiment to the Human Genome Era*, ed. Paul Lombardo (Bloomington: University of Indiana Press, 2011), 142–3.

45 UAA, Pathology Report, 22 January 1959, signed by Le Vann.

46 UAA, Provincial Training School Operative Report, 19 January 1959. The surgeons appointed to undertake these surgeries worked for an annual honorarium of $1,500, and took their direction directly from the Eugenics Board. According to provincial law, they could not be held liable for any action arising from the operations; see UAA, letter from Donovan Ross, Minister of Health, to Lieutenant Governor in Council, 7 January 1958.

47 UAA, Provincial Training School Clinical Record, General Summary of Case, [date unclear on the record].

48 A paucity of available records now makes it impossible to substantiate a direct link between the numbers of individuals sterilized and the numbers of patients discharged.

49 UAA, Physical Examination, Anthropometric Data and General Examination, 8 August 1955.

50 UAA, letter from Mrs R.C. Carlyle, RN, and G. Hulley, MD, to Medical Officer, Provincial Training School, 29 April 1966.

51 UAA, letter from Le Vann to Mrs R.C. Carlyle, RN, and G. Hulley, MD, 19 May 1966.

52 UAA, letter from Hulley and Carlyle to Le Vann, 18 May 1966.

53 UAA, letter from Le Vann to Hulley and Carlyle, 11 May 1966.

54 UAA, letter from John Dickson to Le Vann, 4 October 1971.

55 UAA, letter from Le Vann to John Dickson, Doctors Medical Clinic, Victoria, BC, 12 October 1971.
56 "Mentally retarded should be sterilized, suggest doctors," *Edmonton Journal*, 28 September [year unknown], in UAA, Leilani Muir files, newspaper clippings.
57 Ibid.
58 UAA, letter from McTavish to Faulkner, 8 September 1975.
59 UAA, Court of Queen's Bench of Alberta, Judicial District of Calgary, File No. 8701-20014, DLW (Plaintiff) and Her Majesty the Queen in the Right of Alberta as represented by the Minister of Social Services (defendant), 1 December 1987.
60 UAA, letter from Carole Carver, articled student at Dinning, Crawford, Valance, Hunter and Loster, to Mrs Leilani M. Muir, 30 December 1987.
61 UAA, letter from Frances Zinger, Barrister and Solicitor, to Leilani M. Muir, 11 August 1988.
62 UAA, letter from Amy Anne Scorah [previously went by Marie], "To Whom it May Concern," 12 September 1988.
63 UAA, letter from Lenore B. Harlton, Price Harlton Barrister and Solicitor, to Frances Zinger, 24 October 1988.
64 UAA, letter from James J. McCormick, Director of Social Services, to Lenore B. Harlton, 4 November 1988.
65 History of LEAF taken from its website: http://leaf.ca/about-leaf/history/, accessed 10 April 2011.
66 Valerie Korinek, *Roughing It in the Suburbs: Reading Chatelaine Magazine in the Fifties and Sixties* (Toronto: University of Toronto Press, 2000), 309. For more on Doris Anderson, her single-motherhood, and her work-life balance, see Doris Anderson, *Rebel Daughter: An Autobiography* (Toronto: Key Porter Books, 1996).
67 UAA, Leilani M. Muir LEAF Case Proposal, 14 September 1989.
68 Ibid.
69 Ibid.
70 See, for example, Gibbons, "True [Political] Mothers of Tomorrow."
71 UAA, letter from Annie Bunting, LEAF, to Myra Bielby, Field and Field, 14 February 1990.
72 UAA, letter from Peter Calder, Chartered Psychologist, to Myra Bielby, Field and Field, 28 December 1989 re: Psychological Assessment of Ms Leilani Muir.
73 Ibid., 2.
74 UAA, Discovery Binder, Undertaking 11: Produce Dr Le Vann's qualifications in the area of child psychiatry and his other qualifications in other areas.
75 See trial transcripts.

7. Abortion, Sterilization, and the Eugenics Legacy

1 CHSA, FHH-037, letter from D.M. Hay to the Chairman, Therapeutic Abortion Committee, 18 November 1974.

2 CHSA, FHH, "History and Physical Examination" Jane Doe, for Dr Hay, recorded by C. Robinson, RN, 18 November 1974, 1–2.

3 As Beth Palmer explains, many women from Calgary travelled to the United States to procure abortions; see Beth Palmer, "'Lonely, tragic, but legally necessary pilgrimages': Transnational Abortion Travel in the 1970s," *Canadian Historical Review* 92, no. 4 (2011): 637–64.

4 CHSA, FHH, "Foothills Hospital, Referral for Consideration by Therapeutic Abortion Committee," [n.d.], 1–2.

5 CHSA, FHH, "(Women) Cornell Medical Index Health Questionnaire," [n.d.], 1–2.

6 Ibid., 3–4.

7 CHSA, FHH, "Social History," 20 November 1974, 1–11.

8 CHSA, FHH-037, Therapeutic Abortion Committee, "Therapeutic Abortion," [n.d.], 4.

9 For more on the topic of illegitimacy and its medicalization, see Rickie Solinger, "Race and 'Value': Black and White Illegitimate Babies, in the USA, 1945–1965," in *Women and Health in America*, 2nd ed., ed. Judith Walzer Leavitt (Madison: University of Wisconsin Press, 1999).

10 CHSA, FHH-037, "Section 237 of the Criminal Code Prior to the Amendment," document used by the Foothills Hospital, received 18 February 1970, 1.

11 Ibid., 2.

12 Ibid.

13 Christabelle Sethna, "All Aboard? Canadian Women's Abortion Tourism, 1960–1980," in *Gender, Health and Popular Culture: Historical Perspectives*, ed. Cheryl Krasnick Warsh (Waterloo, ON: Wilfrid Laurier University Press, 2011), 90–1.

14 CHSA, Alberta Hospital Services Commission, "Therapeutic Abortions in Hospitals in Alberta, 1972" (October 1973), 1. The numbers for 1970, 1971, and 1973 (6 months), respectively, were: Newfoundland, 25, 80, 77; Prince Edward Island, 18, 39, 27; Nova Scotia, 263, 645, 398; New Brunswick, 72, 146, 83; Quebec, 541, 1,903, 1,386; Ontario, 5,657, 16,244, 9,878; Manitoba, 248, 864, 594; Saskatchewan, 217, 760, 512; Alberta, 1,172, 3,169, 1,864 [4,002 was the total for 1973]; British Columbia, 2,981, 7,090, 3,974; and Yukon, 6, 9, 24. These statistics were published in the report, but generated by Statistics Canada.

15 CHSA, FHH-037, Foothills Hospital Memorandum, "Therapeutic Abortions and Sterilization Committee," 19 April 1973, 1.
16 Ibid., 2. These findings match the interpretations offered elsewhere by Christabelle Sethna and Beth Palmer.
17 CHSA, CGH-100, Alberta Hospital Services Commission, "Therapeutic Abortions in Hospitals in Alberta in 1975," 1975, 2.
18 Ibid., 3.
19 See subsequent annual reports of the Alberta Hospital Services Commission, 1973 and 1975.
20 CHSA, FHH-037, Don Husel, Chief, Department of Obstetrics and Gynecology, "Brief relating to: Sexual Sterilization & Therapeutic Abortions in the Royal Alexandra Hospital" (presented to the Board of Governors, [1970?]), 3.
21 Ibid., 4.
22 Ibid., 6. Of the sterilized women, 10 were between the ages of 15 and 19; 61 were between 20 and 24; 157 were between 25 and 29; 206 were between 30 and 34; 208 were between 35 and 39; 114 were between 40 and 44; and 14 were over age 45. Also, 51 abortions were performed on girls under age 15, but none of these was sterilized (7).
23 CHSA, FHH-037, Alberta Hospital Services Commission, "Therapeutic Abortions in Hospitals in Alberta, January to June 1973," 1973, 6.
24 Ibid., 7.
25 Sethna, "All Aboard?," 98–9.
26 Christabelle Sethna and Steve Hewitt, "Clandestine Operations: The Vancouver Women's Caucus, the Abortion Caravan and the RCMP," *Canadian Historical Review* 90, no. 3 (2009): 463–95.
27 See Sethna, "All Aboard?"
28 Palmer, "'Lonely, tragic, but legally necessary pilgrimages.'"
29 For more on Morgentaler, who is an extremely important figure in these debates, but is the subject of studies elsewhere, see Catherine Dunphy, *Morgentaler: A Difficult Hero* (Toronto: John Wiley & Sons Canada, 2003).
30 This definition continues to be used by the World Health Organization; see its website: http://www.who.int/about/definition/en/print.html, accessed 2 July 2013.
31 CHSA, FHH-037, clippings file, [n.d.].
32 Ibid.
33 CHSA, FHH-037, letter from Murray Ross, Executive Director, Alberta Hospital Association, to R. Alan Hay, Executive Director, Ontario Hospital Association, 16 January 1970.
34 CHSA, FHH-037, memo from R.A. Slute, Director, Association Services Division, Ontario Hospital Association, to all members, 19 August 1969, 1.

35 Ibid.
36 CHSA, FHH-037, memo from R.B. Ketcheson, MD, Ad Hoc Chairman, to Chairman and Members of the Foothills Hospital Board, 12 May 1970 [not for circulation] re: indications or criteria for therapeutic abortions at the Foothills Hospital.
37 Ibid.
38 See, for example, Schoen, *Choice and Coercion*, 168.
39 CHS, FHH-037, letter from Harry Brody to L.R. Adshead, Secretary of the Hospital Board, Foothills Hospital, 7 October 1970, 1.
40 Ibid.
41 Ibid., 2.
42 Walter Nagel, "Doctors seek new policy on therapeutic abortions," *Calgary Herald*, 3 November 1970, 1–2.
43 Stephani Keer, "Abortion becoming freer," *Calgary Herald*, [exact date unknown] October 1970, 4.
44 For more on this image of the women, see Molyneaux, "Controlling Conception," 81.
45 CHSA, FHH-037, minutes of a meeting of the Ad Hoc Committee to Study Effects of Increased Demands for Therapeutic Abortions, Royal Alexandra Hospital, Edmonton, 15 September 1970, 3.
46 Ibid., 4.
47 Harry Brody, Stewart Meikle, and Richard Gerritse, "Therapeutic Abortion: A Prospective Study, I," *American Journal of Obstetrics and Gynecology* 109, no. 3 (1971): 347.
48 Ibid., 352–3.
49 CHSA, FHH-037, minutes of a meeting of the Ad Hoc Committee to Study Effects of Increased Demands for Therapeutic Abortions, Royal Alexandra Hospital, Edmonton, 15 September 1970, 4–5.
50 Ibid., 8.
51 Ibid.
52 CHSA, FHH-037, letter from H. Brody, MD, Director, Department of Obstetrics and Gynecology, to L.R. Adshead, Administrator, 21 December 1970, 1.
53 Ibid.
54 CHSA, FHH-037, letter from Brody to Ralph Coombs, Assistant Administrator, 16 December 1970.
55 Ibid.
56 Ibid.
57 Brenda Cheevers, "Abortion Centre is optimistic about future progress in city," *Calgary Herald*, 8 January 1971.

58 Ibid.
59 As quoted in Ibid.
60 CHSA, CGH-100, CGH Medical, Therapeutic Abortions, 1972–75, letter from G.V. Chablani, MD, to E.H. Knight, Executive Director, Calgary General Hospital, 15 April 1975.
61 CHSA, FHH-037, memo from Dr K.I. Pearce to R. Coombs, 25 October 1973, 2.
62 CHSA, FHH-037, memo from R. Coombs, 19 November 1973, re: Abortions.
63 CHSA, FHH-037, letter from Oscar Sommerfeld, President, Pro-Life, to Justice E. Patrick Hartt, Law Reform Commission of Canada, 1 June 1973.
64 Ibid.
65 D.E. Zarfas, "Psychiatric Indications for the Termination of Pregnancy," *Canadian Medical Association Journal* 79, no. 4 (1958): 230.
66 Ibid., 231.
67 Ibid., 232. For more on the logic behind using sterilization to assuage mental symptoms, see Braslow, *Mental Ills and Bodily Cures*, 51–70.
68 Zarfas, "Psychiatric Indications," 232.
69 Ibid.
70 Ibid.
71 Daniel Cappon, "Psychiatric Indications for the Termination of Pregnancy – Comments," *Canadian Medical Association Journal* 79, no. 4 (1958): 236.
72 Dickens, "Eugenic Recognition in Canadian Law," 558.
73 Ibid., 563–4.
74 CHSA, CGH-100, Minutes of the meeting of the Therapeutic Abortions Committee, 18 June 1974.
75 CHSA, Grace Hospital (GRA)-011, letter from Dr Norman Brown, Canadian Medical Protective Association, to Dr Ian Burgess, Vice-President, Salvation Army Grace Hospital, Calgary, 2 November 1978, 1.
76 Ibid., 2.
77 Ibid.
78 Ibid., 3.
79 "Sterilization ban is sought," *Calgary Herald*, 9 December 1979.
80 See also "Protect mentally ill from sterilization, says law reform commission," *Calgary Herald*, 9 December 1979, B3.
81 Law Reform Commission of Canada, "Sterilization," 121.
82 Ibid., 122.
83 CHSA, GRA-011, letter from Jeffrey N. Thom, Fenerty, Robertson, Prowse, Fraser & Hatch, to David Luginbuhl, Salvation Army Grace Hospital, Calgary, 8 April 1980, 1.
84 Ibid., 3. See also Statutes of Alberta, 1976, Chapter 63, Dependent Adults Act, section 1(h) and section 1(h)(ii).

85 CHSA, GRA-011, letter from David Luginbuhl to Lieutenant-Colonel D. Routly, Women's Social Services Secretary, Salvation Army Headquarters, 16 May 1983, 1–2.

86 CHSA, GRA-011, Grace Hospital Medical Staff: Sterilization Committee, Records and Correspondence, 1971–87, Medical Executive Sterilization Committee, consent form and case file.

87 CHSA, GRA-011, Grace Hospital Medical Staff: Sterilization Committee, Records and Correspondence, 1971–87, Medical Executive Sterilization Committee, 1983.

88 CHSA, GRA-011, Grace Hospital Medical Staff: Sterilization Committee, Records and Correspondence, 1971–87, letter from Calvert to Motta, 2 May 1985.

89 CHSA, GRA-011, Grace Hospital Medical Staff: Sterilization Committee, Records and Correspondence, 1971–87, letter from Wren to Office of Public Guardian, 28 November 1983.

90 CHSA, GRA-011, Grace Hospital Medical Staff: Sterilization Committee, Records and Correspondence, 1971–87, letter from Social Services and Community Health to Wren, 16 February 1984.

91 CHSA, GRA-011, Grace Hospital Medical Staff: Sterilization Committee, Records and Correspondence, 1971–87, letter from Wren to Sterilization Committee, Grace Hospital, 14 January 1983.

92 CHSA, GRA-011, Grace Hospital Medical Staff: Sterilization Committee, Records and Correspondence, 1971–87, letter from Wren to social worker, 2 September 1983.

93 CHSA, GRA-011, Grace Hospital Medical Staff, Therapeutic Abortions Committee, 1971–87, Policy: Sterilization, 2 May 1985; and Policy: Sterilization, 19 February 1987.

94 CHSA, GRA-011, Grace Hospital Medical Staff: Sterilization Committee, Records and Correspondence, 1971–87, letter from Wren to Major David Luginbuhl, Executive Director, Grace Hospital, 23 July 1987.

95 As cited in Ingrid Makus, *Women, Politics, and Reproduction: The Liberal Legacy* (Toronto: University of Toronto Press, 1996), 134.

8. Conclusion

1 PAA, Peter Lougheed Papers, 72.59/154, letter from Jan Weijer to Peter Lougheed, 21 March 1969, 2.

2 This newspaper article was included as an attachment in the materials forwarded to Lougheed, 12 April 1968, but the newspaper, article title, and page number are unknown.

3 Dickens, "Eugenic Recognition in Canadian Law," 558.

4 Canada, Parliament, House of Commons, Private Member's Bill, M-312, accessed 1 October 2012, available online at http://www.stephenwoodworth.ca/canadas-400-year-old-definition-of-human-being/motion-312.

5 "How the abortion debate has reared its head in Parliament," CBC News online, 26 April 2012, available at http://www.cbc.ca/news/canada/story/2012/04/26/f-abortion-woodworth-motion-parties.html, accessed 11 June 2012.

6 Mike Schouten, "Harper is paying the price for shutting down the abortion debate," *National Post*, 25 May 2012, available online at http://fullcomment.nationalpost.com/2012/05/25/mike-schouten-harper-is-paying-the-price-for-shutting-down-the-abortion-debate/, accessed 11 June 2012. Schouten is campaign director for weneedaLAW.ca, a group that advocates for federal abortion legislation in Canada.

7 See, for example, "Rona Ambrose resignation petition hits 6,100 signatures after abortion vote," *National Post*, 28 September 2012, 1, available online at http://news.nationalpost.com/2012/09/28/petition-calling-for-status-of-women-ministers-job-after-abortion-vote-garners-6100-signatures/, accessed 1 October 2012.

Bibliography

Primary Sources

Calgary Health Services Archives, Calgary General Hospital.
Calgary Health Services Archives, Foothills Hospital.
Calgary Health Services Archives, Grace Hospital.
Centre for Addiction and Mental Health Archives, "Mental Hygiene of the
  Province of Alberta, Canadian National Committee for Mental Hygiene,"
  October–November 1921; additional surveys were conducted in 1928 and 1947.
City of Edmonton Archives, Emily Murphy Scrapbooks.
Legislative scrapbooks.
Provincial Archives of Alberta, Premier's Papers.
Provincial Archives of Alberta, Attorney General Files.
Provincial Archives of Alberta, "Mental Health Surveys in Alberta."
Public Library of Red Deer, clippings file on Doreen Befus.
Red Deer & District Archives, Doreen "Ellen" Befus Files.
Robert Lampard papers, personal collection, "Medical History of Dr. L.J.
  Le Vann," curriculum vitae.
Saskatchewan Archives Board, Violet McNaughton Papers.
United Farm Women of Alberta, Convention Meeting Minutes.
United Farmers of Alberta, Annual Reports.
University of Alberta Archives, Eugenics Board, Meeting Minutes.
University of Alberta Archives, Field Law Papers, Re: Leilani Muir.
University of Alberta Archives, Leilani Muir Papers.

Secondary Sources

Alberta. Department of Public Health. Vital Statistics Branch. *Annual Report*.
  Edmonton, various years, 1927–66.

Allen, Richard. "The Social Gospel and the Reform Tradition in Canada, 1890–1928." *Canadian Historical Review* 49, no. 4 (1968): 381–99.

Allen, Richard. *The Social Passion: Religion and Social Reform in Canada, 1914–28.* Toronto: University of Toronto Press, 1971.

Allen, Richard. *The View from Murney Tower: Salem Bland, the Late Victorian Controversies, and the Search for a New Christianity.* Toronto: University of Toronto Press, 2008.

Anderson, Doris. *Rebel Daughter: An Autobiography.* Toronto: Key Porter Books, 1996.

Andrews, Jonathan, and Anne Digby, eds. *Sex and Seclusion, Class and Custody: Perspectives on Gender and Class in the History of British and Irish Psychiatry.* Amsterdam: Rodopi Press, 2004.

Ansari, J.M.A., and H.H. Francis. "A Study of 49 Sterilized Females." *Acta Psychiatrica Scandinavica* 54, no. 5 (1976): 315–22.

Arnold, T. "Wave of anger, outrage greets proposed law: a time line." *Edmonton Journal,* 11 March 1998.

Avrich, Paul. *Sacco and Vanzetti: The Anarchist Background.* Princeton, NJ: Princeton University Press, 1996.

Backhouse, Constance. *Petticoats and Prejudice: Women and Law in Nineteenth-Century Canada.* Toronto: Women's Press/Osgoode Society, 1991.

Baillargeon, Denyse. *Babies for the Nation: The Medicalization of Motherhood in Quebec, 1910–1970.* Trans. W. Donald Wilson. Waterloo, ON: Wilfrid Laurier University Press, 2009.

Baragar, C.A., Geo. A. Davidson, W.J. McAlister, and D.L. McCullough. "Sexual Sterilization: Four Years Experience in Alberta." *American Journal of Psychology* 19, no. 2 (1935): 897–923.

Barnes, Allan C., and Frederick P. Zuspan. "Patient Reaction to Puerperal Surgical Sterilization." *American Journal of Obstetrics and Gynaecology* 75, no. 1 (1958): 65–71.

Batten, Jack. "Is There a Male Conspiracy against the Pill?" *Chatelaine,* July 1969.

Baumeister, Alan A., Jay A. Sevin, and Bryan H. King. "Neuroleptics." In *Psychotropic Medication and Developmental Disabilities: The International Consensus Handbook,* ed. S. Reiss and M.G. Aman. Columbus: Ohio State University, 1998.

Befus, Doreen. "Who Says 'Impossible'?" *Decision,* March 1990, 16–17.

Black, Edwin. *War against the Weak: Eugenics and America's Campaign to Create a Master Race.* New York: Four Walls Eight Windows, 2003.

Black, W.P., and A.B. Sclare. "Sterilization by Tubal Ligation – A Follow-up Study." *Journal of Obstetrics and Gynaecology in the British Commonwealth* 75, no. 2 (1968): 219–24.

Blackwell, Tom. "Canadians airbrush the truth about Tommy Douglas's enthusiasm for eugenics: MD." *National Post*, 14 March 2012. Available online at http://news.nationalpost.com/2012/03/14/tommy-douglas/.

Blair, W.R.N. *Mental Health in Alberta: A Report on the Alberta Mental Health Study, 1968* [The Blair Report]. Edmonton: Ministry of Human Resources and Development, 1969.

Blake, Raymond. *From Rights to Needs: A History of Family Allowances in Canada, 1929–1992*. Vancouver: UBC Press, 2009.

Bock, Gisela. "Racism and Sexism in Nazi Germany: Motherhood, Compulsory Sterilization, and the State." *Signs* 8, no. 3 (1983): 400–21.

Bowker, Marjorie Montgomery. "Brief on Mental Retardation for a Special Legislative and Lay Committee appointed by the Legislative Assembly of Alberta for the Study of Preventative Health Services in Alberta." December 1965.

Boyer, Yvonne. "First Nations, Métis and Inuit Health and the Law: A Framework for the Future." Thesis, University of Ottawa, 2011.

Brandt, Allan M. "Racism and Research: The Case of the Tuskegee Syphilis Study." In *Sickness and Health in America*, 3rd ed., ed. Judith Walzer Leavitt and Ronald L. Numbers. Madison: University of Wisconsin Press, 1997.

Braslow, Joel. *Mental Ills and Bodily Cures: Psychiatric Treatment in the First Half of the Twentieth Century*. Berkeley: University of California Press, 1997.

Brennan, Brian. *The Good Steward: The Ernest C. Manning Story*. Calgary: Fifth House, 2008.

Broberg, Gunner, and Nils Roll-Hansen, eds. *Eugenics and the Welfare State: Norway, Sweden, Denmark, and Findland.* East Lansing: Michigan State University Press, 2005.

Broberg, Gunnar, and Mattias Tydén. "Eugenics in Sweden: Efficient Care." In *Eugenics and the Welfare State: Norway, Sweden, Denmark, and Finland*, ed. Gunnar Broberg and Nils Roll-Hansen. East Lansing: Michigan State University Press, 2005.

Brody, Harry, Stewart Meikle, and Richard Gerritse. "Therapeutic Abortion: A Prospective Study, I." *American Journal of Obstetrics and Gynecology* 109, no. 3 (1971): 347–53.

Bromberg, W. "Schizophrenic-like Psychosis in Defective Children." *Proceedings and Addresses of the Annual Session*, American Association for Mental Deficiency, 39 (1934): 226–57.

Brown, T.E. "Cesarean Section in Lethbridge." *Alberta Medical Review* 16, no. 2 (1951): 18–20.

Burnett, Kristin. *Taking Medicine: Women's Healing Work and Colonial Contact in Southern Alberta, 1880–1930*. Vancouver: UBC Press, 2011.

Busfield, Joan. "The Female Malady? Men, Women and Madness in Nineteenth Century Britain." *Sociology* 28, no. 1 (1994): 259–77.

Campbell, Nancy. *Discovering Addiction: The Science and Politics of Substance
Abuse Research.* Ann Arbor: University of Michigan Press, 2007.

*Canada Year Book 1939: The Official Statistical Annual of the Resources, History,
Institutions, and Social and Economic Conditions of the Dominion.* Ottawa:
King's Printer, 1939.

Cappon, Daniel. "Psychiatric Indications for the Termination of Pregnancy –
Comments." *Canadian Medical Association Journal* 79, no. 4 (1958): 234–6.

Caulfield, Timothy, and Gerald Robertson. "Eugenic Policies in Alberta: From
the Systematic to the Systemic?" *Alberta Law Review* 35, no. 1 (1996): 59–79.

Cellard, André, and Marie-Claude Thifault. "The Uses of Asylums: Resistance,
Asylum Propaganda and Institutionalization Strategies in Turn of the
Century Quebec." In *Mental Health and Canadian Society: Historical Perspec-
tives,* ed. David Wright and James Moran. Montreal; Kingston, ON: McGill-
Queen's University Press, 2006.

Chapman, Terry L. "Early Eugenics Movements in Western Canada." *Alberta
History* 25, no. 4 (1977): 9–17.

Cheevers, Brenda. "Abortion Centre is optimistic about future progress in
city." *Calgary Herald,* 8 January 1971.

Christian, Timothy. "The Mentally Ill and Human Rights in Alberta: A Study
of the Alberta Sexual Sterilization Act." Thesis, University of Alberta, 1974.

Christie, Nancy. *Engendering the State: Family, Work, and Welfare in Canada.*
Toronto: University of Toronto Press, 2000.

Cook, Ramsay. *The Regenerators: Social Criticism in Late Victorian English
Canada.* Toronto: University of Toronto Press, 1985.

Cowan, Ruth Schwartz. *Heredity and Hope: The Case for Genetic Screening.*
Cambridge, MA: Harvard University Press, 2008.

Darwin, Leonard. *What Is Eugenics?* London: Watts and Company, 1928.

Davenport, Charles. "The Nams: The Feeble-minded as Country Dwellers."
Survey 27 (1912): 1844–5.

Devereux, Cecily. *Growing a Race: Nellie L. McClung and the Fiction of Eugenic
Feminism.* Montreal; Kingston, ON: McGill-Queen's University Press, 2006.

Dickens, Bernard. "Eugenic Recognition in Canadian Law." *Osgoode Hall Law
Journal* 13, no. 2 (1975): 547–77.

Dickinson, Robert L. "Sterilization without Unsexing: 1. Surgical Review with
Especial Reference to 5,820 Operations on Insane and Feeble-minded in
California." *Journal of the American Medical Association* 92, no. 5 (1929): 373–9.

Dodds, Donald J. *Voluntary Male Sterilization.* Toronto: Damian Press, 1970.

Douglas, Tommy C. "The Problems of the Subnormal Family." MA thesis,
McMaster University, 1933.

Dowbiggin, Ian. *Keeping America Sane: Psychiatry and Eugenics in the United States and Canada, 1880–1940.* Ithaca, NY: Cornell University Press, 1997.

Dowbiggin, Ian. *The Sterilization Movement and Global Fertility in the Twentieth Century.* Oxford: Oxford University Press, 2008.

Duffin, Jacalyn. *History of Medicine: A Scandalously Short Introduction.* Toronto: University of Toronto Press, 1999.

Dugdale, Richard. *The Jukes: A Record and Study of the Relations of Crime, Pauperism, Disease and Heredity.* New York: G.P. Putnam Sons, 1874.

Dummitt, Christopher. *The Manly Modern: Masculinity in Postwar Canada.* Vancouver: UBC Press, 2007.

Dunphy, Catherine. *Morgentaler: A Difficult Hero.* Toronto: John Wiley & Sons Canada, 2003.

Ellison, R.M. "Psychiatric Complications following Sterilization of Women." *Medical Journal of Australia* 2 (1964): 625–8.

Enoch, M. David, and Keith Jones. "Sterilization: A Review of 98 Sterilized Women." *British Journal of Psychiatry* 127, no. 6 (1975): 583–7.

Fancher, R.E. "Henry Goddard and the Kallikak Family Photographs." *American Psychologist* 42 (1987): 585–90.

Feldberg, Georgina. "On the Cutting Edge: Science and Obstetrical Practice in a Women's Hospital, 1945–1960." In *Women, Health, and Nation: Canada and the United States since 1945,* ed. Georgina Feldberg, Molly Ladd-Taylor, Alison Li, and Kathryn MacPherson. Montreal; Kingston, ON: McGill-Queen's University Press, 2003.

Fiamengo, Janice. *The Women's Page: Journalism and Rhetoric in Early Canada.* Toronto: University of Toronto Press, 2008.

Fisher, Thomas. "Legal Implications of Sterilization." *Canadian Medical Association Journal* 91, no. 26 (1964): 1363–5.

Fisher, Thomas. "Medico-Legal: Sexual Sterilization." *Canadian Medical Association Journal* 76, no. 9 (1957): 785–7.

Fleming, Meredith, and Terrence C.R. Joyce. "Elective Sterilization of the Human Male (Vasectomy)." *Canadian Hospital* 445, no. 6 (1968): 1–3.

Foucault, Michel. *Birth of the Clinic: An Archaeology of Medical Perception.* Trans. A.M. Sheridan. 1973. New York: Vintage Books, 1994.

Foucault, Michel. *Madness and Civilization: A History of Insanity in the Age of Reason.* New York: Vintage Books, 1965.

Frost, E. Mary. "Sterilization in Alberta: A Summary of the Cases Presented to the Eugenics Board for the Province of Alberta from 1929 to 1941." MA thesis, University of Alberta, 1942.

Gagan, David, and Rosemary Gagan. *For Patients of Moderate Means: A Social History of the Voluntary Public General Hospital in Canada, 1890–1950.* Montreal; Kingston, ON: McGill-Queen's University Press, 2002.

Galton, Frances. *Inquiries into Human Faculty and Its Development*. London: J.M. Dent and Sons, 1907.

Garrison, Paul L., and Clarence J. Gamble. "Sexual Effects of Vasectomy." *Journal of the American Medical Association* 144, no. 4 (1950): 293–5.

Gavreau, Michael, and Nancy Christie. *A Full-Orbed Christianity: The Protestant Churches and Social Welfare in Canada, 1900–1940*. Montreal; Kingston, ON: McGill-Queen's University Press, 2001.

Gibbons, Sheila. "The True [Political] Mothers of Tomorrow: Eugenics and Feminism in Alberta." MA thesis, University of Saskatchewan, 2012.

Gibson, David. "Involuntary Sterilization of the Mentally Retarded: A Western Canadian Phenomenon." *Canadian Psychiatric Association Journal* 19, no. 1 (1974): 59–63.

Goddard, Henry. *The Kallikak Family: A Study in the Heredity of Feeble-Mindedness*. New York: Macmillan, 1912.

Goffman, Erving. *Asylums: Essays on the Social Situation of Mental Patients and Other Inmates*. Garden City, NY: Anchor Books, 1961.

Goodman, Jordan, Anthony McElligott, and Lara Marks, eds. *Useful Bodies: Humans in the Service of Medical Science in the Twentieth Century*. Baltimore: Johns Hopkins University Press, 2003.

Grant, James Russell. "Propfschizophrenia: A Clinical and Physiological Essay." *Alberta Medical Review* 21, no. 3 (1956): 6–9.

Grant, James Russell. "Results of Institutional Treatment of Juvenile Mental Defectives over a 30-Year Period." *Canadian Medical Association Journal* 75, no. 11 (1956): 918–21.

Grekul, Jana. "Social Construction of the Feeble-Minded Threat." PhD diss., University of Alberta, 2002.

Grekul, Jana. "Sterilization in Alberta, 1928–1972: Gender Matters." *Canadian Review of Sociology* 45, no. 3 (2008): 247–66.

Grekul, Jana, Harvey Krahn, and Dave Odynak. "Sterilizing the 'Feeble-minded': Eugenics in Alberta, Canada, 1929–1972." *Journal of Historical Sociology* 17, no. 4 (2004): 358–84.

Grob, Gerald. *The Mad among Us: A History of the Care of America's Mentally Ill*. New York: Free Press, 1994.

Hanisch, Carol. "Struggles for Leadership in the Women's Liberation Movement." In *Leadership and Social Movements*, ed. Colin Barker, Alan Johnson, and Michael Lavalette. Manchester, UK: Manchester University Press, 2001.

Harris-Zsovan, Jane. *Eugenics and the Firewall: Canada's Nasty Little Secret*. Winnipeg: J. Gordon Shillingford Publishing, 2008.

Hazelgrove, Jenny. "The Old Faith and New Science: The Nuremberg Code and Human Experimentation in Britain, 1946–73." *Social History of Medicine* 15, no. 1 (2002): 109–35.

Hernstein, Richard J., and Charles Murray. *The Bell Curve: Intelligence and Class Structure in American Life*. New York: Free Press, 1994.

Herzberg, David. *Happy Pills in America: From Miltown to Prozac*. Baltimore: Johns Hopkins University Press, 2008.

Hoffer, Abram. "Effect of Atropine on Blood Pressure of Patients with Mental and Emotional Disease." *Archives of Neurology and Psychiatry* 71 (1954): 80–6.

Hoffer, Abram. "Objective Criteria for the Diagnosis of Schizophrenia Exemplified by the Atropine Test." *Confinia Neurologica* 14, no. 6 (1954): 385–90.

Hudson, Geoffrey. "Regions and Disability Politics in Ontario, 1975–1985." Paper presented at the conference "Putting Region in Its Place," University of Alberta, Edmonton, 26–28 October 2007.

Huxley, Julian. *Essays of a Biologist*. London: Chatto and Windus, 1923.

Jackson, L.N. "Vasectomy in the United Kingdom." *Practitioner* 203, no. 215 (1969): 320–3.

Jackson, Mark. "Changing Depictions of Disease: Race, Representation and the History of 'Mongolism.'" In *Race, Science and Medicine, 1700–1960*, ed. Waltraud Ernst and Bernard Harris. London: Routledge, 1999.

Jackson, Mary Percy. "Midwifery among the Metis." *Alberta Medical Review* 14, no. 3 (1949): 11–14.

Jahn, Penelope. "Legal Crusade of the Eternal Children." *Maclean's*, 30 November 1981, 20.

Jasen, Patricia. "Race, Culture, and the Colonization of Childbirth in Northern Canada." *Social History of Medicine* 10, no. 3 (1997): 383–400.

Johnsrude, Larry. "Province revokes rights; Government opts out of Charter, limits sterilization victims' right to sue for compensation; Alberta's Sterilization Solution." *Edmonton Journal*, 11 March 1998.

Jones, Edgar, and Shahina Rahman. "Framing Mental Illness, 1923–1939: The Maudsley Hospital and Its Patients." *Social History of Medicine* 21, no. 1 (2008): 107–25.

Kater, Michael H. *Doctors under Hitler*. Chapel Hill: University of North Carolina Press, 1989.

Keer, Stephani. "Abortion becoming freer." *Calgary Herald*, [exact date unknown] October 1970.

Kelm, Mary Ellen. *Colonizing Bodies: Aboriginal Health and Healing in British Columbia, 1900–1950*. Vancouver: UBC, 1999.

Kelm, Mary Ellen. "Diagnosing the Discursive Indian: Medicine, Gender, and the 'Dying Race.'" *Ethnohistory* 52, no. 2 (2005): 371–406.

Kevles, Daniel. *In the Name of Eugenics: Genetics and the Uses of Human Heredity*, 2nd ed. Cambridge, MA: Harvard University Press, 1995.

Kevles, Daniel. *In the Name of Eugenics: Genetics and the Uses of Human Heredity*, new ed. Cambridge, MA: Harvard University Press, 2004.

Klausen, Susanne. *Race, Maternity, and the Politics of Birth Control in South Africa, 1910–1939*. New York: Palgrave Macmillan, 2004.

Kline, Wendy. *Bodies of Knowledge: Sexuality, Reproduction, and Women's Health in the Second Wave*. Chicago: University of Chicago Press, 2010.

Kline, Wendy. *Building a Better Race: Gender, Sexuality, and Eugenics from the Turn of the Century to the Baby Boom*. Berkeley: University of California Press, 2001.

Kluchin, Rebecca. *Fit to Be Tied: Sterilization and Reproductive Rights in America, 1950–1980*. New Brunswick, NJ: Rutgers University Press, 2009.

Korinek, Valerie. *Roughing It in the Suburbs: Reading Chatelaine Magazine in the Fifties and Sixties*. Toronto: University of Toronto Press, 2000.

Ladd-Taylor, Molly. "Sterilizing the 'Retarded': Contraceptive Surgery and Eugenics in the 1970s and 1980s." *Canadian Bulletin of Medical History*. Under review.

Lampard, Robert. "The Sexual Sterilization Act of Alberta: An Introduction, 1928–1972." In *Alberta's Medical History: Young and Lusty, and Full of Life*. Red Deer, AB: Robert Lampard, 2008.

Law Reform Commission of Canada. "Sterilization: Implications for Mentally Retarded and Mentally Ill Persons." Working Paper 24. Ottawa: Law Reform Commission of Canada, 1979.

Leavitt, Judith Walzer. *Make Room for Daddy: The Journey from Waiting Room to Birthing Room*. Chapel Hill: University of North Carolina Press, 2009.

Lechat, Robert. "Intensive Sterilization for the Inuit." *Oblate Fathers of the Churchill-Hudson Bay Diocese*, Fall / Winter 1976/1977, 5–7.

Lederer, Susan E. *Subjected to Science: Human Experimentation in America before the Second World War*. Baltimore: Johns Hopkins University Press, 1995.

Le Vann, L.J. "Clinical Comparison of Haloperidol with Chlorpromazine in Mentally Retarded Children." *American Journal of Mental Deficiency* 75, no. 6 (1971): 719–23.

Le Vann, L.J. "A Clinical Survey of Alcoholics." *Canadian Medical Association Journal* 69, no. 6 (1953): 584–8.

Le Vann, L.J. "A Concept of Schizophrenia in the Lower Grade Mental Defective." *American Journal of Mental Deficiency* 54 (1950): 469–72.

Le Vann, L.J. "The Evaluation of Auditory Hallucinations." *Alberta Medical Review* 15, no. 1 (1950): 25–6.

Le Vann, L.J. "Haloperidol in the Treatment of Behavioural Disorders in Children and Adolescents." *Canadian Psychiatric Association Journal* 14, no. 2 (1969): 217–20.

Le Vann, L.J. "Neuleptil – A New phenothiazine." *Modern Medicine of Canada* 27, no. 9 (1972): 681–6.

Le Vann, L.J. "A New Butyrophenone: Trifluperidol: A Psychiatric Evaluation in a Pediatric Setting." *Canadian Psychiatric Association Journal* 13, no. 3 (1968): 271–3.

Le Vann, L.J. "A Pilot Project for Emotionally Disturbed Children in Alberta." *Canadian Medical Association Journal* 83, no. 10 (1960): 524–7.

Le Vann, L.J. "Thioridazine (Mellaril) a Psycho-sedative Virtually Free of Side-effects." *Alberta Medical Review* 26, no. 4 (1961): 144–7.

Le Vann, L.J. "Trifluoperazine Dihydrochloride: An Effective Tranquilizing Agent for Behavioural Abnormalities in Defective Children." *Canadian Medical Association Journal* 80, no. 2 (1959): 123–4.

Le Vann, L.J., and R.E. Cohn. "Clinical Evaluation of Norbolethone Therapy in Stunted Growth and Poorly Thriving Children." *International Journal of Clinical Pharmacology, Therapy and Toxicology* 6, no. 1 (1972): 54–9.

Lindee, Susan. *Moments of Truth in Genetic Medicine*. Baltimore: Johns Hopkins University Press, 2005.

Lombardo, Paul. "Anthropometry, Race, and Eugenic Research: 'Measurements of Growing Negro Children' at the Tuskegee Institute, 1932–1944." In *The Uses of Humans in Experimentation*, ed. Erika Dyck and Larry Stewart. Forthcoming.

Lombardo, Paul. "Return of the Jukes: Eugenic Mythologies and Internet Evangelism." *Journal of Legal Medicine* 33 (2012): 207–33.

Lombardo, Paul, ed. *A Century of Eugenics in America: From the Indiana Experiment to the Human Genome Era*. Bloomington: Indiana University Press, 2011.

Lombardo, Paul. "Davenport's Dream: 21st Century Reflections on Heredity and Eugenics." *Quarterly Review of Biology* 84, no. 2 (2009): 178.

Lombardo, Paul. *Three Generations No Imbeciles: Eugenics and Supreme Court, and Buck v. Bell*. Baltimore: Johns Hopkins University Press, 2008.

Lu, Therese, and Daphne Chun. "A Long Term Follow-up Study of 1,055 Cases of Postpartum Tubal Ligation." *Journal of Obstetrics and Gynaecology in the British Commonwealth* 74, no. 6 (1967): 875–80.

Lunbeck, Elizabeth. *The Psychiatric Persuasion: Knowledge, Gender, and Power in Modern America*. Princeton, NJ: Princeton University Press, 1994.

Lux, Maureen. "Care for the 'Racially Careless': Indian Hospitals in the Canadian West, 1920–1950s." *Canadian Historical Review* 91, no. 3 (2010): 407–34.

Lux, Maureen. *Medicine that Walks: Disease, Medicine, and Canadian Plains Native People.* Toronto: University of Toronto Press, 2001.

MacLean, R.R., and E.J. Kibblewhite. "Sexual Sterilization in Alberta: Eight Years' Experience, 1929 to May 31, 1937." *Canadian Public Health Journal* (1937): 587–90.

MacLean, Randall. "Procedures to Be Followed in Obtaining the Admission of a Patient to a Provincial Mental Hospital." *Alberta Medical Review* 7, no. 4 (1942): 23–9.

Makus, Ingrid. *Women, Politics, and Reproduction: The Liberal Legacy.* Toronto: University of Toronto Press, 1996.

Mandelbaum, David G. *Human Fertility in India: Social Components and Policy Perspectives.* Berkeley: University of California Press, 1974.

Marshall, David. *Secularizing the Faith: Canadian Protestant Clergy and the Crisis of Belief, 1850–1940.* Toronto: University of Toronto Press, 1992.

Maynard, Steven. "Maple Leaf (Gardens) Forever: Sex, Canadian Historians, and National History." *Journal of Canadian History* 36, no. 2 (2001): 70–105.

Mazumdar, Pauline. *Eugenics, Human Genetics and Human Failings: The Eugenics Society, Its Sources and Its Critics in Britain.* London: Routledge, 1992.

McCoy, David R. "The Emotional Reaction of Women to Therapeutic Abortion and Sterilization." *Journal of Obstetrics and Gynaecology in the British Commonwealth* 75, no. 10 (1968): 1054–7.

McLaren, Angus. "'Keep Your Seats and Face Facts': Western Canadian Women's Discussion of Birth Control in the 1920s." *Canadian Bulletin of Medical History* 8, no. 2 (1991): 189–201.

McLaren, Angus. *Our Own Master Race: Eugenics in Canada, 1885–1945.* Toronto: McClelland & Stewart, 1990.

McLaren, Angus, and Arlene Tigar McLaren. *The Bedroom and the State: The Changing Practices and Politics of Contraception and Abortion in Canada, 1880–1980.* Toronto: McClelland & Stewart, 1986.

Michel, Matthew A. "The new marriage act." *Prairie Messenger*, 19 July 1933, 11.

Mitchinson, Wendy. *Giving Birth in Canada, 1900–1950.* Toronto: University of Toronto Press, 2002.

Mohan, R.P. "Factors to Motivation towards Sterilization in 2 Indian Villages." *Family Life Coordinator* 16 (1967): 35–8.

Molyneaux, Heather. "Controlling Conception: Images of Women, Sexuality and the Pill in the Sixties." In *Gender, Health and Popular Culture: Historical Perspectives*, ed. Cheryl Krasnick Warsh. Waterloo, ON: Wilfrid Laurier University Press, 2011.

Nagel, Walter. "Doctors seek new policy on therapeutic abortions." *Calgary Herald*, 3 November 1970.

Nagel, Walter. "Male birth control: vasectomies on increase in city, doctor says." *Calgary Herald*, 7 April 1970.

Nagel, Walter. "Sterilization conditions spelled out for trustees." *Calgary Herald*, 18 April 1970.

National Film Board of Canada. *The Sterilization of Leilani Muir*. Dir. G. Whiting. Ottawa, 1996.

Norris, A.S. "An Examination of the Effects of Tubal Ligation: Their Implications for Prediction." *American Journal of Obstetrics and Gynaecology* 90, no. 4 (1964): 431–7.

O'Neil, John D. "Self-determination, Medical Ideology and Health Services in Inuit Communities." In *Northern Communities: The Prospects for Empowerment*, ed. Gurston Dacks and Ken Coates. Edmonton: Boreal Institute for Northern Studies, 1988.

O'Reilly, B.X. "The doctor has a chance to do much good." *Prairie Messenger*, 19 June 1929, 7.

Palmer, Beth. "'Lonely, tragic, but legally necessary pilgrimages': Transnational Abortion Travel in the 1970s." *Canadian Historical Review* 92, no. 4 (2011): 637–64.

Palmer, Howard. *Patterns of Prejudice: A History of Nativism in Alberta*. Toronto: McClelland & Stewart, 1985.

Palmer, Howard, and Tamara Palmer. *Alberta: A New History*. Edmonton: Hurtig Publishers, 1990.

Penfold, Steven. "'Have You No Manhood in You?' Gender and Class in the Cape Breton Coal Towns, 1920–1926." *Acadiensis* 23, no. 2 (1994): 21–44.

Pichot, André. *The Pure Society: From Darwin to Hitler*. Trans. David Fernbach. London: Verso, 2009.

Poffenberger, Thomas. "Two Thousand Voluntary Vasectomies Performed in California: Background Factors and Comments." *Marriage and Family Living* 25, no. 4 (1963): 469–74.

Poffenberger, Thomas, and Shirley Poffenberger. "Vasectomy as a Preferred Method of Birth Control: A Preliminary Investigation." *Marriage and Family Living* 25, no. 3 (1963): 326–30.

Pressman, Jack D. *Last Resort: Psychosurgery and the Limits of Medicine*. Cambridge: Cambridge University Press, 1998.

Primeau, Paul. "A Social History of the Eugenic Movement: The Enactment of the Sexual Sterilization Act S.A. 1928 and its effect on Indian and Metis People." Thesis, Lakehead University, 1998.

Proctor, Robert. *Racial Hygiene: Medicine under the Nazis*. Cambridge, MA: Harvard University Press, 1988.

Reagan, Leslie. "Crossing the Border for Abortions: California Activists, Mexican Clinics, and the Creation of a Feminist Health Agency in the 1960s." In *Women, Health and Nation: Canada and the United States since 1945*, ed. Georgina Feldberg, Molly Ladd-Taylor, Alison Li, and Kathryn McPherson. Montreal; Kingston, ON: McGill-Queen's University Press, 2003.

Reagan, Leslie. *When Abortion Was a Crime: Women, Medicine and Law in the United States, 1867–1973*. Berkeley: University of California Press, 1998.

Reaume, Geoffrey. "Patients at Work: Insane Asylum Inmates' Labour in Ontario, 1841–1900." In *Mental Health and Canadian Society: Historical Perspectives*, ed. James E. Moran and David Wright. Montreal; Kingston, ON: McGill-Queen's University Press, 2006.

Rennie, Bradford. *The Rise of Agrarian Democracy: The United Farmers and Farm Women of Alberta, 1909–1921*. Toronto: University of Toronto Press, 2000.

Revie, Linda. "More than Just Boots! The Eugenic and Commercial Concerns behind A.R. Kaufman's Birth Controlling Activities." *Canadian Bulletin for Medical History* 23, no. 1 (2006): 119–43.

Richardson, Angélique. *Love and Eugenics in the Late Nineteenth Century: Rational Reproduction and the New Woman*. Oxford: Oxford University Press, 2003.

Rodgers, David A., Frederick J. Ziegler, Patricia Rohr, and Robert J. Prentiss. "Sociopsychological Characteristics of Patients Obtaining Vasectomies from Urologists." *Marriage and Family Living* 25, no. 3 (1963): 331–5.

Rotskoff, Lori. *Love on the Rocks: Men, Women, and Alcohol in Post–World War II America*. Chapel Hill: University of North Carolina Press, 2002.

Rudy, Jarrett. *The Freedom to Smoke: Tobacco Consumption and Identity*. Montreal; Kingston, ON: McGill-Queen's University Press, 2005.

Russell, Bertrand. *Marriage and Morals*. New York: Liveright, 1929.

Rutherdale, Myra. "'Canada is no dumping ground': Public Discourse and Salvation Army Women and Children, 1900–1930." *Social History* 40, no. 79 (2007): 115–42.

Rutherdale, Robert. "Fatherhood, Masculinity, and the Good Years during Canada's Baby Boom, 1945–1965." *Journal of Family History* 24, no. 3 (1999): 351–73.

Samson, Amy. "Coercion, Surveillance and Eugenics." PhD dissertation, University of Saskatchewan, in progress.

Samson, Amy, "Eugenics in the Community: Alberta's Sexual Sterilization Act, 1928–1972." *Canadian Bulletin of Medical History*. Under review.

Schilder, P. "Reaction Types Resembling Functional Psychoses in Childhood on the Basis of an Organic Inferiority of the Brain." *Mental Hygiene* 19 (1935): 439–46.

Schmidt, John. "Unifarm." *Calgary Herald*, 27 March 1973.

Schoen, Johanna. *Choice and Coercion: Birth Control, Sterilization, and Abortion in Public Health and Welfare*. Chapel Hill: University of North Carolina Press, 2005.

Schoen, Johanna. "Reassessing Eugenic Sterilization: The Case of North Carolina." In *A Century of Eugenics in America: From the Indiana Experiment to the Human Genome Era*, ed. Paul Lombardo. Bloomington: University of Indiana Press, 2011.

Schouten, Mike. "Harper is paying the price for shutting down the abortion debate." *National Post*, 25 May 2012; available online at http://fullcomment.nationalpost.com/2012/05/25/mike-schouten-harper-is-paying-the-price-for-shutting-down-the-abortion-debate/.

Seaman, Barbara. *The Doctor's Case Against the Pill*, 25th anniversary ed. Alameda, CA: Hunter House, 1995.

Sethna, Christabelle. "All Aboard? Canadian Women's Abortion Tourism, 1960–1980." In *Gender, Health and Popular Culture: Historical Perspectives*, ed. Cheryl Krasnick Warsh. Waterloo, ON: Wilfrid Laurier University Press, 2011.

Sethna, Christabelle, and Steve Hewitt. "Clandestine Operations: The Vancouver Women's Caucus, the Abortion Caravan and the RCMP." *Canadian Historical Review* 90, no. 3 (2009): 463–95.

Shannon, T.W., Samuel Fallows, and W.J. Truitt, eds. *Eugenics or Nature's Secrets Revealed: Scientific Knowledge of the Laws of Sex Life and Heredity*. Marietta, OH: S.A. Mullikin Company, 1917.

Shevell, Michael. "A Canadian Paradox: Tommy Douglas and Eugenics." *Canadian Journal of Neurological Sciences* 39, no. 1 (2012): 35–9.

Shorter, Edward. *A History of Psychiatry: From the Era of the Asylum to the Age of Prozac*. New York: John Wiley & Sons, 1997.

Shorter, Edward, and David Healy. *Shock Therapy: A History of Electroconvulsive Treatment in Mental Illness*. New Brunswick, NJ: Rutgers University Press, 2007.

Showalter, Elaine. *The Female Malady: Women, Madness and English Culture, 1830–1980*. New York: Virago Press, 1987.

Shute, D. "Subtotal Hysterectomy in Southern Alberta." *Alberta Medical Review* 17, no. 2 (1952): 23–4.

Singh, Ilina. "Not Just Naughty: 50 Years of Stimulant Drug Advertising." In *Medicating Modern America: Prescription Drugs in History*, ed. Andrea Tone and Elizabeth Siegel Watkins. New York: New York University Press, 2007.

Smith, Matthew. "Putting Hyperactivity in Its Place: Cold War Politics, the Brain Race and the Origins of Hyperactivity in the United States, 1957–1968." In *Locating Health: Historical and Anthropological Investigations of Health and Place*, ed. Erika Dyck and Christopher Fletcher. London: Pickering & Chatto, 2011.

Snyder, Sharon L., and David T. Mitchell. *Cultural Locations of Disability.* Chicago: University of Chicago Press, 2006.

Solinger, Rickie. "Race and 'Value': Black and White Illegitimate Babies, in the USA, 1945–1965." In *Women and Health in America*, 2nd ed., ed. Judith Walzer Leavitt. Madison: University of Wisconsin Press, 1999.

Spitz, Vivien. *Doctors from Hell: The Horrific Account of Nazi Experiments on Humans.* Boulder, CO: Sentient Publications, 2005.

Stern, Alexandra Minna. *Eugenic Nation: Faults and Frontiers of Better Breeding in Modern America.* Berkeley: University of California Press, 2005.

Stern, Alexandra Minna. "From Legislation to Lived Experience: Eugenic Sterilization in California and Indiana, 1907–79." In *A Century of Eugenics in America: From the Indiana Experiment to the Human Genome Era*, ed. Paul Lombardo. Bloomington: Indiana University Press, 2011.

Stiker, Henri. *A History of Disability.* Trans. William Sayers. Ann Arbor: University of Michigan Press, 1999.

Stote, Karen. "An Act of Genocide: Eugenics, Indian Policy, and the Sterilization of Aboriginal Women in Canada." PhD diss., University of New Brunswick, 2012.

Struthers, James. *The Limits of Affluence: Welfare in Ontario, 1920–1970.* Toronto: University of Toronto Press, 1994.

Szasz, Thomas. *The Myth of Mental Illness: Foundations of a Theory of Personal Conduct.* 1960. New York: Harper Collins, 1974.

Tallin, G.P.R. "The Legal Implications of the Non-Therapeutic Practices of Doctors." *Canadian Medical Association Journal* 87, no. 5 (1962): 207–15.

Taylor, Georgina. "Ground for Common Action: Violet McNaughton's Agrarian Feminism and the Origins of the Farm Women's Movement in Canada." PhD diss., Carleton University, Ottawa, 1997.

Thifault, Marie-Claude, and Isabelle Perreault. "Premières initiatives d'intégration sociale des malades mentaux dans une phase de pré-désinstitutionnalisation: l'exemple de Saint-Jean-de-Dieu, 1910–1950." *Social History* 46, no. 88 (2011): 197–222.

Tomes, Nancy. "Feminist Histories of Psychiatry." In *Discovering the History of Psychiatry*, ed. Mark S. Micale and Roy Porter. Oxford: Oxford University Press, 1994.

Tone, Andrea. *Devices & Desires: A History of Contraceptives in America*. New York: Hill and Wang, 2001.

Turda, Marius. *Modernism and Eugenics*. Basingstoke, UK: Palgrave Macmillan, 2010.

Urquhart, M.C., and K.A.H. Buckley, eds. *Historical Statistics of Canada*. Cambridge: Cambridge University Press, 1965.

Valverde, Mariana. *The Age of Light, Soap and Water: Moral Reform in English Canada, 1885–1925*. Toronto: Oxford University Press, 1991.

Van der Heyden, J. "Dangers of birth control told at Dutch congress." *Prairie Messenger*, 25 August 1929, 1.

Wahlsten, Douglas. "Leilani Muir versus the Philosopher King: Eugenics on Trial in Alberta." *Genetica* 99, no. 2–3 (1997): 185–98.

Wailoo, Keith. *Dying in the City of the Blues: Sickle Cell Anemia and the Politics of Race and Health*. Chapel Hill: University of North Carolina Press, 2001.

Waiser, Bill. *Saskatchewan: A New History*. Calgary: Fifth House, 2005.

Waldram, James B. *Revenge of the Windigo: The Construction of the Mind and Mental Health of North American Aboriginal Peoples*. Toronto: University of Toronto Press, 2004.

Wallace, R.C. "The Quality of the Human Stock." *Canadian Medial Association Journal* 31, no. 4 (1934): 427–30.

Watkins, Elizabeth. *On the Pill: A Social History of Contraceptives, 1950–1970*. Baltimore: Johns Hopkins University Press, 1998.

Weikart, Richard. *From Darwin to Hitler: Evolutionary Ethics, Eugenics, and Racism in Germany*. New York: Palgrave Macmillan, 2004.

Weindling, Paul. *Health, Race and German Politics between National Unification and Nazism, 1870–1945*. Cambridge: Cambridge University Press, 1989.

Woodsworth, J.S. *Strangers within Our Gates*. Toronto: Doreen Stephen Books, 1909.

Woodsworth, J.S. *Strangers within Our Gates*. 1909. Reprint, Toronto: University of Toronto Press, 1972.

Zarfas, D.E. "Psychiatric Indications for the Termination of Pregnancy." *Canadian Medical Association Journal* 79, no. 4 (1958): 230–4.

Index

Aberhart, William, 12, 115
Aboriginal people: 1920s medical surveys, 62–6; and Alberta's eugenics program, 12, 13, 22–3, 54, 55–83; case of George Pierre, 20, 22–3, 55–6, 62, 80–2, 232; and the CNCMH, 39; First Nations, 13, 54, 56, 57, 59, 61, 65, 74, 75, 77, 82; First Nations activism, 57, 83; and informed consent, 20, 22, 55–6, 59, 62, 75, 77, 80–2; Inuit, 12, 13, 59, 118; and IQ ranking, 60; Métis, 46, 56, 57, 59–60, 61, 65, 67, 83; and the notion of race degeneration, 56, 57, 58, 67, 74, 83; and poverty, 23, 63, 64, 67; racism towards, 55–6, 57–8, 59–62, 83; reports about childbirth, 67; and residential schools, 57; as targets of sterilization, 54, 56–8, 59–60, 62, 75, 83; women, 57, 58, 59, 60, 64, 67, 83, 206
abortion, 198–225; and 1892 Criminal Code, 89, 91, 202; and 1980 amendment to the Criminal Code, 224; Abortion Caravan protest, 205, 206; case of Jane Doe, 25, 198–201, 205, 208, 214, 225; and

the Catholic Church, 95, 101–2, 104, 204, 231; current debates over, 226–9; decriminalization of, 17–18, 21, 25–6, 89, 109, 171, 188, 201–6, 210, 224–5; and definition of health risks, 201, 208–15; and disability, 25–6, 202, 206–8, 215–24, 225; legal history in Canada, 202–8; pro-choice, 18, 26, 227, 228, 229, 233–4; pro-life, 18, 214–15, 228, 229, 233–4; for psychiatric reasons, 212–13, 215–17; and voluntary sterilization, 204–5
Alberta Medical Association (AMA), 208, 210–11, 212; articles on sterilization in the *Alberta Medical Review*, 23, 80, 106–7, 108–9
alcoholism, 8, 104, 260n69
Allen, Richard, 98
Ambrose, Rona, 228
American Medical Association (AMA), 102, 117
Anderson, Doris, 193, 194
Association for Voluntary Sterilization, 138
Asylum for the Insane in London, Ontario, 97–8